HEALTHCARE FROM THE TRENCHES

An Insider Account of the **Complex Barriers** of U.S. Healthcare from the **"Providers"** and **Patients' Perspective**

ALEJANDRO BADIA, M.D., F.A.C.S.

CONTRIBUTORS

Dr. Julio Gonzalez

Dr. Philip Forno

Dr. George Balfour

Dr. Mark Rekant

Dr. A.J. DiGiovanni

Dr. Laurent Dreyfuss

Dr. Roger Khouri

Dr. Jose Lamas

Dr. Stefano Lucchina

A South Florida Pediatrician

Dr. Rios-Ruh

Dr. Scott Sigman

Dr. Robert Terrill

Dr. Gregorio Caban

Dr. Aileen Marie Gonzalez

John Kastanis

Nancy Williams, R.N.

Dr. Kay Kirkpatrick, Georgia State Senator

Cindy Papale-Hammontree, Medical Office Manager/Author

Uva de Aragon, Retired University Professor/Author

A Pennsylvania Medical Malpractice Defense Attorney

Kerry Anderson, Restaurant Worker/Patient

Kristin Forno, O.T., C.H.T.

Lina Peterson, D.P.T.

Kimberly Light, Regulatory Affairs Executive

Erica Pacey, Jewelry Designer/Patient

Justin Irizzary, Co-Founder and CFO, OrthoNOW®

DEDICATION

To my deceased great uncle, Dr. Cesar Carvallo,
the last physician in my family lineage from Cuba.

To my parents, Cristobal and Maria, and my stepmother, Carmen,
who brought me to the United States and gave me every opportunity
to follow my dreams and the path of prior family physicians.

To my only sibling, Susana Rylander, who for the past
20 years has supported me through the additional role of
executive assistant and weathered many storms and my
never-ending "new projects."

To my children, Alessia and Alessandro,
my primary reason for living.

To my grandparents, Cristobal, and Consuelo, who like so many
immigrants, took care of me when my youthful parents had to
work/study and taught me the meaning of compassion and empathy.
It was my grandmother's crippling rheumatoid arthritis that lead to
me pursue a career of treating pain while restoring function.

To my patients, the reason I still enjoy being
a physician and surgeon.

CONTENTS

Foreword

Julio Gonzalez, M.D. J.D.

Orthopedic Surgeon Board Certified and Fellowship Trained in Joint Reconstruction

To the layperson, the doctors' lounge is a mysterious place. Few can enter it, and fewer still are allowed to eat the stale food that's usually served there. But if you get through its doors, you will immediately be exposed to the ills that torment medicine. There, you will hear stories of the colleague struggling against a frivolous lawsuit whose futility is clearly visible to all except the plaintiff's attorney. You will also hear about the insurance company that, refusing to cover the recommended treatment, demands a "peer-to-peer." When the physician calls, he is met by a voice that is obviously from the Far East and belonging to one who is not a member of the discussed specialty, claiming to be a "peer". Of course, the proposed treatment is rejected.

You will hear the story of the patient, who midstream through therapy with an expensive, life-saving cancer medication has her funding cut off by the third-party payer until such time her doctor, a renowned oncologist, tries an outdated, cheaper medication the literature has already demonstrated will not work.

And these are the simpler problems. Just down the road, a physician with 30 years under her belt is selling her practice to the hospital because she can no longer make ends meet. She is the seventy-second doctor to be hired by the hospital to provide purely outpatient services. Then there is the cardiologist who, lured by increasing Medicare reimbursements, mortgaged his home to build a world-class cardiothoracic suite only to have Medicare change its mind about the reimbursement for cardiac catheterizations. Now, he is declaring bankruptcy and getting hired by a hospital. And there are the two medical partners who have been trying to dissolve their practice for the past two years but are unable to come to terms. Whenever they see each other, it looks like they will come to blows. In the meantime, their respective attorneys make their way to the bank each week to cash the checks each is cutting for representing them.

As the conversation grows ever darker and the future appears grimmer, someone laments not having practiced decades earlier when physicians were respected, and their orders were truly... well... orders. Another shakes his head regretfully in recognition of the world that today's residents will inherit. "It'll be worse for them," observes one. To which another quips, "Maybe not. They'll be employed."

There will finally be a pause where the only sound heard is from the anchor on CNN blaring from the television hanging on the wall opposite the lounge's door. The consternation hangs heavily over a room that used to be tarnished with the smell of cigarettes.

Suddenly a doctor breaks the silence. "Sarah, he says. "I've been meaning to talk to you about this case. I saw this lady of yours with absence seizures. Her MRI is really interesting..."

And all the sudden, the doom melts away, and all is well again as if medicine and science could provide some shield to the cataclysm that will surely come.

This is the world Dr. Badia brings to you in *Healthcare from the Trenches*. It is a world that is often distressing, but it is the world in which your doctor lives. It is the world that each of us tries to navigate in taking care of our patients, and believe me, it's a world that every one of us could do without. But Dr. Badia's is a necessary visit because it offers the first step in solving problems; an understanding of what the problems actually are. For far too long policymakers and reformers have made the mistake of trying to manipulate healthcare without first engaging in the world Dr. Badia exposes; without undergoing the difficult process of understanding.

Healthcare from the Trenches may be one small volley in a long, involved, and complicated conversation about our healthcare system's future, but its effects can be colossal.

Introduction

I did not want to write this book.

Why would a busy single practice orthopedic surgeon like me, who also engages in academic writing, be inclined to take on the additional task of writing a book for the purpose of giving "providers" and patients a forum to describe the real-life challenges of providing and obtaining healthcare in the United States? A reluctant healthcare entrepreneur, I had already invested my time, money, and energy to embark upon my OrthoNOW® journey, something I will discuss in more detail later.

Unlike many of my medical peers, I have always had an innate understanding of business, which has served me well in many ways. However, the "curse" of being an entrepreneur means that whenever you identify a problem, you want to fix it. And with consistent diligence, hard work, and a bit of luck, you can achieve your goal of a successful startup, or reap a financial windfall that makes all your efforts worthwhile. However, this is quite a different challenge in the healthcare arena.

In terms of U.S. healthcare, we face some serious problems – not only with skyrocketing costs but also patient access and efficient delivery. Yes, our healthcare system is fraught with challenges…and as a foolhardy, obstinate physician with an entrepreneurial soul, I believed I could somehow make an impact in my own specialty of orthopedics and musculoskeletal medicine. Despite the barriers and frustrations, I still enjoy caring for my patients. Wait, let me rephrase that: I *love* being a surgeon, relying upon my core knowledge in physiology and anatomy, and healing my fellow man.

But somewhere during this past decade, my noble calling transformed into an oppressive burden. I began to notice that the majority of physician discussions – whether in the surgeon's lounge, on an email list-serve or on a conference lunch break—centered more around the major hurdles we dealt with when treating our patients (according to the Hippocratic Oath we had taken), instead of the exchange of ideas regarding a difficult case, or a new technique for a particular procedure.

Where did it all go wrong?

I can't say with pinpoint accuracy, but based on my own experience, it was a gradual buildup that took place some years after I went into private practice…and has devolved into a bureaucratic nightmare since the implementation of the Affordable Care Act, which most people recognize as "Obamacare." What began as incremental interference in the relationship between doctor and patient is now an almost impenetrable wall comprised of governmental and insurance industry busybodies. These nonmedical forces contribute to increased costs, inefficiencies, and delays that, at best, needlessly exacerbate a patient's pain and suffering, and at worst, aggravate the initial injury and/or illness until they may be no longer reparable.

Given these harrowing developments, any medical professional who accepts the challenge of seeing patients every day must go into "survival mode." But it is not just doctors and nurses; nowadays, even the end-users, the patients, realize something must give if we are to continue to provide healthcare that is the envy of the world.

So, why *did* I write this book?

To give a voice to the key participants in every healthcare transaction: the ones who provide and the ones who receive. If you pay attention to the news and current events, you might have noticed something odd whenever the topic of optimizing healthcare delivery in the U.S. is debated and discussed. Neither the doctor, nor the patient gets the opportunity to share their experiences and offer their solutions. Instead, public policy, the popular media, and even organized healthcare focus exclusively on the opinions and talking points generated by the insurance industry, Big Pharma, and so-called, "healthcare systems," otherwise known as "hospitals."

Why is it that those who devote nearly their entire lives to their chosen profession, who have sacrificed years to the pursuit of a medical education and residency, and who dedicate themselves to the care of others – often at the expense of quality time with their loved ones – rarely get a say in any substantive healthcare discussion?

I mean, these are only the *purveyors* of medical care to patients. No need to involve them, right?

As for patients, many are rightly frustrated by the mounting inefficiencies and barriers to receiving care, including Kerry, who shares her harrowing experience with the workers' compensation system in Florida in a later chapter. Yet while patients complain and voice their concerns, there is no real improvement in sight to the complex problems that plague U.S. healthcare and affect them personally. No, I do not pretend to have a "quick fix" for everything. However, I believe with firm conviction that to make any positive changes to our healthcare system, clinicians who are "in the trenches" must have their say, and patients' challenges must be given thoughtful consideration. After all, we are not statistics or numbers on a P&L statement: we're human beings who deserve a role in solving what is soon to become an existential crisis in the United States as the population ages.

Via a series of anecdotes and stories from medical professionals and patients, along with my own journey as an orthopedic surgeon and healthcare disruptor, this book sheds light on the biggest barriers in actual clinical practice, including:

- The Behemoth Hospital System
- Big Government
- The Big Business of Health Insurance
- Medical Malpractice & Tort Reform
- Ambulance-Chasing Trial Lawyers
- Popular Media (the Marcus Welby days are over and Fake News rules)

All these factors have contributed to an ever-increasing epidemic that some have termed "burnout" but is best described as "moral injury." Practicing medicine with our hands tied behind our backs and the constant threat of looming medical malpractice lawsuits have dire consequences.

Defined as "perpetrating, failing to prevent, bearing witness to, or learning about acts that transgress deeply held moral beliefs and expectations," moral injury describes the no-win situation doctors find themselves in when they can't practice medicine according to their conscience. In far too many instances, they are forced to choose between the best interests of their patients and the demands imposed by their employers, insurance companies, and government agencies and dictates. No wonder why an estimated 300 to 400 doctors commit suicide each year – a rate of 28 to 40 per 100,000, or more than double that of the general population!

To "disrupt" any industry, one must go against the grain and be willing to upset the status quo which will naturally anger many of the current stakeholders. This is perhaps most evident in healthcare where *multiple* entities, processes, and people are involved, amplified by the fact that healthcare inherently is a sensitive subject, as it well should be. The problem is that the current methodology has become needlessly cumbersome and extremely expensive. It is simply not sustainable. This is most evident in the U.S., but many other industrialized, western countries suffer the same issues to a lesser scale and should take note.

While my goal is not to offend or attack anyone, I will portray the issues through a series of anecdotes and actual occurrences via physicians, allied healthcare professionals, administrators and even patients, that will clearly illustrate the problems. Even telling the stories may ruffle some feathers, but my goal is to let the reader determine if perhaps the problem could be handled in a more cost-effective, and yes, *humane*, manner. Obtaining care should not involve jumping through multiple hoops and triggering bureaucratic hurdles, but rather connecting the patient in need with the most appropriate caregiver. Not only is this more cost-effective, it is the "right" thing to do. Most of us in the healing profession sacrificed much to obtain the societal trust to intervene and help our fellow man.

In Section I, I discuss the journey, often from a tender age, of how a physician comes to occupy that place in society. We are not afraid of hard work; however, we did not anticipate the myriad of barriers that would be placed in our path between patient assessment and definitive treatment. Many of these obstacles involve peripheral people who have somehow been injected into the process, oftentimes not adding any value. In fact, it is quite the opposite: they tend to hinder the process, which naturally drives up costs.

As physicians, we bear no ill will toward these gatekeepers, yet we must help the public understand in clear terms that they do not add much, if any, value to the process of delivering healthcare. Because the system inserted them into the doctor-patient relationship, they are just performing their job as instructed. Remember that each of these cogwheels represents an additional salary and benefits package, contributing to the overall cost of healthcare. In later chapters, I will discuss the "cottage industry" players – the opportunists who have discovered viable ways to cash in on our dysfunctional healthcare bureaucracy by adding themselves into the equation of healthcare delivery.

Compared to the behemoth that is the insurance industry however, these peripheral players are of minimal consequence. Do the math: United Healthcare alone employs nearly 250,000 people and most of them add little or nothing to the healthcare paradigm. In the 20th Century, the health insurance industry was created to provide financial support for individuals to address their major care expenses to ensure that the pool of insured consumers would cover the patient in need.

In today's ongoing healthcare discussion, rarely does anyone mention that the health insurance industry adds zero value to the delivery of care. There is a conflation of "health care" with "health insurance," so I want to be clear on that point. The purpose of health insurance should simply be to "collect premiums" and reimburse care.

The laughable commercial about how United Healthcare saved an aged biker from a drug interaction clouds the truth: It was certainly a physician, nurse, or perhaps a pharmacist who avoided medical catastrophe, not an insurance adjustor or executive. This does not mean that the insurance company employees are not important; it simply means they DO NOT PROVIDE CARE. It is not their role to do that, much less is it mine to perform an actuarial analysis. Neither possesses the skill set or education for that. While I do not pretend to have a definitive answer as to how to decrease healthcare costs, I will offer a simple solution towards the conclusion of the book that explains how the health insurance industry should be compensated and how to bring it back to its original purpose.

When it comes to reforming the U.S. healthcare system, we as members of our society perform a critical role. By attempting to exact change, we imply that we care. We must not only recognize that healthcare costs are spiraling out of control, we must also assume responsibility for solving the problem. That means we do not care only when we have a fever, or our kid sprains his ankle in soccer, or Grandma presents with chest pain in the middle of the night. It means we make healthcare the priority it deserves to be every single day...not just the moment we need it. How do we do that? By discussing potential solutions and good ideas on social media, pressuring our employers to provide choice, and imploring our local city commissioners, state representatives, congressional representatives, senators, and president. We must seek change at all levels of government.

While presidential candidates may proclaim "Medicare for All," we ought to step in and point out that we have some of the solutions right in front of our noses. Let's discuss them with the same enthusiasm and passion as we do newspaper tabloids, sports stars, or the viral video du jour. Understand that many of our cultural and media distractions represent what the Roman poet Juvenal coined, "Bread and Circuses." Instead of falling into the trap, we must focus our attention on what matters most: the reasonable delivery of healthcare as a human need.

In the following pages, you'll hear from a variety of medical professionals – from surgeons to nurses to occupational therapists – along with patients who have volunteered to share their stories to educate others, begin a dialogue, and pave the way to restoring and preserving the world's best healthcare system. Together, we can resolve the healthcare crisis for ourselves and future generations.

The Hippocratic Oath

I swear to fulfill, to the best of my ability and judgment, this covenant:

I will respect the hard-won scientific gains of those physicians in whose steps I walk, and gladly share such knowledge as is mine with those who are to follow.

I will apply, for the benefit of the sick, all measures [that] are required, avoiding those twin traps of overtreatment and therapeutic nihilism.

I will remember that there is art to medicine as well as science, and that warmth, sympathy, and understanding may outweigh the surgeon's knife or the chemist's drug.

I will not be ashamed to say, "I know not," nor will I fail to call in my colleagues when the skills of another are needed for a patient's recovery.

I will respect the privacy of my patients, for their problems are not disclosed to me that the world may know. Most especially must I tread with care in matters of life and death. If it is given me to save a life, all thanks. But it may also be within my power to take a life; this awesome responsibility must be faced with great humbleness and awareness of my own frailty. Above all, I must not play at God.

I will remember that I do not treat a fever chart, a cancerous growth, but a sick human being, whose illness may affect the person's family and economic stability. My responsibility includes these related problems if I am to care adequately for the sick.

I will prevent disease whenever I can, for prevention is preferable to cure.

I will remember that I remain a member of society, with special obligations to all my fellow human beings, those sound of mind and body as well as the infirm.

If I do not violate this oath, may I enjoy life and art, respected while I live and remembered with affection thereafter. May I always act so as to preserve the finest traditions of my calling and may I long experience the joy of healing those who seek my help.

Written in 1964 by Louis Lasagna, Academic Dean of the School of Medicine at Tufts University, and used in many medical schools today.

SECTION I

THE HIDDEN JOURNEY
OF A MEDICAL PROFESSIONAL

Chapter 1 – Preparation: The Long Journey

*"I swear to fulfill, to the best of my ability, this covenant:
I will respect the hard-won scientific gains of those
physicians in whose steps I walk, and gladly share such
knowledge as is mine with those who follow."*

I am a proud immigrant. I was born in Cuba and came to the United States with my parents in 1964. My father is a native of Valencia Spain. He was studying engineering in Havana when he met my mother, who lived across the street in the modest neighborhood known as "Ampliacion de Almendares."

My mom descends from a long lineage of physicians. I discovered just how long that lineage was several years ago, when I gave a lecture for the Cornell Entrepreneurial Network (CEN) and decided to research my family history a bit more. What I discovered was simply amazing. One of my relatives, Dr. Nicolas Gutierrez (1800-1890), was a co-founder of the Cuban Academy of Medical, Physical and Natural Sciences He was my great, great, great, great grandfather and was credited with being the first physician to splint a long bone fracture. Yes, we are talking orthopedics, but back then it was not called orthopedics; they were all general doctors. He attained many accolades including publishing the first medical journal in Cuba, after the Cholera epidemic of 1833, and was the official Cuban physician for the King of Spain, Chancellor of the University of Havana, etc.

My maternal great uncle, Cesar E. Carvallo de Aragon, was the closest physician relative to me and was one of a group of Cuban physicians who studied at Le Sorbonne, in Paris. I had the honor of repairing his painful shoulder rotator cuff tear when he was in his 80s and he was an exemplary and grateful patient. He was also the godfather to my only sister, Susana. Between him and Dr. Nico Gutierrez there were three other physicians and surgeons who remain the source of great family pride. While I knew little detail of their lives, there was always a subliminal presence for me.

Naturally, the profession of medicine influenced my upbringing. As an immigrant in New Jersey, Mom worked doing inhalation therapy and assisting the anesthesiologist. Back then, of course, there was not quite as much emphasis on titles, but because she possessed an inherent ability to perform the job, she worked her way up. Her position involved a significant amount of patient care. As a four-and-five-year-old child, I heard her stories when my dad and I picked her up at the hospital at the end of a shift. That was before my parents divorced a few years later. Regardless, from a young age, I felt a strong motivation to follow in my family's medical footsteps.

How did I decide to become a hand surgeon?

It was a gradual process, but the exact moment I discovered hand surgery existed is seared in my memory. Since both my parents had to work, my paternal grandparents stayed home with my sister and me. My grandmother suffered from crippling rheumatoid arthritis, to the point where her hands were totally deformed – the typical deformity that accompanies that disease. When I was eight years old, I accompanied my grandparents to Columbia Presbyterian to see a doctor who turned out to be a hand surgeon, a specialist. I didn't realize back then, but at the time he was only one of two gentlemen in the entire city of New York who focused exclusively on hand surgery, a new specialty at the time. I recall sitting in that office, my legs dangling from the chair, glancing back and forth between the doctor and his degrees as I heard him talk to my grandmother. "This is something I could do," I thought to myself. And I never looked back.

You might say that practicing medicine is in my blood.

While that pivotal memory remains etched in my mind, here's the most interesting part: about 25 years later, I realized the doctor's name was Bob Carroll. After he passed at age 92, there was a full-page obituary in the New York Times. A decade or more after I first met Dr. Carroll as a child, he trained a gentleman named Joseph Imbriglia – who would end up being my main mentor in hand surgery in Pittsburgh, Pennsylvania. So, in many ways, Bob Carroll was like my grandfather for hand surgery in an ironic twist of fate. To this day, my grandmother's sewing machine – the old Singer with the foot control – stands in my office, perpendicular to the desk where I sit and work, a constant reminder of that defining moment in my medical journey.

While my choice might seem a little premature, the truth is that for most physicians, the decision to study medicine occurs well before college. Before you set foot on a college campus, you deal with an incredible amount of pressure to achieve excellent grades in high school and a great score on the infamous SAT. Every student and would-be doctor became serious about his or her chosen field well before junior high, when they realize they must attend a reputable university as a prerequisite for acceptance into medical school. It is a domino effect of overachievement.

Long before you ever earn the "M.D." after your name, you cope with constant stress. When I decided to become a hand surgeon, I knew the road ahead would be difficult. I attended public school the entire way and achieved high enough grades to be accepted into Cornell University. What a huge blessing that was for me. When I first got to Cornell, I remember all my peers were either majoring in pre-law or pre-med. That is just the way it was. I would meet people all the time and they would remark, "Well, I'm a relatively intelligent person; I'm going to law school or medical school." For me, just being there was special. I flourished at Cornell, but my grades were not handed to me on a platter. I recall endless nights making this chart in biochemistry or studying a subject in-depth. I worked hard for it. I have no regrets.

Early on, there is already a significant amount of stress and sacrifice. For example, most students who receive athletic scholarships are not pre-med, but will attend a school with a top-level football program. When a pre-med student athlete does attend a good school, everyone makes a big deal out of it because it is unusual. For most individuals that aspire to be a medical doctor, they must forego the pursuit of a sport, even if they excel in it, to focus on achieving the grades they need to be accepted into a good undergraduate university. In my case, I was a swimmer, but not a good enough swimmer to earn a scholarship.

As a young and curious child, I was exposed to many influences even as I considered pursuing medicine. My early career interests usually centered around the natural sciences, and like most kids with a scientific slant, I first fell in love with dinosaurs. However, for me it was not only simple awe for their size or magnificence, but rather a true passion for understanding their timeline, classifications, and theories surrounding their demise. My initial interest in paleontology soon morphed into an interest in archeology – supported by my dad's *National Geographic* magazines, which aided my pursuit of knowledge and gave me a great excuse to read everything in sight. It cultivated my interest in learning and my proficiency in rote memorization of cultures and time periods, a useful skill for later studies. Fortunately, there was no Indiana Jones at that time, as my fate might have been sealed!

As I grew, my passion for reptiles and cultures of the past soon waned, and I became interested in the contemporary animal kingdom. I also relished the memorization of phyla, genomes, and species, which transformed into an interest in the anatomy of species, highly relevant in terms of understanding evolution via the concept of "Ontology recapitulates phylogeny." Simply put,

I soon developed a real passion for the understanding of structure and func-tion in living things. Apart from a brief foray into veterinary pursuits, I soon realized that my love for anatomy was tied to my vocation for medicine. It became clear to me, even at around age eight, that related sciences were just a stepping-stone to my pursuit of becoming a physician.

Furthermore, my early interest in medicine was intertwined with the con-cept of surgery, the ultimate expression of anatomy. I remember this well, though I have *no* inkling as to why a such a young child would become com-mitted to a career choice, although many kids that age express an unwavering desire to become astronauts, police officers, and baseball players. Still, I could not have anticipated or appreciated the incredible amount of studying that would later be required, or the sacrifices I would be forced to make during my young adulthood. What I can say with certainty is that my mind was made up. Throughout middle school and high school, I knew which path lay ahead of me in terms of college and professional school.

I cannot say the same about entrepreneurism. While the debate rages about whether entrepreneurs are born or made, I can report that there were few, if any influences on me in this area growing up. Because there were no business-owners in my family, I was never exposed to the inherent challenges of creating and nurturing an enterprise from a concept to a thriving company; therefore, I can only assume I was born with an entrepreneurial spirit. I will share more about my entrepreneurial curse later. Suffice it to say, at this point in my journey my sole focus was getting into medical school and pursuing my professional dream – one that, in my mind, encompassed much more than just a "job." It was a vocation.

One of my early memories involves my admiration for my sixth-grade teacher, Ms. Coniglio, at Abraham Lincoln Elementary School in Elizabeth New Jersey. She, too, had an interest in dinosaurs and commissioned me to paint a large mural for her boyfriend of some of the great creatures of the Jurassic Period. Or was it Cretaceous? At the time, I had also demonstrated an aptitude for art in the form of drawing and painting animals and, of course, dinosaurs. Nonetheless, this project stemmed from my having drawn a similar mural just outside our classroom, with several helpers -- much like Michelangelo enlisting apprentices to paint his Sistine Chapel. I recall the thrill of being able to skip class to further the project and my teacher culti-vating my interest in paleontology. This soon led to other projects, such as dissecting an animal in front of my entire class. I clearly recall making an incision and pointing out key anatomic structures in a fish I had come across in my neighborhood…or was it a frog? That detail I don't recall, but I do remember enjoying the experience of teaching and sharing, perhaps foreshadowing a later interest that would culminate in my co-founding of the then largest cadaveric surgical lab in the world, the DaVinci Center, later renamed MARC (Miami Anatomic Research Center)

All of this was a bit ironic considering I was a shy kid, all the way until junior high school. Nonetheless, under the guidance of Mrs. Consiglio, this brief teaching exposure placed me in a situation where I could espouse anatomy or animal facts, while feeling perfectly comfortable – and even invigorated. However, as any frustrated patient can attest, being a good doctor is more than understanding science or anatomy. My junior high years were key to my development as a person; one who could relate to people, hold a conversation, and perhaps even lead.

Sports is a great confidence builder for youth, and I was no exception. I seemed to have an innate ability as a swimmer and one of my few regrets in life is that I did not pursue it earlier, despite my parents placing me in the YMCA's learn-to-swim program. Sure, I could already swim underwater, hold my breath, and get across one of those stand-up pools we all recall from our neighborhoods. After all, my dad taught me and often crossed the length of the pool with me on his back, Flipper style. Little did I appreciate that neither he, nor my mom, really knew how to swim in deep water! For a five-year-old, that three-foot pool was enough coupled with some Jersey Shore, and later, Florida, vacations. However, at the YMCA they taught me how to dive; the subtleties of the frog kick; and how to turn my head when breathing during freestyle.

For whatever reason, the instructor realized that I was at home in the water and learned easily. Then, he asked me to try out for the actual YMCA swim team…what a thrill for a kid who was often chosen near last during kickball team selection! In the sport of swimming, someone recognized real aptitude in me. Nevertheless, disappointment followed later: when I attended the first practice, I realized the kids were all much bigger and more proficient at swimming because they had already been attending practices. Instead of sticking to it, I felt so intimidated after the first practice that I resigned myself to not pursuing the sport. Sadly, my parents did not push me to continue and not "sticking it out" became a rallying call for me in the future. Yes, I learned from that experience, but I do wonder to this day if I might have predated

Pablo Morales, the Cuban American Olympic gold medalist, as a champion in the men's butterfly of "Natacion."

At the "advanced" age of 15, I took up swimming again during high school, when most highly competitive swimmers are seeking Junior Olympics fame or deciding where to swim for college. Nonetheless, I managed to win a "Most Improved Swimmer" award my junior year and soon owned high school records in the individual medley, representing my diverse interests, and the freestyle relay, suggesting an affinity for teamwork and synergy. This was not a great team, being a middle of the road public high school, but it did instill confidence. Relatedly, my sophomore year I managed to represent the fine state of New Jersey in the Junior Superstars, an all-around athletic event that was an offshoot of the famous ABC Sports show, "The Superstars," where pro athletes competed with each other in a variety of disciplines. My swimming prowess helped propel me to the regional championships in Boston, where I managed a fourth place since I was still a lousy miler, and a worse yet sprinter. Nevertheless, it was an enriching experience for which I must thank my coaches, Bruce Peragallo and Mike Scarpato. The latter was also my swim coach, and one of the three men who most influenced my life.

Coach Scarpato taught me not to make excuses and that there is little substitute for hard work. His voice rings clear when I recall one of his favorite lines, "Forget the riffraff." He was referring to those kids in tough inner-city high schools, who might distract you along the way. I knew he was right and never forgot his teachings, although I still somewhat resent the browbeating he gave me when I got touched out during a 200 IM swim, to then follow minutes later by barely completing the 100 butterfly. You see that day the diving event – which was always my chance to rest between those arduous disciplines – was cancelled. Consequently, the 50 freestyle represented my only chance to recover, and that lasted all of…oh…about 25 seconds. During the final lap, I could barely lift my arms out of the water, and there was Coach Scarp, yelling at me from poolside as he walked – no, slumbered – along the pool edge, taking me towards the finish. When I was disqualified, I recall in detail the expression of disappointment on his face, not so much his apparent anger.

Ironically, what stands out most clearly in my memory is how I told myself I would never quit again, and that it is more important not to let oneself down. Such thoughts often crossed my mind during frequent on-call nights at the trauma hospital, or in the midst of an arduous microsurgical replantation where I was still "under the microscope" 12 hours later and the digit was still ischemic (lacking adequate blood supply). Nope, I would redo the micro anastomosis yet again if the finger had not "pinked up" but NEVER quit. Although I owe a debt of gratitude to many people for instilling that commitment in me, Coach Scarpato remains top of mind.

No doubt that participation in sports teaches discipline and commitment, but interpersonal skills are paramount to becoming a good and trusted clinician. I must confess that I am the only person I have ever heard of that counted both rugby and ballroom dancing as valued hobbies…at the same time!! You see, I was fortunate in that I had two parents, albeit divorcing during my tender age of eight, who were excellent dancers. One must think it is the Cuban culture and roots, but I remember my mother starting formal ballroom dancing after her divorce as an excellent way to socialize and meet new friends in the area. Simultaneously, John Travolta gained fame as the confident dancer in the transformational film, Saturday Night Fever. Recognizing that I was perhaps a bit shy, I recall when Mom suggested I take a ballroom dance class in her studio and she found me a partner. While I was fourteen and the "older woman" dance partner was perhaps an uneven match, it was certainly a confidence builder. I am not sure if Elena continued dancing, but I recall loving it and ended up being my mom's partner for the next level: intermediate ballroom at Roger's Dance Studio in Upper Montclair, New Jersey, near where I grew up. Soon after, I went on to dance with my then high school sweetheart, also a bit older than I, and we even managed to compete in the Nationals, and later, North American Ballroom Dance Championships. We were part of a formation dance team and I recall having to lie about my age since this was not the under 18 Juniors competition. Nonetheless, it helped me to develop more confidence. Since then, dancing has forever been a part of my life and an important element of who I am. Late nights in the O.R. are often accompanied by a quick demo, sterile of course, if the right music comes on.

High school consisted of maintaining my grades, although without a huge amount of studying, coupled with swim practice, often in the early morning, and after-school training. Throw in some ballroom or hustle dance class/competition training, and I kept myself busy. That is a good thing; I do not regret growing up without the challenges of mobile technology, social media, and the ubiquitous gaming that youth and parents now must contend with. In earlier years, we played touch football or street hockey, YES, in the street.

The communication of, "Car!" was vital, but most of the time, I maintained a sharper focus than my classmates or friends. The ability to focus would serve me well as I was about to be thrown into a completely different environment from my high school days: Cornell University.

I often feel that my medical destiny took fruition upon my acceptance to Cornell. I could not have imagined that as a simply "good student" I could gain admission into an Ivy League school of that stature having come from, as mentioned, a large inner-city public school within a working class and immigrant community. Of course, I had the drive, desire, and family background that could steer me into this career choice, but I often harbored doubts about whether I would "get in," medical school. Cornell or any other college is merely a stepping-stone to obtaining professional school admission. Not to belittle my university days, as they are now perhaps my most cherished memories, but I had a singular goal: admission into med school.

I remember opening my acceptance letter and perhaps even doubting its validity for a nanosecond. In a strange foreshadowing, I had received an acceptance letter from N.Y.U. a few weeks earlier but was most smitten with the idea of a Cornell education. Why? I had already experienced its beautiful campus on the idyllic setting of the Western New York Finger Lakes Region. For two consecutive summers, I attended the Cornell swim camps. Much like my academics in later years, Cornell forged my swimming skills into contention for local dominance during my high school days. I will never forget the first time I stepped onto the Arts Quad, during a rare break from thrice daily swim sessions. I felt awestruck by the academic grandeur, the statues, and the classical architecture adorned with climbing ivy. Never had I seen anything so breathtaking.

The Quad itself was stunning, with its crisscrossing pathways that led to the entrances of storied buildings enmeshed in just enough trees to provide areas of shade and beauty, with well-placed open areas that merged with blue skies, under which students engaged in games of frisbee, hacky sack or simply sat in a circle amongst scattered books and socks. "This is idyllic," I thought to myself as I imagined myself as a Cornell student someday. However, in a mindset befitting my grounded character, I did not think I would ever return to the campus with dry hair and a backpack full of books, instead of a Speedo®.

Nevertheless, the memory remained etched in my mind, and I asked Mr. Heinz, my assigned guidance counselor, about the possibilities. He was quick to point out that nearby Bloomfield College also had an excellent premed program and suggested I investigate it. Whether it was the school's proximity or its more modest academic reputation that inspired his lowball recommendation, I cannot say for sure. All I do know is that his response sent me hurtling back to earth, wondering if similar level colleges could gain me admission to medical school. I told my mom right away about Mr. Heinz and his suggestion, to which she bellowed, "Oh, no. We will see about that. Let me ask what your chances are for shooting high."

Mom consulted our dermatologist, who as it turned out, was a proud member of a long family lineage of Cornellians, the Abels and Stackpoles. His son, Carter, was a member of my high school class and in hot contention for valedictorian (he later beat out Nancy Cohen in the closing weeks for the honor). I thought, "This is WAY above my level." However, Dr. Robert Abel educated my mother on the nuances of elite college admission and advised her that if my SAT scores were satisfactory and my class standing sufficed (maintaining the top four percent among nearly 800 students), I might "have a chance." He also reassured her that kids with diverse interests and a commitment to outside endeavors might hold some sway with the admissions committee.

When Mom relayed this information to me, I believed I had a shot. I am not sure if it was the swim camp experience or my unusual hobbies, but I somehow made it in. In my mind, my acceptance to Cornell represented the most monumental step towards reaching my goal – even to this day – but I also remember thinking it was only the beginning…boy, was I right.

The Cornell University College of Arts and Sciences was a true pressure cooker. In the days before classes began, as we settled into the dorms, I met a multitude of people from various states in the union, and countries near and far who appeared quite impressive to me. Many came from prep schools or long Cornell legacies like my Elizabeth High classmate, Carter. Others were members of prominent families or had older siblings at Harvard or Princeton. I wondered, "What am I doing here?" although I never doubted for a minute my ability or worth – until my Psych 101 midterm! With fierce competition (it seemed that every other student I met was of the driven, "premed" variety) and endless steps in the journey, I felt relieved to have been assigned a freshman pre-med advisor named Nelly Maseda, who helped put me at ease.

Like me, Nelly had a Latin background and a public-school education. With thoroughness and clarity, she explained the process that I was about to embark upon. As we discussed my freshman year schedule, I understood the importance of every exam and every hurdle and stepping-stone. I remember how hard I studied for my first major college exam: The Psych 101 midterm. While I thought I had prepared adequately for this first test of my collegiate worthiness, I was not prepared for the result. Despite hours of study and preparation, I only managed a C+. I soon realized that this represented an average result. Since grades were calculated on the infamous curve, it was simply an indication of a middle-of-the-road grade in a school populated with intelligent kids, many of them with a superior pre-college education/preparation than mine.

However, the grading curve explanation brought me little solace, given my pre-med status. I thought, "How am I going to achieve my goals if I already scored just an average grade in a critical course despite my seemingly very best effort?" It was a serious wake-up call. I remember calling Nelly with the news, and she managed to muster some words of encouragement, but I KNEW I had to bring my game to a new level. Up to that point I had been attending water polo practice in the hope of learning and mastering this new and demanding sport. After practice – which often involved treading water for nearly 15 minutes while holding a brick, or even a chair completely out of the water, shoulders exposed – I returned to the dorm exhausted. I realized I could not continue on that path and decided to immerse myself in fraternity life, where I could participate in sports via the interfraternity intramural league, but keep studies my priority while gaining a home away from home: Rockledge, a frat house.

The Cornell Iota chapter of Alpha Sigma Phi was a terrific support system. While many of the brothers were in the engineering school, there were several other pre-med students who served as a tremendous resource. The rush process began during the latter half of my first semester; precisely when I needed to focus on improving that psychiatry grade, along with all my other courses that initial freshman semester. Yet it also taught me a valuable lesson in time-management, a vital skill that would serve me throughout my career. I managed an A- during that final Psych exam, garnering me a B+ for the course which was certainly acceptable. Moreover, I learned from the experience that with simple focus, I could overcome adversity and achieve my goals. Cornell has a way of doing that to you.

My later Cornell years were the most memorable of my life. While I embraced the "work hard, play hard" adage that so many deem a cliché, I learned to enjoy the journey and not simply fixate on the future. The pre-med track was difficult and organic chemistry was the infamous "weed out" course that I fortunately excelled in. I would later use this analogy of excessive competition, rather than collaboration, between colleagues. The rivalry started there...

I went on to choose the physiology concentration within the biological sciences major because I felt I would have the best affinity to this discipline, and with this approach, would achieve the best grades. It wasn't the easiest curriculum, but I enjoyed it so much I managed to become a teaching assistant for the core course during my junior year, thanks to my sophomore-year performance. This gave me my first exposure to teaching. The experience of delivering a lecture to my peers, some of whom were senior to me, was both a challenge and a tremendous preparation for the future in academia, even outside traditional academic practice. Being a teaching assistant instilled confidence and humility, as there were often fellow undergrad students who knew some of the material better than I. This experience certainly represented foreshadowing.

During my freshman year, I tried to continue my ballroom dancing hobby. I even managed to come home to New Jersey to enter a competition with my dance partner, who was disappointed in my lack of focus. Another decade would pass before I'd hustle, swing, waltz, or foxtrot across the dance floor, but I always knew I'd take it up again someday.

While I was never a 4.0 student, I was determined to earn the necessary grades to achieve my goal of entering medical school while I enjoyed my college experience to the fullest. The latter half of my freshman year I began to play rugby, a sport that encouraged camaraderie and forced me to maintain my fitness level. I hit the weight room and got my cardio by running outside on the beautiful roads surrounding the "gorgeous" Cornell gorges. I played intramural sports and reveled in our frat house's social environment, where I met some of the most interesting people I would ever encounter. A few, such as Rohit Bakshi, Alexander Counts, Ralph D'Onofrio, John Latella, and Jose Santini would become lifelong friends. Others, like Craig Stanley, helped me get through Computer Science 100 and became my finals week study partners. After all, not everyone can keep up with a study "tool."

Senior year brought the stress of studying for the MCAT, the Medical College Admission Test, the one playing field leveler that existed in the application journey. My grades were good but not stellar; however, my college life was well-rounded, and I felt that was more important in becoming a

"good doctor." I enrolled in the Kaplan course to review the chemistry, physics, biology, and other subjects that would ensure an acceptable MCAT grade
and propel me into the next chapter of my life. It was somewhat ironic that
this exam took place in the Cornell Law School, in what now feels like a
foreshadowing of the other challenges I would encounter in my future professional life. By the way, remember Pablo Morales, the Cuban American
Olympic medal winner for the butterfly? After retiring from Olympic sports,
he pursued his J.D. Degree at Cornell Law School and walked those same
Anibel Taylor halls!

MCAT grades soon came and my application was complete. I had to write
an essay, of course, in which I stated with conviction that I was hoping to
"use my hands as tools." To this day, that phrase elicits guttural laughter from
my frat brother and fellow physician, Dr. Rohit Bakshi, my primary proof-
reader. Although I was expressing my early desire to enter a surgical field, I
must confess that I will not forgive Dr. Bakshi, who is now a Harvard neu-
rology professor, for allowing me to use that simplistic phrase.

For reasons unexplained, I do not have clear recollection of receiving my
med school acceptance letters. Perhaps their arrival was anticlimactic, since
SO much had gone into the process and the prior preparations. The first
acceptance I received was from UMDNJ (New Jersey's medical school in
Newark) – a major relief since it confirmed that I would somehow achieve
my goals. It represented my best shot because state universities focus on admitting their own residents. While I felt pleased, it did not compare to the
emotion I experienced they day I received my N.Y.U. acceptance letter.

The New York University medical campus was not on Washington Square,
site of the undergrad campus where I had been accepted four short years prior,
but rather in midtown Manhattan. I was fully aware that the primary teaching
hospital was Bellevue, a storied institution among public hospitals, and the
location where Dr. William A. Nolan had trained. A general surgeon, Dr.
Nolan wrote the book, *The Making of a Surgeon*, a major influence for me
during my younger days in this journey, as I have mentioned. It felt apropos
that I would soon be walking the same halls and wards my mentor had travelled.
How exhilarating to achieve this major milestone in my path to becoming a
physician, and perhaps a surgeon as well!

While admission to medical school is possibly the most significant hurdle
in a physician's career path – assuring the student that their dream will be soon
realized - it simply represents the start of an intense decade of study and struggle

all medical students must endure on our path to becoming healers. Although I was well on my way, I scarcely imagined what I was about to experience.

DOING THE STUDENT "SIDE-HUSTLE" TO SURVIVE

The life of an undergraduate student is challenging in many ways. However, unless one comes from an affluent family that offers full support, the economic pressures can be significant. Most students must live somewhat austere existences in dorms, frat houses, or simple shared apartments, remaining forever cognizant of their spending habits. An almost inexorable and expected rite of passage, if you are a medical student, you must be willing to continue the college student lifestyle well into and beyond medical school and the residency training years. Well accustomed to living on a budget, my solution was to work two-to-three jobs during every summer break – and the summer before my first year of medical school was no exception. The romantic notion of backpacking through Europe was not a luxury a child of middle-class parents could afford (although I would later make up for that in a big way). I went back to lifeguarding during the day and driving a palette jack in a produce warehouse at night. I also mixed in some shifts teaching Nautilus (familiar to fitness enthusiasts older than age 50) at a hotel gym. In short, I did anything I could to save up some pocket money to keep me going during my first year of medical school in Manhattan, where the cost of living is high.

Aside from cost-of-living issues, I had to contend with the skyrocketing cost of tuition, which is amplified at private universities. How was I, an immigrant to the United States and the son of divorced, middle-class parents fortunate enough to attend an Ivy League university, followed by a top-tier private medical school? With a lot of help…for which I will always be grateful. Although my dad was an electrical engineer, he once remarked to me that he never made more than $50,000 a year. True, this was 30 years ago but even at that time, it was not a huge salary. It could not support a Cornell education for me and a Rutgers University education for my sister during the same period I attended N.Y.U. Med.

My father used to lament that the union electricians at his company often made more money than he once they accumulated some overtime wages, which is symbolic of many troublesome issues I will raise later in the book. *How can the person who sacrificed years and expenses to obtain the education and knowledge that supports what the technician performs, make less than that person?*

What does that tell an aspiring professional who faces daunting expenses and makes untold personal sacrifices to prepare for a position that knowledge – as opposed to rote handiwork – is NOT the employment currency? This is not at all to belittle a respected tradesman, like an electrician or plumber, but our society must reward those who invest years in an education while others earn money right after their high school graduation. Education and innovation propel a populace forward.

I recall my father discussing the beauty of partial differential equations as his eyes rolled back in his head and I could literally see his brain power grinding away. Does that not have a value to society? If intelligence and accumulation of knowledge are not rewarded, what message does that send to our culture? In fact, Dad was an aspiring PhD student when he broke down from sheer exhaustion from caring for two young children at home while my mother worked evening shifts as a hospital technician. Of course, in the daytime he HAD to work too before attending engineering school in the late afternoon. However, once he realized he would be "overqualified" for many engineering jobs, he gave up the doctorate track and settled on completing his master's thesis. Now it's even worse. What does that say to our young people? Apart from issues I will discuss in healthcare remuneration for the best trained and educated, there is a growing sentiment that college educations may not be a good economic investment. Coupled with the nearly linear cost increases, this ought to be of paramount concern to us all.

Despite my family's limited resources, I managed to attend Cornell due to my mother's tenacity and stubbornness. The financial aid package that followed my acceptance letter to N.Y.U. made it quite doable for me to attend that undergraduate school. On the other hand, Cornell's financial aid package left much to be desired. It seemed they wanted me to attend their university with minimal financial assistance, which deflated the euphoric feeling I had when I opened their acceptance letter. Undeterred, my mother phoned the university financial aid office to schedule an appointment with the dean of admissions who oversaw financial aid, in lieu of asking questions.

Within a week, we drove the four hours to the beautiful Finger Lakes region of New York and parked in front of the admissions building on 410 Thurston Avenue – a lovely old, wooden home that was the nucleus of Cornell future brainpower. During our meeting Dean Scanlon appeared to be understanding and accommodating, yet when we left, we were still uncertain of the outcome, much like the application process itself. Within 10 days we received a letter that outlined a combination of grants and low interest loans that would make it feasible for me to attend. I will never forget that gesture, along with my mother's unwillingness to accept an unfair decision. She taught me the power of discussion, tenacity, and compromise at an early age.

The N.Y.U. School of Medicine offered a similar type of package...without the need for any arm wrestling. The late Dean Brienza, who oversaw admissions and financial aid, was regarded as a nearly mythical figure among students. I remember well his kindness and steady affect because he treated each student who came to him with their hardships as if they were his only concern.

Consequently, I did not graduate with an overwhelming burden of debt, despite attending two private universities. While I consider myself fortunate, I am concerned about current challenges students face and my prospects of funding both of my own children's educations. We will certainly not qualify for financial aid (nor should we), but the rising cost of tuition has become unmanageable for many people unless they do qualify for significant aid.

Forbes presented data proving that the price of higher education has increased eight times faster than wages since the 1980s, a clear indication that few parents can pay for their children's schooling with average job earnings. Bloomberg illustrated that tuition expenses have climbed 538% percent, while medical costs, the subject of this book, have increased 286% – an absurd amount, considering that the C.P.I. (consumer price index) has only risen 121% in the corresponding three decades. Much has changed in the past 35 years since I began my long journey at Cornell. These developments elicit serious concern for the future of health professions, starting with allopathic and osteopathic medical school education and beyond.

To provide contrast, consider the testimonial of another first-generation immigrant, Alphonse J. DiGiovanni, retired general and vascular surgeon, who attended medical school several decades ago:

"In 1956, the cost of medical school was not excessive. On the other hand, some of my tuition and expenses were paid for by the GI Bill after my service in the U.S. Army, which I appreciated. Although it was partial, it carried me through the first two-and-a-half years at Hahnemann University in Philadelphia. I made up the difference by working at night at different places as a junior intern. And I met my expenses even though I had a young, growing family – a wife and three children, before I entered a four-year surgical residency program.

"Back then, a college student and a medical school student could work a few jobs to cover their tuition and expenses because costs were reasonable. I had no choice but to pay for my undergraduate education and my medical school education as the son of hardworking immigrants who arrived in the United States from Italy as a young married couple. My father was a tailor and my mother a seamstress. I was grateful for the opportunity to pursue my dreams, thanks to military service and later, several odd jobs. Today, it's just not possible for students to do that and I think it's a shame."

Medical school graduates are not the only ones facing immense challenges regarding the high cost of education, followed by underwhelming salaries. According to 20-year pharmacist Aileen Gonzalez, today's pharmacy school graduates cope with an oversaturated market exploited by corporate America:

"In Cuba, my grandmother was a pharmacist, so I followed in her footsteps. However, now I tell everyone that if anybody in their family that wants to study pharmacy, I advise against it, unless it is truly in their heart. But to be a doctor because your father was a doctor? I would not do it. The New York Times published an article about pharmacists being overworked and stressed, but other than that nobody mentions it. What is interesting is that in Miami and South Florida at least – I am not sure about the rest of the nation – they have opened many pharmacy schools. Twenty years ago, when I first graduated and got a job, I received a sign-on bonus. Now, because of the influx of pharmacy school graduates, there are no more sign-on bonuses.

"Worse, while inflation has gone up, salaries have remained stagnant. Pharmacists make anywhere from $50 to $65 to a max of $70 per hour…and even that is rare. I do not even think a $70 per hour wage exists anymore, and wages overall are going down to $35 or $40 an hour. I took a $70,000 loan to attend Nova Southeastern University, a private school. Currently, Nova and the many private pharmacy schools that have opened have increased their tuition to $150,000. And that is only the academic part of it. If students need money for housing and living expenses, they take out even more money in loans. Some of them graduate from pharmacy school with $200,000 to $300,000 in debt, and they cannot get a job.

"Aware of their predicament, American corporations take advantage of them. They will hire a pharmacist for $35 or $40 per hour, yet the pharmacist must pay back enormous loans. I am still paying mine 20 years after my graduation, although I took a break a few years ago from my profession to buy condos and flip properties, which helped me pay off a chunk of it. Even so, I still owe about $14,000 and I send the minimum payment of $120 per month. It is painful. My income does not even support the lifestyle that I live. I am a single mom with a daughter. I like to live comfortably and give my daughter a good life because I grew up in a high middle-income family. It has been a rough couple of years, but I do not look at situations as negative. I think they are all there to learn from and they just made me more powerful, like 'Bring it on.' Give me an issue and I will deal with it, but I am also going to learn from it. There's always a message in everything you encounter."

Keep in mind that many personal fitness trainers, or specialized mechanics, will make well over $100 an hour. Put that in perspective when considering what Aileen makes as a pharmacist, despite the critical role she plays in managing healthcare and the extensive background she must have in science and pharmacology to safely deliver that care.

Lest you think I am all gloom and doom, let me share some positive developments. In 2018, right around the time I began to ponder writing this book, N.Y.U. School of Medicine made a startling announcement: attendance at their medical school would be tuition free – for all. Not surprisingly, the applications surged nearly 50 percent in 2019 and the applicant pool is more diverse, a concern among medical schools since the average graduate is white, yet many are asked to practice in underserved communities of color. The goal is also to encourage graduates to ignore reimbursements when choosing less lucrative specialties. Much of this funding comes from private sources, including the Langone namesake. During this time, I was also named to the medical school's board of governors, prior to my 30th graduation reunion. Like many private institutions, successful graduates are expected to contribute to the future viability of the school.

MEETING MY CADAVER

The first year...no, the first *day* of medical school is an immersive experience thanks to one critical course: anatomy. On your first day of classes, they introduce you to your "cadaver." Some students name him, but I do not recall if I named mine. However, I do remember that the professors assign six first-year students to each body. You pair up with another student, then rotate three shifts in following the class assignment as we dissect the specific body parts and commit to memory all the relevant anatomic structures and, most importantly, understand the topographical relationship of these structures to each other.

Perhaps as a further foreshadowing, I recall in vivid detail that we began with the anatomy of the right shoulder. As the first to make the incision on our cadaver, it was evident that I was geared for surgery. This type of three-dimensional learning on an actual human being cannot be replaced by any book or even computerized graphic images. I mention this because anatomy is one of the subjects that is undergoing drastic alterations with today's major shifts in medical education via technologies, such as virtual reality and cyber-learning. For countless reasons, it has been given less priority; in many institutions, students do not receive exposure to it at all. I will expand upon current changes in medical education later.

During that first semester, my five co-anatomy partners almost become family. I often found them dissecting away at midnight when I decided to stop by the lab and review my retroperitoneal structures. Like running into your kid brother in your home's kitchen at midnight, fixing himself a sandwich, these spontaneous encounters soon forged a crucial bond between my classmates and me. We realized we were in it together – a completely different mindset from my undergrad days of vigorous competition in organic chemistry. In an ideal world, this sense of camaraderie would last forever, but that is not the case. While anatomy cultivated teamwork, many other basic science courses engendered fierce competition, because many of us would later seek competitive residency slots. This is yet another reason why physicians confront many struggles in "the real world." You see, the race never ends. I would soon learn that others take clear advantage of that fact.

Near the completion of the second medical school year, which is the "basic science" curriculum, all U.S. medical students sit for the National Board exam. Part one of the first exam focuses solely on the basic health sciences, including biochemistry, pathology, pharmacology, etc. The competition is fierce, and the tension is palpable. I recall traveling to the N.Y.U. law school, ironically, to study in a less stressful environment, away from my med school classmates. This was yet another critical hurdle, whereby my grade would be used as the most accurate barometer of my knowledge and aptitude to then compete for certain residency positions. At N.Y.U. Medical School, our grades were essentially pass/fail; hence there was little else to compare other applicants by. For me, the exam was critical. I already knew I would be pursuing a surgical residency, most likely in orthopedics, which was one of the most competitive slots. As was typical for me, I managed a good, but not terrific, score. However, good enough was my goal.

Between my first two years of med school, I took a job doing research in a non-invasive cardiology lab at N.Y.U. Dr. Mariano Rey, the Director and

Lead Researcher, was also a Cuban- American. Due to his gentle teaching style and our shared ethnic heritage, he became a mentor. It was unusual to meet a Latino faculty member at N.Y.U., let alone one with a Cuban background. Dr. Rey had been one of the "Pedro Pan" immigrants, young children who left Cuba alone, without their parents, to escape communism. Decades later in Miami, I would meet many more community and industry leaders with the same background as Dr. Rey.

As my mentor, he provided my first exposure to clinical research, when we examined the cardiac stress test results of a specific demographic: NFL referees who happened to be mostly middle-aged men performing a stressful activity once a week. The position did not pay much, but my goal was to develop a well-rounded resume to set me up for success when I applied for the residency match later (have I mentioned the race for success never ends in the medical profession?). I needed exposure in clinical research and co-authoring a study was critical fodder for that application. I already had some basic science research experience, assisting Dr. Joseph LeDoux, a prominent neurobiologist, in a lab at Cornell Med during a college summer. That involved a daily commute to "The City" from my New Jersey home during that hardworking "break". This was another example of doing whatever it took to round out my future med school application because research was a critical component.

To make some money to support myself during my first med school summer, I took a position as a waiter at one of those Manhattan restaurants that have sidewalk tables. I had some prior experience as a busboy and later, a banquet waiter in various New Jersey restaurants during my late high school years and summers off from college. It provided me with critical pocket money, so I figured I would work at this restaurant during my third semester as a med student, due to its proximity. My employment did not last too long, however. I will never forget the day when the owner, a mean-spirited lady who was the matriarch of the family business, fired me for the offense of requesting a week off just before classes resumed. I wanted to spend time with my girlfriend and her family at their Jersey Shore home, but it was too much for a struggling student who was working several jobs to ask: how dare I enjoy some much-needed R & R before re-immersing myself into the grind? It felt symbolic when *The Back Porch*, located on the mythical corner of 33rd and 3rd (pronounced with a *New Yawk* accent), closed its doors. I experienced an interesting mix of emotions when I heard the news.

With part one of the National Board exam behind me, I threw myself into the clinical years of medical school, which encompassed not only book work, but real-life challenges in becoming a physician. With only a knowledge of basic sciences, I had to concentrate on both to develop an understanding about clinical medicine. Traditionally, the third-year med school curriculum consists of five clinical subjects: the "majors" of medicine and surgery; and the" minors" of pediatrics, psychiatry, and ob-gyn. Each rotation lasted several months, with a group of fellow students assigned to each rotation and location. Ironically, of the eight or so students in my surgery rotation, all but one wanted to pursue a surgical career – ensuring the continuation of the competition. Each time our resident surgeon asked who wanted to insert a central line or place a foley catheter, multiple hands shot up in unison. Despite the challenges, I felt fulfilled in the surgical rotation. While I enjoyed the intellectual pursuit of internal medicine rounds, I did not like the often-tentative nature of the decision-making process. Psychiatry was worse: most of the time, there was little we could do for these hapless patients. Pediatrics was like veterinary medicine: patients could not converse with you and describe their problem with clarity. Dealing with their anguished and stressed parents made it worse. Obstetrics and gynecology involved caring for only half the population. Through these experiences, I realized that I enjoyed treating the gamut of patients: young, old, male, female, sick, or relatively healthy. Surgery afforded that opportunity and, as I stated in my essay, I yearned to "use my hands as tools." (Hmm, I still cannot believe "Roho" let me use that phrase!).

While each clinical discipline soon had its enthusiasts, the fourth year of med school allowed one to pursue those fields – or more crucially, other specialties – in more detail. Many areas were given virtually no exposure during the third year; therefore, it is a vital year of learning and discovery.

For example, how would any med student know they had an interest in ophthalmology when our only introduction to it was a two-hour session on how to do a fundoscopic examination during the medicine clerkship? The fourth year was a way to explore clinical interests in such fields as radiation oncology, pathology, or dermatology. It also gave students a chance to see how other institutions and even other cities' healthcare systems functioned. The fourth year provided an opportunity to travel and cultivate one's chosen area of clinical interest. Naturally, I chose orthopedic surgery.

One of the most common questions people ask me is, "Why hand surgery?" I imagine many physicians get this type of question from friends, family, or even patients. Like any lifelong decision, it is comprised of many factors. My third-year surgery rotation confirmed my interest in pursuing a surgical career. The specific choice of orthopedics stemmed from many influences, beginning with the childhood experience of going to the hand surgeon with my grandmother, and in subsequent years, the impact Dr. Nolan's book had upon my psyche. In addition, I had the opportunity to meet and observe orthopedic residents and surgeons in the N.Y.U. medical campus gym. Located in the gallows of our old dormitory, Coles Hall, it was open 24 hours with cardkey access.

Due to their demanding schedules, I would often encounter an orthopedic surgical resident at odd hours of the night. I noticed how satisfied these specialists seemed to be with their career choice, and how their outlook often contrasted with the exhausted complaining of the general surgery or ob-gyn residents. In a testament to their interest in physical fitness and health, the orthopedic faculty also came down to the gym often to work out - hence, the jokes about how an orthopedist typically bench presses more than their board scores, or how if one wants to hide money from an orthopedic surgeon, place it in a book!

These light-hearted digs at our specialty reflect a certain truth: the profile of an orthopedic surgeon whose interests extend beyond the scholastic. Although that resonated with me, the reality of board scores and grades cannot be overstated. As I mentioned before, orthopedics is one of the toughest residencies to obtain; our board scores, grades, and research experience must be near the pinnacle.

Another contributing factor in my decision to pursue orthopedics was a critical experience I had during my third-year surgical clerkship, when my med school permitted us to choose a surgical specialty and spend one week on that service. It soon crystallized my decision to pursue further rotations during my fourth year.

Possibly due to my curiosity about the city of San Francisco, I managed to obtain a visiting fourth-year orthopedics rotation at the San Francisco General Hospital, a trauma center and city hospital much like Bellevue. I lived around the corner from the University of California-San Francisco (UCSF), the parent academic institution. While doing a rotation at that private facility would have likely been much easier from a logistics and time perspective, I chose the more grueling site: the county hospital in "The Mission District." It involved getting up at 5 a.m. every day, driving a beat-up VW beetle that a gal lent me, and parking on the street outside in time to do "pre-rounds." I had to see every patient on the inpatient service before making the rounds with the resident, then repeating same process with the attending orthopedic physician. By 8 a.m., I had seen every patient three times, and the team had generated an arms' length list of tasks for me to complete. Since the prize was the privilege of going into the operating room with one of the junior residents to assist, efficiency was a must. One of my first surgeries was a routine hip fracture that the resident essentially walked me through! In the moment, I could scarcely believe I was the one making the incision, delving through anatomy I had only recently dissected and studied, and inserting metal hardware. The operation allowed the patient, a little old lady, to begin taking steps again just a few days later, and the immediacy of her recovery left an indelible imprint. My career suspicions were confirmed: I would indeed pursue an orthopedic surgery residency. Let the competition begin anew!

When I returned to New York, I did a full month rotation at my parent service, the Bellevue Orthopedic Surgery Department. I had to ensure that they, too, saw my commitment and aptitude since my classmates and I would soon prepare our "match" applications. In yet another foreshadowing, I travelled to Miami to do a clinical rotation at the Jackson Memorial Hospital, where I devoted a week to four different services: spine, trauma, pediatric, and hand. Soon, it became obvious which subspecialty I preferred, and I even managed to meet (albeit briefly) the chief of the hand surgery division, Dr. William Burkhalter, who in another ironic twist, would soon serve as the primary mentor for my future hand surgery partner in Miami.

While the fourth-year clerkship allows a medical student to explore and possibly even confirm an area of personal interest, it also allows them to decide where to forge a life. Due to my love of the ocean and my Cuban roots, Miami was a natural choice. Having spent my second medical school summer in the city often termed "The Capital of Latin America," my fourth-year clerkship cemented my decision.

Based on the ongoing need to round out my resume, I pursued further research – this time in basic science – at the Mount Sinai Hospital of Miami Beach. Two years before my fourth year visiting clerkship, I spent a summer in Dr. Charlie Weiss's lab doing bench research on the inhibition of scar formation with hyaluronic acid. Not only did the experience provide me with the opportunity to perform surgical procedures again (this time on rabbits), it also introduced me to some genuine friends and future contacts for my subsequent move to Miami. With any lifelong pursuit, there are multiple forks in the road that require an individual to decide which one to pursue. For me, that summer in Miami, which was followed by a clinical rotation two years later, made a life-altering impact.

I remember going knee-boarding and water skiing one afternoon with some step-cousins, distant family who also influenced my choice to make Miami my home. As we boated in the area between the Venetian Islands and Hibiscus/Star Islands, it hit me that we were water skiing within minutes of skyscrapers in a metropolitan area. We were not in some remote bay or the tranquil Florida Keys, but rather the fast-growing yet immature city of Miami, where beautiful waterfront homes were minutes away from big city life.

Unlike my only sibling, Susana, I fully recognize that I am a city boy. However, I loved the concept of being able to enjoy these types of leisure and water activities within eyeshot of a downtown environment. During one of those moments, I made a bold declaration to my cousins: "Someday I am going to live in one of those houses on the water, guys!" They say a pitcher must visualize the pitch with clarity before hurling the baseball and a soccer player must recreate the penalty kick in their mind before stepping towards the ball. The same principle applies to career and life choices.

Hence, my fourth year of medical school was truly formative. After the orthopedic rotations in San Francisco and Miami, I spent time back at my home institution of N.Y.U., where I did an additional rotation at the granddaddy of all public hospitals, Bellevue Hospital. Having completed my internal medicine rotation during the AIDS crisis, I was already familiar with the storied halls of this great city hospital (I had also done pediatrics and psychiatry there). Psychiatry seems to be the most well-known service in the eyes of the public, thanks in part, to the old television series, *The Honeymooners*. Those who watched and remember the show can relate to Ralph Kramden (played by the late actor Jackie Gleason), bellowing about how he was sending his friend, Ed Norton, to Bellevue because he thought his friend was crazy. If Bellevue's psychiatry service was infamous, the trauma slot there was downright folkloric. I somehow felt at home, and it may be partly due to the stories and anecdotes I read in Dr. Nolan's book.

The Residency "Match Day" is a monumental, but nerve-wracking day for all fourth-year medical students around the country. On this day, you find out where you will train for the next three, five, or perhaps 10 years. This will be the institution, or conglomerate of hospitals, where you will begin to practice the art and science of medicine. It is also where you will live, sort of, and maybe even establish some roots during those harrowed years. Yes, it is a significant milestone in a new doctor's life.

However, my Match Day turned out to be rather anticlimactic, due to a simple interaction that took place while I was walking between Bellevue and N.Y.U. University Hospital, something all of us did several times a day. Suddenly, I heard someone exclaim, "Congratulations!" When I turned around, I saw the orthopedic department secretary grinning from ear to ear. "You got in", she announced with great enthusiasm. My reaction was one of angst and bewilderment: this was not the way I was supposed to learn of this news, nor was it necessarily what I was hoping for. In other words, this staff member had violated a long-standing tradition that medical students were not to find out the results of the residency matching until the same moment, in this case in the afternoon of Match Day.

"Are you okay? Aren't you pleased?" she asked.

I experienced mixed emotions. Of course, I was happy that I managed to obtain an orthopedic residency at a premier institution, but sometimes one has deep aspirations that are not easy to explain. I had really loved San Francisco with its prestigious research hospital, U.C.S.F., and had also envisioned living in the tropical, Latin climate of Miami, with a similar public-renowned hospital. When she noticed the tears welling up in my eyes, she apologized. Not wanting to hurt her feelings, I assured her I was indeed grateful and excited. To be honest, that was the last time I felt much regret. While I had looked forward to a change of environment and clinical atmosphere, I knew I would receive tremendous training. So, I buckled up and prepared to spend another half decade in "The Big Apple."

In that moment, I simply regretted the fact that someone ruined my Match Day surprise. No longer would I regard this milestone in every medical student's life as "The Big Day." That afternoon, as I opened my envelope among 150 other soon-to-be doctors who were screaming, crying, and jumping, Ralph Kramden again came to mind. "Oh, WHAT a surprise!" I yelled. While I refused to ruin anyone's moment, I later confided in some friends what had happened, and why I could not fully partake in their elation. Regardless, it was time to look ahead. Despite the Match Day mishap, I was about to walk the same halls as Dr. William A. Nolan, M.D., and incarnate *The Making of a Surgeon*. And that was something to celebrate.

Chapter 2 – The Residency: Doctor Bootcamp

*"I will apply, for the benefit of the sick, all measures
[that] are required, avoiding those twin traps
of overtreatment and therapeutic nihilism."*

There are few parallels to describe the phenomenon and experience of surgical residency. While it is akin to a U.S. Marine boot camp, it does not last for 13 weeks but rather five years…or six…or even seven in subspecialties like neurosurgery that require fellowship training post residency. The infamous "Decade with Dave," referred to the typical 10 years spent under tutelage of Chairman Dr. David Sabiston, a legendary figure in the history of American medicine, at Duke Cardiothoracic surgery program.

One out of every six general surgery residents quit residency training. Conversely, 89 percent of Marine recruits complete what is arguably the most challenging of military training programs. The latter is far more demanding in short-term physical requirements, but the sheer length of time, stress, and demands upon one's personal life to become a surgeon is unmatched. True, many other residencies present challenges; speaking from personal experience, it is the surgical programs that often require every other night on-call. That simply means you do not sleep in your bed at home every second night…for years.

The point here is not to whine or complain. On the contrary, most of us would have it no other way, a topic I will delve into later. What is important for the public to understand, however, is that few honored professions or trades demand this much in terms of time to enter the ranks of fully trained professionals and colleagues. Therefore, someone who chooses medicine makes the sacrifice because they understand it is necessary. It is the price they must pay to assimilate the amount of knowledge and hands-on experience required for a successful future practice, yet they hold onto the hope that there are rewards at the end. These days, however, the prevailing sentiment among physicians of most specialties is that the prestige, income, potential, and independence of their profession is no longer commensurate with the sacrifices they had to make to achieve it. This attitude may not pose a problem now, but my overriding concern – shared by many of my peers – is that the brightest and most talented young people will reject the notion of making similar sacrifices to become part of this honored profession. Our anecdotes will illustrate the enormous challenges we faced in training, and how they now seem to pale in comparison to our current challenges. No, I'm not referring to endless hours and dismal pay (although they are a contributing factor), but the lack of control and the multitude of daily stressors physicians deal with when they apply their education and clinical experience to the daily treatment of patients.

I began my surgical internship, the first year of residency, on the wards of what was to be for my entire training period: Orthopedic surgery. The general surgery residency consists of multiple monthly rotations where the intern is quite the work horse on every respective service: vascular surgery, neurosurgery, urology, cardiothoracic, etc. Weeks after completing medical school, I was one of two interns that fulfilled the daily tasks required for 40-to-60 patients on the Bellevue Hospital Orthopedic Surgery service.

Within days of starting my surgical internship, I faced a traumatic event: my co-intern resigned to return to internal medicine – a dramatically different experience. He had already completed a one-year internal medicine internship at the prestigious, private New York Hospital, a classic affluent hospital located up the avenue from Bellevue in Manhattan. I am not sure why he changed his mind. What I do know is that a surgical service with multiple patients requires a certain passion and interest. Internal medicine, although demanding in its own way, is an entirely different animal. They are two challenging, but completely different, fields of medicine. I imagine my co-intern possessed the excellent grades and board scores to secure an orthopedic residency and probably figured it was an excellent specialty for future practice since it is hard to come by. However, given its relentless demands, you must love it. Prestige alone is not reason enough to stay the course in orthopedics. He likely made the right choice for himself by moving on.

My co-intern's abrupt departure left me with an entire service to manage because the second-year residents and above spend most of their time in the operating room or certain clinics like pediatric ortho or hand surgery. This entails the hands-on (no pun intended) management of every patient on the service – from drawing blood (in the pre-phlebotomist era) and checking those labs, to ordering follow up X-rays and chasing down the films in the infamous X-ray file room. Described as "scut" work, or menial and routine labor, the term originated in the 1960s. Its etymology is unclear but likely began as medical jargon – probably by an overworked intern!

Lucky for me, within two weeks Dr. Bernard Miot came to my rescue. He was brought on by our department chairman, who had put the word out that there was a cherished ortho residency slot now available. Bernie was a terrific guy with a tendency to work at a steadier and more relaxed pace. It would be a challenging yet rewarding start to my training, and I would forever call Bernie my savior. The rest of my surgical internship remains a blur except for select incidents and patients that will linger forever in the recesses of my memory.

The sickle-cell AIDS patient who would come into the ER weekly (always at 2 a.m.) and often required admission due to her unfortunate sickle crises and pain management issues, or an abscess that needed draining. The steady gaze of Dr. Richard Goldfrank, renowned E.R. physician and expert in poisons who authored THE definitive text, Toxicologic Emergencies, kindly asking me to see the prisoner who shattered both ankles jumping off a prison balcony. Or another prisoner who disrespected the nurse and doctors so much that I sent him up to the prison ward with a long leg cast – featuring little pink bears and balloons on a yellow background from the pediatric area. Let his fellow inmates have fun with that…

However, certain cases made an indelible impact on my psyche. Thanks to the strength and scope of their impressions, I can recollect almost the entire course of care for each one.

A Not-So-Happy New Year

On New Year's Eve, 1989, we experienced a quiet peacefulness in the Bellevue Hospital trauma slot, the emergency room section where severe injuries or catastrophic cases were rapidly worked up and treated, often while the patient was either unconscious or screaming. It turned out to be the lull before the storm. As a relatively new intern on the trauma service, I was forewarned about what this festive night would imply for Manhattan's most important Level 1 trauma center. While I waited, I paced the floor and reached for yet another coffee…but nothing. At one point, I even laid down on a gurney that was in a small room used for acute labor and delivery cases that presented through the E.R. Still, *nada*. Just an eerie silence. Then, an hour after the clock struck midnight, I heard the familiar intercom announcement, "Trauma 4344, 4344," which was the in-hospital phone extension for the trauma slot. It usually produced a Pavlovian response in those of us on the trauma team. I can still remember those digits clearly and I experience a similar gut reaction when I hear a quiet knocking on a door, reminiscent of that 5:30 a.m. wake-up knock during my swimming camp days. *Knock, knock, knock… 4344!*

Following my brief nap on the E.R. gurney, I found myself up on the general surgery floor responding to some nursing inquiries. I remember rushing back down and, as I entered the trauma slot, seeing a youngish African American gentleman who was dressed somewhat well, compared to our usual trauma slot denizens, but not particularly for a New Year's Eve event.

Since our patient was unresponsive, the trauma team flew into action. We cut off his clothing and then began the usual drill of inserting large gauge IV catheters to proceed with fluid resuscitation protocols. The highly professional New York City paramedics, known as E.M.S., gave us a quick report that included the vital information that a gunfight had broken out in the coat-check area of a major New York City nightclub. With IV fluids pouring into his veins, the trauma chief yelled, "Let's turn him!" We had to inspect the back area because we had seen no signs of trauma, let alone a bullet wound. At first, nothing was noted. Our focus shifted to intubating him as he was going downhill fast, with barely perceptible blood pressure. However, something had to explain this rapid decompensation, so once again, we turned him.

At that point one of the trauma nurses shouted, "There it is!" I looked and in his right flank, near the kidney region, was a small hole – the entry site of a small caliber handgun bullet. The coordinated team jumped into action to wheel him to the elevator designated to bring him straight to surgery. The gurney blasted through the double doors and would enter OR room one, a large suite designed to handle major trauma. By then, his blood pressure was barely palpable, and his EKG leads soon revealed flatline. With the defibrillator paddles used in shock care, we managed to get a heart rhythm again. But as we made another attempt to transfer him onto the O.R. bed, we again lost the heart rate. We began chest compressions, with intermittent cardiac defibrillations, and the loud utterances of "All clear!" This went on for what seemed to be an hour…nobody wanted to give up. We had already administered multiple units of blood with no pressure response. Nobody wanted to "call it."

Time passed in a blur of endless instructions, protocols, compressions, and intermittent yelling. After what seemed an eternity, the chief of trauma and the anesthesiologist "lucky" enough to be on call that night, agreed to pronounce the patient. We were floored. A cold silence gripped the room as we all acknowledged the fact that a young man had lost his life – all with a single penetration of a small caliber bullet in an obscure, barely visible location. He was never stable enough to even "lap him." An open laparotomy incision would have revealed a belly full of blood. Uncontrolled internal hemorrhage created so much instability that we could not even transfer him, let alone make an incision to find and stave off the bleeding.

I left the O.R. room and sat just outside the main O.R. office, adjacent to the double doors we had recently entered with a man who had depended on us to save his fleeting life. Dumbfounded, I gathered the energy to go back to the ER. That is when I heard it. The screams of a family member, or maybe a spouse, friend, girlfriend…someone. Delivering the news was never easy, of course, and for some reason, this case stands out in my mind. I soon found out that aside from New Year's Eve, the man had also been celebrating a personal achievement: passing the NY Bar exam. He had chosen a somewhat seedy, but popular club when a random, senseless fight broke out in the coat-check area. He got hit and here we were. As I quietly sobbed, I bowed my head. I can only remember a few incidences during my intern year in which I cried out of genuine emotion. I cannot even explain why this case affected me to such a degree but in an ironic twist, I discovered sometime after that this man was the son of the chief of another major trauma center in Brooklyn. It is hard to imagine the scene that unfolded when someone broke the news to his father – a medical professional who likely had multiple experiences with similar tragedy involving other patients. This time, the deceased patient was his own son, a man cut down in the prime of his life, when he was about to embark upon his own chosen law profession.

Cardiac Chaos

While the trauma service led me to encounter mortality on occasion, this threat of death was omnipresent amid the cardiothoracic surgery service. Heart surgery inspires awe among lay people, kind of like neurosurgery ("brain surgery"), as it should. Opening a chest and replacing small blood vessels on the surface of the heart, which is often beating, or replacing a valve are feats that inspire genuine wonder. On the flip side, cardiac surgical and/or post-op patients present arduous challenges, which fall under the domain and responsibility of the CV (cardiovascular) intern. These fragile and often very sick patients are on this service to reclaim their lives in a literal sense, and although the senior residents and cardiothoracic surgery fellows bear the brunt of responsibility for them, they tend to place much of the work burden on the interns. These interns must answer to the resident and cardiac fellow, who in turn, answers to the CV surgeon attendings – the physicians who spend most of their time doing surgery, reviewing cardiac cath images to plan, and seeing patients in the office. The interns and residents do the "work."

Early in my intern year, I was assigned to the C.V. Blue Service at the prestigious University Hospital (N.Y.U. Medical Center), later renamed Tisch Hospital, and more recently, Langone Medical Center. It really depends on who writes the bigger check…but more on that later. That service was run by the chief of the cardiothoracic division, Dr. Frank Spencer – who also happened to be the Chairman of the Department of Surgery and one of the three or four most powerful people on the entire medical campus, this infamous service was grueling. Dr. Spencer, affectionately (or so we assume) known as "The Boss," descended from what was known as the golden era of surgery.

A co-author of the definitive textbook, *Principles of Surgery*, Dr. Spencer enjoyed close relationships with multiple chairmen around the country. Remember "Decade with Dave?" Well, in a similar manner, The Boss was above reproach and inspired confidence. One of the most charismatic men I have ever met, he spoke with a southern drawl, having grown up in North Texas and attended medical school at Vanderbilt University in Nashville Tennessee. This accent remained despite decades in the big apple.

During my medical school surgery rotation, Dr. Spencer impressed students with his ability to recall all our names during the initial introduction to the service and field of surgery. However, for an intern, he was a man to be feared, although he was reasonable and fair (usually). Every night, without fail, the C.V. senior fellow, someone who had already been in surgical training for near a decade, would have to do "Boss rounds." This entailed taking a phone call at 10 p.m. sharp at the far side of the C.V. surgery recovery room, most often next to a table strewn with left-over Chinese food – a frequent "gift" from one of the infectious disease consultants, who was asked to see one of our patients in trouble, or from one of the many cardiologists.

The Boss call was stressful on many fronts. The fellow was expected to have ALL the information and numbers regarding Dr. Spencer's patients, including lab results, chest X-rays, and consultant impressions. Who obtained that body of data for him? The intern. There were only two of us for a service of upwards of 60 patients. The information had to be precise, organized and above all, timely. That call always came at 10 p.m.: you could set your Swiss, or maybe even Atomic, watch to it. What happened after the Boss call? The intern was given permission to go home – usually. Understand this was the first intern, the one who had been on-call the previous night and worked throughout the next day, only to be held till the Boss call so that the fellow could feel he had backing, "Hold on, Dr. Spencer, let me get you that white count or chest film…" The intern was within striking distance, but not too close.

The other intern, whom I will call "Intern B," was upstairs, busy on the wards, or likely the C.V.C.U. (cardiovascular intensive care unit) putting out fires. Constantly. While Intern A was hoping the Boss call went well, and no further tasks were needed, intern B was compiling data for morning rounds, in between the extinguishing of crises. That could be a patient with tachycardia (racing heartbeat) or an abnormal blood test result that needed correcting (please administer 2 more runs of K+ … potassium, nurse X). Once all the scut was near completed (and it never is), Intern B would now TRY to sleep. This mental/physiological function was attempted in a small room known as "The Doghouse," comprised of a bunkbed next to a desk in what was likely a converted janitor's closet. The walls and ceiling adjacent to the bunkbed were covered with graffiti consisting of memorialized ridiculous calls a past intern had received, usually from a floor nurse. "Doctor the patient's potassium is 3.9. What should I do?"

While this may not sound humorous, when we know that a normal potassium level is about 4.0, and the well-meaning nurse woke you up at 4 a.m. to "inform" you that it is 3.9, it *is* funny. Or tragic…but you had to laugh to keep from crying. You see, the intern, on every other night call as you might have surmised, will only get to sleep about 45 minutes. It typically began at around 3:45 because by 5 a.m., one must be awake to get data collected for the pre-rounds with the resident and then the C.V. fellow. Frequent interruptions mean that the total amount of sleep (most of it, REM), will be well under an hour. Subsequently, all patient care decisions are made by 7:45 a.m. since the surgeons, NOT the interns, must be down in surgery before 8 a.m.

The cycle of work begins. These repetitive rounds, during which each patient might be seen three times, generates a lot of scut work. Turns out, C.V. surgery is the only service where the intern dreads hearing the words, "You are needed in O.R. X." Why? This order has several ramifications. They will tell you to scrub in, then ask you to hold the heart in an unnatural position to allow the fellow or the attending surgeon to get a stitch into, for example, the back wall of the heart.

This might sound exciting, but to reach into a sterile field with your arm completely outstretched and your shoulders against two surgeons' backs, or flanks, is not a comfortable feat. You cannot even see what they are doing, and you cannot move your hand or arm, because that could be the precise moment when the surgeon passes the needle through the 2 mm lumen of the tiny vein graft. Pure torture. In fact, one morning I held this position for what seemed an eternity, an inexact period that followed barely an hour of sleep some hours prior. As I struggled, I promised God I would give up my firstborn child if he simply allowed me to retract my arm and perhaps close my eyes. At last came the words I longed to hear, "Badia, take a breather but don't go anywhere." I scrubbed out and sat on an OR stepping stool, resembling a metal, 10- inch high bench, where I promptly fell asleep, my back against the green tile OR wall below the X-ray viewer. Thank you, God. Fortunately, I forgot my promise many years later with the precious birth of my first, a daughter.

Interns like me repeated this frenetic activity and relived these scenes repeatedly for a month...or two if you happened to draw two C.V. rotations back to back, like a buddy of mine did. C.V. surgery internship was truly the epitome of the folkloric, grueling surgical internship experience; the stuff of urban (medical) legends that had been memorialized by my inspiring literary hero, Dr. Nolan. I remember leaving the hospital (yes, after Boss rounds) and walking back to my Tudor City apartment, ten blocks up First Avenue. However, I would typically go north on 2nd Ave so that I could witness some non-medical human activity as young people walked between bars and café restaurants – and because I would grab a slice or two of pepperoni pizza along the way. By contrast, 1st Ave. had neither pizza, nor many people. While I yearned to see that normal life activity, after several weeks I entered a dazed, robotic existence where I would see those same people, but strangely enough, not miss it. That was when I became a bit worried: How could I think this was a normal, expected routine? I arrived at my 15th floor micro apartment, with no recollection of ever hitting the bed and waking up six hours later, only to repeat the cycle again: 42 on, 6 off. 42 on 6 off, and then...every other Sunday completely off. *Yippee.* Fortunately, the rotation ended before I made a complete transformation into a Zombie, and I would be off to my next adventure, like vascular surgery. Not quite as bad...but close.

Now, you must be thinking, "How in God's name can a surgeon provide good, safe care with no sleep?" The simple answer is, "They can." Out of motivation, drive, and simple necessity, it is amazing what a human being can accomplish. Never underestimate the power of adrenaline, combined with a desire to perform. I just read a story where an ultra-marathoner broke a speed record of running the Appalachian trail by four days! Over the course of 41 days, he ran the equivalent of two marathons a day on demanding trails, with minimal sleep and the most extreme demands on his body. Navy Seals embark on missions that permit minimal sleep for days on end. While surgical internship is demanding, it does not compare to running up a mountain at sunrise or being immersed in frigid water for hours...besides, interns do not really do the surgery.

You simply cannot place a value on the continuity of care and the amassment of knowledge that results from not doing "shift work," – and as Malcolm Gladwell explains in his book, Outliers, "ten thousand hours is the magic number of greatness." In medicine, there is no substitute for singular devotion to caring for patients on a surgical ward or ICU, not to mention the hours required gain the knowledge and manual skills to perform surgical tasks. Yes, after internship, it does get better as you advance in residency. Chief residents sleep, and therefore, operate the most in a typical surgical service. However, many people set out to disrupt this long-standing process of surgical training and achieved their goals in a classic example of "Be careful what you wish for."

FAKE NEWS AND THE FUTURE OF MEDICINE

In early 1984, an 18-year-old college student named Libby Zion was admitted to the affluent New York Hospital (yup, a Cornell teaching hospital) with a fever and intense earache. Eight hours later, she would die on a regular nursing floor. Despite providing little information about the myriad of psychotropic and pain medications she had acquired via "doctor shopping" for months prior, this clearly troubled teen also failed to disclose that she had used cocaine earlier that evening. Although a tired intern (an oxymoron) was likely involved in the case, the media glossed over the fact that nurses and other healthcare professionals also administered care to Libby. You see, her father was a prominent New York City journalist. Few people know that he was also an attorney – a former New Jersey federal prosecutor, the office my mother worked with for years as a federally certified interpreter. The urban legend goes that he was the publisher of the New York Times.

Due to Libby's extreme agitation and discomfort, Demerol was ordered, as is often done in these circumstances. In this case, the patient experienced a rare and fatal reaction from the drug's interaction with Nardil, one of the many outpatient drugs she'd been taking. The years following her tragic death were characterized by a public, legal, and journalistic spectacle, which led to the creation of the Bell Commission, chaired by Dr. Bertrand Bell, an ambulatory care director at Jacobi Hospital in the Bronx. In 1987, the Commission crafted recommendations that resident hours be restricted, and in 1989 – the year I began my grueling surgical internship, one month after my lovely Washington Square graduation from N.Y.U. School of Medicine – the New York State Health Department adopted them. I had taken The Hippocratic oath, central to this book in many ways, at the acclaimed Carnegie Hall in midtown Manhattan and embarked upon a career whose origins had been forged in my childhood. For the past two decades I had worked tirelessly to achieve this milestone, and in that moment of euphoria, the Bell Commission findings were the last thing on my mind.

However, I remember the day I learned about the ruling while I was on the infamous cardiac surgery service. The New York Post (not exactly a beacon of responsible journalism sans the sport section), published a headline entitled "NO-SLEEP DOCTORS" (yes, in all caps and bold font.) Underneath the headline was a photo of a surgeon and his team operating on a patient. Mind you, the kyphotic back slump of the surgeon revealed in an instant that this was no 20-something resident physician. As I stood in the doorway of "the doghouse" about to enter the cardiac CVCU, I reviewed the article, "Exhausted interns endanger patients as hospitals break law."

"How dare they?" I seethed. "What does some journalist know about what we are experiencing and accomplishing here?"

On page five, it described the now iconic whistleblower: "The resident – we'll call him Dr. Y – has a recurring nightmare," etc. The truth is, the resident was neither male, nor an intern who would enter a surgical profession that requires late-night consults and trips to the O.R. Rather, it was a female resident who was going into the ENT field. In those days, two years of general surgery was required. I mention her sex not to slight female doctors, but to point out the misleading nature of the news article ("fake news" may be a popular term today, but it's not a new problem). Furthermore, this resident's concern – while understandable – should never have been sensationalized by the New York Post. From accounts I have heard about my colleague-whistleblower, this article paved the way for many adverse changes in my own training, which I will recount later. The case of Libby Zion, while dramatic and unfortunate, elicited a knee-jerk reaction from politicians and bureaucrats. Sound familiar?

This incident illustrates one of the stark realities about the practice of medicine: current healthcare regulations and processes are instituted by folks with little knowledge about the actual delivery of care, or at best, armchair physicians. In this case, Dr. Bell was tasked with running ambulatory care services in the outpatient department of a large city hospital. He was not in charge of the trauma or ICU services, and if he were practicing today, he would likely not be called to lead a Covid19 unit with multiple dying patients on ventilators. While Dr. Bell had good intentions, the medical professionals that administer care that requires around-the-clock attention should have been involved in the formation of sensible rules that do not disturb necessary processes.

The New York Post article went on to say that the health department "has already cited 20 major New York Hospitals including N.Y.U. Medical Center, Lenox Hill, Bellevue, and Montefiore for violating Regulation 400 and FORCING their young doctors to work excess hours."

"Wow," I thought. "I'm training at two of those hospitals." However, my concern had nothing to do with my own welfare or the determination of whether this was just or unjust. Rather, it was focused on the question of why bureaucrats hundreds of miles away in Albany had the authority to make such sweeping statements when my colleagues, mentors, and I were the ones making 6 a.m. rounds outside the I.C.U. I did not realize it at the time, but the entire incident formed the foundation of the frustrated sense of injustice brewing within me. Early in my training I had been exposed to the process of outside forces making unilateral decisions that would affect my profession and, moreover, our patients. Reading the newspaper that morning was a pivotal moment for me. By the way, I keep the "Late City Final" copy of the paper, weathered and yellowed, within the pages of my N.Y.U. graduation photo album, one of the rare mementos I've saved, along with a 911 headline.

The remainder of my internship remains somewhat a blur. The Bell Commission rulings cast a shadow over the remainder of that year, but I sensed that we all knew we were doing the right thing – preparing for a unique profession that required a solid, unwavering commitment. As physicians, we know that the public holds us to a higher standard, and within our profession, there is a code (although imperfect) that dictates how the torch must be passed. Fatigue and lack of sleep were not among the factors causing angst. I suspect none of my readers take issue with the rigorous training Navy Seals must endure – especially if a committed terrorist shows up in their neighborhood. *Why do they make them jump into a pool with an 80-pound backpack, or spend the night in wet clothes, with minimal sleep, while on surveillance mission?* To get the job done, at all costs. I tell my patients, "If you ever walk into a surgeon's waiting room and it's empty... run." I am being facetious, of course, but we all want the best trained and most practiced surgeon to operate on us or a loved one. And that level of expertise comes at a price.

The real challenges of surgical internship may not even be the extended hours and near sleepless nights, but rather, the singular dedication that inevitably affects other aspects of your life. In my case, maintaining a relationship was next to impossible because I had not gotten married during my decade of education. I have no regrets, given the high divorce rate among medical professionals, most notably those who marry in the early stages of their careers.

True, marriage can provide a support system and someone to come home to at the end of your shift. However, for the other spouse, it can be tough to endure their husband's or wife's long absences. It is even worse if both partners are enslaved to some difficult years of true, singular apprenticeship. I found it difficult to maintain contact with friends – whether the few from my high school days or my almost mythical college experience. While I yearned for that companionship and camaraderie, I was just "too busy." And forget med school buddies. Keeping in touch with them was impossible because many of them had left New York City and were in the same predicament. Remember, this took place long before cell phones came along. If you're old enough to remember pay phones, I'm sure you can relate when I tell you I never seemed to have a quarter in my pocket when the thought came to mind, "Let me call so and so." After all, it's not like I was home much.

Money was an even greater concern. During my intern year, I earned a total salary of $25,000. That was it. No moonlighting, no odd jobs, no pyramid scheme to generate additional income. Keep in mind, this was the late-1980s New York standard of living with its consequential consumer price index. My dad had helped me put a down payment on a truly quaint and lovely one-bedroom, one-bathroom corner apartment in a nearby pre-war development named Tudor City. The development had recently renovated a large cache of old apartments, which they were selling requiring only five percent down payments. That was unreal for New York back then. I got into my new residence for well under $10,000 dollars, feeling fortunate to have a decent bathroom with a shower to myself; a separate kitchenette (okay, it was really a closet with French doors); and a couch and TV in another room (albeit five feet away) -- quite a contrast from every other shoebox apartment I looked at before. I was elated.

Now, how I spent my free time was another matter. Given my schedule, no fancy gym memberships were feasible. Socializing might consist of meeting friends at a *Happy Hour* (usually closer to the *Sad Hour* time) and holding on to the same beer most of the night. I peeled off many a bottle label as I chatted with friends, fought to stay awake, and maybe eyed a certain vixen that caught my attention. It was difficult to find time for a subsequent date, due to my hours, and even scheduled meetings were jeopardized, depending on the surgical service I was on and the cases that came in. Many evenings simply consisted of ordering a pizza, perhaps some modest wine or beer, and watching a film on the weathered VCR machine (thankfully, there was a video rental shop on the first floor of my building). In the pre-Blockbuster days, it allowed for flexibility and spontaneity for a meager investment and epitomized the typical intern date.

Then there was the matter of fine New York City dining. Although the Big Apple is famed for its ubiquitous restaurants, most of them were out-of-reach of most residents' budgets. On rare occasions, we might enjoy being taken out by a pharmaceutical rep, and later, by an orthopedic implant company. These unique occasions gave us an opportunity to savor a nice meal and learn something outside of a book or the O.R. lounge, while fulfilling the basic human need to socialize. How ironic that decades later, this custom is restricted by the regulators – as if politicians and bankers did not have business lunches. Or dinners. Or both. One thing I can state with conviction: the term "Martini lunch" was not coined by a medical resident or a well-meaning medical device rep eager to capture the attention of a busy, hungry physician-in-training, if only for a few moments. To this day, I still cannot fathom why this is a problem.

In a decade of training amid the glorious, gastronomic Manhattan, one amazing meal at the renowned Four Seasons stands out in my memory. I had met a young lady from Berkeley California who was working on a project for Merrill Lynch. While the details are a bit sketchy, I remember she picked me up with a limousine and whisked me off to the iconic restaurant, synonymous with the New York *power lunch*, whose successes largely depended upon the financial markets. It remains my singular memory of an upscale dining experience, far removed from the typical pizza, late-night hospital cafeteria food, and occasional Chinese food outside the cardiac recovery room.

There were many memorable experiences, and patients, during the arduous intern year. Much of the year is a fog, but I was able to recall some specific cases that are deeply engraved in my memory.

I remember taking care of a young man who was struck by a bus when crossing the avenue with his mother. He took the brunt of it and had an open tibia fracture that, as often occurs, became infected leading to what we call osteomyelitis. To avoid amputation, we must infuse many weeks of IV antibiotics through a large bore IV. Due to the toxicity of this to peripheral small veins, and to avoid multiple painful needles sticks, nurses would infuse this through a "central line", a large diameter catheter that was inserted in the neck, the internal jugular vein that would dump into the vena cava, then the heart. The intern would change these catheters every three days, via a sterile process over a guidewire to avoid re-sticking the patient and prevent infection of the indwelling catheter. It was tedious work but often allowed me to get to really know some patients as I reassured them throughout the procedure, poking tubes at their neck and then suturing them in so as not to be pulled out inadvertently.

Danny was one of the lead bartenders at the Copacabana, the famed midtown Latin nightclub frequented by celebrities like Sinatra, Sammy Davis Jr, and even the mob during NY mafia "glory days" as profiled in a scene in the film, Goodfellas. Barry Manilow further immortalized it with his pop hit, *Copacabana*: "At the Copa, Copacabana" also refers to the famed Havana nightclub of same name, one I visited during my only trip to my home country, for an international orthopedic congress.

Well, Danny needed his central line changed Q72 hours, and I soon got to know him well. Once discharged (and we did save his leg), he and the nightclub manager were so grateful to me that I not only never waited in line to enter the club, but many a cocktail was "on the house." For a starving resident, this was worth more than gold. I would later meet my girlfriend Maritza of my residency days there and we often danced the night away, despite my tight budget.

Danny died some years later from AIDS complications, but he, like many patients from that year, touched my heart and soul.

While some might consider internship a rite of passage, I suspect most dedicated surgeons view it quite another way. The most quoted result of that challenging year sounds something like, "We learned to take care of sick patients." To a layperson, a sick patient may sound a bit redundant, but for us it describes the patients whose lives are in our hands in the I.C.U., or the ones who take a sudden downturn on the ward right when they are about to be discharged. During the current COVID-19 pandemic, it may mean something else. What you learn from such patients affects the care you give to others for the rest of your professional life. Whether you sign off at midnight or 8 a.m., it does not give you the experience you need to be engaged in every step of that patient's recovery…or demise. No matter how exhausted we felt, we did not want to disengage from their care because we understood the nuances and history of that patient's clinical course. Sure, we supported each other and relied on our senior residents, fellows, and attending surgeons but we wanted to see the job through. And that is the type of physician a patient wants. That is my takeaway from my surgical internship experience.

Orthopedic Residency: Learning How to Reconstruct the Body

General surgery internship bridged the divide from medical student to clinician. While I often dealt with stressful clinical situations, accompanied by the necessity to multi-task, the experience did not bring me much closer to becoming a surgeon. On occasion, a surgical resident would "take me through a case" which means that they would walk me step-by-step through a procedure while my hands did the bulk of the manual work. Medical students interested in a surgical discipline would often tie endless knots with sewing thread on the post of their bed, or the arm of a chair. As with many things manual, increasing speed and dexterity is achieved with practice and repetition. Whether a surgeon's knot, sliding knot, or slip knot, one-handed or two-handed, lefty or righty, the quick and reproducible action is akin to perfecting a free throw shot in basketball. Listen up Shaquille... Practice makes perfect. However, while the handiwork of surgery is essential, it is only a small component of the surgical discipline.

Understanding the anatomy and exact steps required to perform a specific surgical intervention is quite another matter. Execution and repetition alone will not suffice since one can do the wrong thing many times and yield poor clinical outcomes. Then there is the critical ability to ascertain the when, how, and why of surgical procedures. Such in-depth knowledge of managing clinical pathology through surgery is the actual goal of surgical training. Orthopedic residency focuses on the complete care of virtually any affliction of the musculoskeletal system. It is just as important to know when NOT to operate as it is to administer the vital pre, intra, and post-operative care. During the intern year, the basic principles of surgery and patient care are ingrained, but the specific management of diverse pathology will be learned via the different surgical residencies. Urology, otorhinolaryngology (the study of diseases of the ear, nose, and throat), plastic surgery, neurosurgery and so on, require full immersion. My training in orthopedic surgery would now begin. For the rest of my existence, it would influence my life and the future care of my patients.

The R2, or second year of training, marks the first year of orthopedic surgery residency, whereas urology, E.N.T. and others may require several years of general surgery exposure. I spent the bulk of my second year in the University Hospital of N.Y.U., where I had my initial exposure during my third-year clinical internship. This time, however, I held major responsibilities. The R2s assumed the role of intern at this academic hospital, with private patients. There was little to no indigent care, and all the admitted patients to the orthopedic service were under the care of one of the attendings: private practice (albeit academic service), orthopedic surgeons. While it came with a great deal of responsibility, the ultimate decisions were made by the patient's surgeon. Although I shouldered much of the responsibility, each patient's surgeon made the final decisions about their care. The system had its pros and cons, but it provided my first exposure of scrubbing in with an experienced surgeon, where we embarked on a "This is how I do it" lesson – in sharp contrast with Bellevue, where the adage of "See one, do one, teach one" was omnipresent. Learning HOW to do many of these procedures in our early stage of training was beneficial. We engrained some good habits and principles we could then take to the busier public hospitals, or even the Manhattan V.A., where residents were indispensable to patient care, due to the high ratio of patient-to-attending staff. No, it is not a perfect system, but it works. I have almost no misgivings about the process, unlike my evolving views of our entire healthcare system.

During the second year, we are also exposed to the various subdisciplines within orthopedic surgery. We went to the Hospital for Joint Diseases (H.J.D.) for our pediatric orthopedic experience, an all-orthopedic hospital with a sizable pediatric service, where we gained additional knowledge and experience in a focused rotation. I also went to Mount Sinai, in Upper East Side Manhattan, where I had in-depth training in orthopedic oncology. As I described at the beginning with the story of my grandmother, childhood influences often gravitate a person to a specific medical discipline. For me, this includes the sensitive issue of orthopedic tumors.

When I was 11 years-old, a close friend and neighbor of my "yayos" (Spanish for "grandparents") was diagnosed with osteogenic sarcoma. By accident, he sat on a sewing needle on his couch (his mom was a seamstress), which penetrated his lower thigh. When the family obtained an X-ray to localize it, it revealed that the needle was a benign issue. However, an incidental and much more serious finding was a destructive bone tumor in his proximal (upper) tibia. Within a week, he presented to the Sloan Kettering Hospital in New York City, where his doctors promptly performed a below-the-knee amputation. Since I was close to the family, this was quite a shock.

A few months later, his medical team revised it to an above-the-knee amputation – in a drastic alteration to his mobility. Such measures signaled the presence of an aggressive tumor, as is most often the case, but in the 1970s chemotherapy protocols were not as advanced as they are today – nor is limb-salvage surgery. Intrigued by the idea of saving his limb, I remember thinking, "Why can't they cut out the diseased tissue, save the leg, and treat him with drugs?"

In under six months, Armandito died from metastatic tumors to his brain, a frequent location for this type of cell. My mom refused to let me see him due to the severity of his illness, which caused his head to become deformed rather quickly. Perhaps it was that tragic experience that somehow led me to consider a career in orthopedic oncology and limb salvage surgery.

However, during this same residency year I experienced my first in-depth exposure to hand surgery – an interest that had been instilled in me two decades prior with my grandmother's visit to Dr. Carroll and galvanized my interest. The second-year rotation of hand surgery was quite novel for us since it was our first real exposure to consistent outpatient and private practice care. Up to this point, almost every patient we saw was in a hospital setting: clinic, faculty offices, surgery, and ward rounds were all in the confines of the hospital walls. It seemed natural and logical that when a patient suffers from an illness or malady, they go to the hospital. Yet I soon realized that much of healthcare could be delivered outside of these huge, cumbersome, and expensive institutions. In the coming years and decades as I moved through my medical career, that feeling amplified within me.

Among my orthopedic mentors, Dr. Charles Melone, a quirky, somewhat eccentric figure, stands out. Ironically, his private practice office was located upstairs from a luxury auto dealership on 34th street, about one block west of the entrance to the Rusk Rehabilitation Institute, which was part of N.Y.U. Medical Center. However, it seemed worlds apart…I recall once seeing "Iron Mike" Tyson checking out the Ferraris and Lamborghinis as I peered in the window, a luxury that felt quite removed and distant for a second-year resident. I would later see Iron Mike on South Beach (Miami Beach), in a Ferrari, and then sit adjacent to him on a flight to Dublin, Ireland on the way to my inauguration into the RCSI (Royal College of Surgeons of Ireland) while he was giving his one-man soliloquy show, "Undisputed Truth". Perhaps he can help me deliver the knockout punch to the current healthcare debacle.

Dr. Melone shared his office with a bright young hand surgeon, Keith Raskin. Dr. Raskin had served as my chief resident during my intern year, so at least I already had some connection to this now foreign concept: the private practice office setting. I recall admiring the efficiency and mechanics of seeing patients in this calm and aesthetic environment. The fact that patients' pathology was limited to the hand, wrist, and elbow meant they were all ambulatory patients. There was no need for hospitalization, and I was soon to discover that principle held true for many of the surgeries I observed. Again, future foreshadowing.

Consequently, I felt a great interest in the practice parameters and pathology. Patients of all ages came in with a staggering variety of clinical issues: inflammation, acute injuries, pain, nerve problems, tumors, congenital deformities, and yes, arthritis. The latter harkened to my prior experience with my Yaya, who had suffered from the classic manifestations of rheumatoid hand: ulnar drift, caput ulnae, Boutonniere thumb, and swan-neck digits (for the hand surgeon readers). Well-known for many components of hand surgery, Dr. Melone was also adept with arthritis reconstruction, which delighted me. In addition, he had earned a distinguished reputation for evolving the management of distal radius fractures (something I would later have a pivotal role in influencing) and athletic injuries of the hand.

At the time, I could not imagine that I would later serve as the inaugural president of ISSPORTH (International Society for Sport Traumatology of the Hand), 1st assist in the surgery of a world boxing champ, Michael Moorer, and meet pitcher Tommy John. I found it rather ironic that a critical ligament reconstructing procedure would be named after one if its famed recipients, instead of its pioneer inventor, Dr. Frank Jobe, but it is a classic example of the role popular culture plays in overshadowing complex medical care, a phenomenon I'll delve into later.

My first year of orthopedic residency laid tremendous groundwork for later years. Having assisted, and on occasion performed a variety of elective and trauma procedures, I looked forward to the days when I would need to rely on my own knowledge and fortitude. They came sooner than I even anticipated.

I spent most of my third year of orthopedic surgical training back at Bellevue. Having just honed some of the needed skills at the private hospital blocks away (but seemingly a world away), I felt somewhat ready to embark upon a plethora of surgeries. The R3 on the Bellevue orthopedic service was the workhorse. We managed the interns – our own internships now feeling as if they had taken place in a prior lifetime – and the renowned Bellevue emergency room. As interns, we ran to the E.R. and followed orders, often consulting with senior colleagues when any significant medical decision was to be made. In our third year, we assessed, managed, and admitted the patients when necessary. Surgeries often came from the E.R. (typically traumatic injuries), or from a myriad of elective subspecialty orthopedic clinics, usually supervised by the attending orthopedic surgeon of that specialty.

The "third year" was responsible for the entire workings of the service, orchestrating the work that the chiefs ordered during the morning rounds on the wards. Surgery took place at all hours, depending on the patient presentation. We slept in the hospital generally every third night – often staying up all night rodding a femur fracture or applying an external fixator to an open tibia fracture, the stuff of city trauma hospitals. But this is where we *learned*, under the guidance of the fourth-year residents who were only one year older than us yet seemed to possess much more knowledge and greater judgement. In general, fifth-year chief residents had nothing to do with these cases because they had already done their share of ubiquitous fracture and trauma reconstruction. Instead, they did a bulk of the larger elective daytime type cases such as joint replacements and routine spinal surgeries, or focused on bringing elective cases in their evolving field of interest from the clinics, e.g. "Guys, find me two total hips from clinic for next week. I want to use the x, y or z prosthesis on it."

At Bellevue, the third-year resident *really* learned how to operate. How to adjust to an unexpected finding, deal with a sudden "bleeder" that maybe hits the ceiling, or when to switch course when the planned reconstruction was simply not going to work. This was the folklore of residency, the gradual evolution of a whole different language, and finally, a comprehensive understanding of what "Standing on the shoulders of giants" meant. The attending surgeons had been influenced by their teachers and mentors. They discussed the complex cases with the chief resident, approved the fourth-year resident's choice of surgical approach, and on occasion, got their hands "dirty" with the lowly third year.

I owe a debt of gratitude to many attending surgeons. During the predominantly trauma-focused rotation of the third year, Justin Lamont truly taught me how to think about a fracture, devise a logical game plan to address it, and then follow through with precise execution. The latter is akin to hitting a fastball, scoring a penalty kick, or building a bridge. Just like pursuing your career, the surgeon must first visualize the process, then focus like a laser beam with attention to detail. I recall Dr. Lamont's pearls of wisdom on the methods involved in exposing and then reducing a fracture, skills that apply to other facets of orthopedic surgery. In medicine, passing on these pearls to up-and-coming surgeons is expected.

The skills I learned from Dr. Lamont were put to an extreme test on the fateful afternoon of April 24, 1992, a gorgeous, sunny spring day in Manhattan. After a rough call night, I had finally left the hospital. Although I had managed to get a couple hours of sleep, it seemed irrelevant as I did my usual uptown walk on First Avenue from Bellevue to Tudor City, soaking up the sunshine. As I strolled along, I contemplated whether I would catch a couple of z's or rollerblade up to Central Park – something I usually did while heading north on either Park Avenue or Lexington. Considering I was a trauma surgeon, it was youthful folly, if also a great way to blow off steam and get much-needed exercise. While I plotted my route in my head, all the sudden, I heard it: the distinct, deafening sound of sirens. No, not the typical police car or ambulance siren; something much bigger and seeming more urgent.

Well before I saw it, I heard it. Later, I learned it was an ambulance bus that came roaring down First Avenue, southbound, eclipsing the velocity of anything on the nearby, parallel East Side Drive. I thought, "This is it. Better go upstairs and get some rest." Granted, I was not on call and I had worked all night, but the sight I had just witnessed was unlike anything I had even seen before. The call came within a few hours: "Badia, we need you to come in. Some old lady apparently plowed into a bunch of people in Washington Square. It's bad…" With no thought of any argument or explanation, I put my scrubs back on and headed south down the avenue.

A 70-plus year-old woman had plowed her car into a crowd of people at Washington Square Park, the epicenter of New York University, the non-medical campus of our affiliated medical school. It was normally a busy area, a bohemian square where college students, locals, and tourists all coalesce, creating a dizzying sea of humanity. Because the undergrads were in the middle of a beautification project with some elderly community groups, the area was even more packed than usual. Yes, the city's most vulnerable population had come together for a benevolent cause: cleaning, painting park benches, and making minor repairs to the common areas of the park on a picture-postcard spring day. The police later determined that the septuagenarian had hit the gas instead of her brake when she dropped off her daughter at an adjacent apartment building.

When I entered the Bellevue E.R., it was utter pandemonium, especially in the trauma area. I saw an older lady in one trauma berth and a young fella in the adjacent gurney.

Both had multiple lines in place and were already receiving units of packed cells (blood). Their clothing had been cut off. Beyond that, my memory gets fuzzy and hovers around being up all night with several polytraumatized patients. One elderly female had bilateral femur fractures and an open tibia fracture, which is enough to kill someone of advanced age. However, we spent hours stabilizing her lower limbs, and consequently, we resuscitated her. We placed titanium rods in her femurs, and a non-reamed nail in her tibia to stabilize her wounds simultaneously. And while the details of another elderly person's injuries escape me, we managed to save them, too.

What I *do* remember in stark detail is the scene I encountered in Room 1, where we bring cardiac surgery patients and some of the more egregious polytrauma cases. Between cases, I went there to check in on my colleagues and as I entered the room, I was greeted with chaos and empty blood bank bags strewn all over the place. Two anesthesiologists and several trauma and vascular surgeons were working on his thorax. I do not recall the exact nature of the injury, but it seemed like forever that this large, hyper-focused team had been working on this kid. I happened to be there when they called it quits… something nobody wanted to do. In fact, in an all-out effort to save his life, the medical team depleted the entire hospital's supply of suitable Rh factor blood.

The young man was only 19, one of the undergraduate students who was in the group painting park benches. He was only halfway through his college days when he was struck by cruel fate. While I did not work on him directly, the moment anesthesia pronounced, "Enough already," is etched in my soul. The surgeon argued and called for another round of Herculean, but fruitless efforts.

In a tragic twist on an expected outcome, that night two young students died, and two elderly patients managed to survive. From a logical, scientific, or even theological point of view, it simply did not make sense. Yes, many of life's injustices are put on display at large city trauma centers, and this incident comprised another chapter. Bellevue had received four of the most gravely injured patients with others going to nearby St. Vincent's, and others to Beth Israel, Cabrini etc.

For me, the story did not end, however. A quarter century later I was walking with my young daughter, Alessia, entering the same park from the south side, adjacent to the N.Y.U. Law school, site of so many nights of study as I escaped the medical campus climate. I was reminded of that sad day and began to recount the story to my cherished daughter, trying to delicately give her a flavor of her dad's experiences, good and bad. Suddenly a gentleman who was a few years older than me stepped up and affirmed, "Yup. That was April 24, 1992. Mrs. Stella Maychick accidentally accelerated into a group of people, young and old. I was a university maintenance supervisor and had been checking some of the buildings when I saw the carnage. I will NEVER forget." He certainly did not. His ironic and timely affirmation lent credence to the story I gently recounted to my impressionable child. I did not know whether to downplay his account or embrace him. We had somehow shared an incredible, life-changing experience, relegated to infamy in New York City lore. I told him that I had participated in saving two of the injured, older patients, and witnessed the eventual demise of one young man. He reminded me that four were killed at the scene and over 25 injured, and that our team was tasked with the most critical. After we snapped a picture together, we went our separate ways. Even Alessia was taken aback by the sheer fateful coincidence. Although it had already been seared in my memory, this man provided another perspective, melancholy as it was.

The Third Year: Finally Touching A Patient

My ability to manage orthopedic trauma was tested again and again. Later, during my third year of training, I began to get a bit anxious about my financial constraints and resulting lifestyle effects. I was in my late 20s, still making barely $30,000 a year and had to be very selective on how to spend my limited free time. Living in The Big Apple, few restaurants were affordable. I visited Little India – a one-block section of Greenwich Village (East 6th Street) – often. There my buddy Ralph and I once counted 19 restaurants – on either side of a single block! We had a laughing attack from that observation as we walked and counted.

Most of my friends were well into their careers and making a comfortable living, especially those from my Cornell days. Some were investment bankers and flying high (it was the early 90s after all) and my lawyer and other professional friends were long finished with school and building a normal life, even while paying off school loans. It was more than a decade after high school.

Although my father helped me pay much of my apartment mortgage payments and maintenance at first, it was not long before I became uncomfortable with that. Little by little, I told him, "It's really my apartment so I'll take over the mortgage payments and the maintenance." On my resident's salary alone, I could have never done it; the only reason I could relieve my father of any financial assistance was because I moonlighted. Like some of my resident colleagues, I worked in the Manhattan V.A. emergency room, which was three blocks past Bellevue, and the site of orthopedic service rotations during three of the five years of training.

Adding several 14-hour nocturnal E.R. shifts to an already busy schedule is no easy task. Yes, it was daunting, but it afforded me the opportunity to have some semblance of a normal life. Those paychecks made a big difference and truly taught me the value of a dollar. It was the first decent money I ever made, although quite meager for being the sole physician in an all-night E.R. I recall it being around $33 dollars an hour. Around that time, a medical school friend (who was then at Yale doing internal medicine) admitted he was doing the same thing. To me, it made more sense for him since he was an internist and not an orthopedic surgeon. Imagine my surprise when I discovered he was making a higher hourly rate than me, even though he was in New Haven and I was in midtown Manhattan!

It made little sense. Armed with this new knowledge, I marched down to the emergency department and demanded a raise. To my surprise, they gave us a sizeable hourly increase that took hold only a few months later. This incident signifies the only time a federal government agency acquiesced to a straightforward request in a timely fashion. It was fair and I was pleased. However, aside from the additional demands on my time, hiding this endeavor from our chairman's sight proved to be a challenge. Yet it paled in comparison to the exhausting weeks when I would sandwich a moonlighting shift between an "every other night" call schedule.

It went something like this: On a Monday, I left my conveniently located apartment at 6 a.m. in a straight-shot, ten-to-twelve block walk to work. Yes, I always walked because cabs were too expensive. To paraphrase an old joke, it may not have been "uphill both ways," but throughout every season, including the freezing cold and snow of winter, I hoofed it – often after many grueling hours on the job – because I couldn't afford any other method of transportation. Tuesday night, I moonlighted at the V.A. Hospital. Thanks to the protective nurses, most of the time I did not have to stay awake all night. Many vets came in at 3 a.m. with chest colds and the nurses would tell them, "We're not going to wake up the doctor," or, "The doctor's busy, you're going to have to wait." Of course, on multiple occasions, I had to be up. Although my shift ran until 8 a.m., they let me sneak out if I had to make rounds on time, so as not to risk my primary job: orthopedic resident. Although the ortho chair did not want us to moonlight (it was against the rules), he was a little clueless and looked the other way. Moonlighting was a necessity because they barely paid us enough to survive in a city with a high standard of living like New York.

Wednesday morning, I went back to make rounds and fulfill my obligation to be on call that night. Guess what? I worked through Thursday and arrived home at 8 p.m. To sum it up, I left my apartment at 6 a.m. Monday morning and returned Thursday night. I had not set foot in my home for three nights. Think about that. It is unheard of for most people. Yet this is how I spent many weeks during the remainder of my training.

Nowadays, thanks to the New York Post article, residents leave. If they make rounds at 6:30 a.m., they go home the next day after morning rounds when everyone goes into surgery. However, back then I worked through the next day, then did afternoon rounds with chief resident to review what was going on with the patients, before leaving around 6 p.m. And yet, I harbor no regrets.

NOT QUITE THE CHRISTMAS MIRACLE I'D PRAYED FOR

The R4 year was the third year of orthopedic training, which often focused on teaching others and taking responsibility. We dealt with more complex pathology, since the more junior residents handled much of the routine patient care issues and "everyday" trauma. It also included more rotations at outside institutions to broaden our experience and skill set. I have a vague memory doing a second tumor rotation, this time at the nearby H.J.D. again, which would later become our partner institution with the formation of the N.Y.U.-H.J.D. program. Today it is called Langone Orthopedics Hospital, erasing over a century of a storied name. If football stadiums have a price, apparently prestigious healing institutions do as well.

The orthopedic oncology program was not nearly as strong as my broad experience at the Mount Sinai Hospital two years prior. Although I had already become quite interested in hand surgery, there was still a lingering possibility of me pursuing this demanding sector of musculoskeletal medicine. I believe those latent ambitions were dashed one fateful Christmas Eve afternoon.

While making my plans to take the New Jersey Transit train to visit my family for a two-day Christmas holiday, I learned of an urgent admission to the H.J.D. tumor service: an adolescent boy from Puerto Rico who presented late in his country for evaluation of a rapid-growing mass just above his knee. Due to the nature of his lesion, they transferred him A.S.A.P. to New York City, where I was to conduct the initial evaluation. When I examined him, I was appalled to see that the tumor had already fungated through the skin and violated any tissue and skin planes that might allow for any limb salvage attempts. I presented the case to the attending, who promptly instructed me to schedule the case for the next day, Christmas Eve. Not being a Christian, he may not have realized the significance of that day to myself and other members of the team, but the advanced extent of this patient's disease compelled me to agree.

The next afternoon, we performed an above-knee amputation on a 14-year-old boy – on Christmas Eve day. Some hours later, I rode the train in a foggy state of mind. I do not remember much more, other than sitting at dinner with family during one of the most important holiday traditions for Latinos, and I could not get this young boy out of my thoughts. All I could think about was that he was spending his Christmas Eve in a hospital minus his right leg. That marked the exact day I decided to proceed with applying for a hand fellowship, yet another prolonged selection process, that would commence in the spring. It takes a special kind of physician to face death or life-shattering events on a regular basis in their normal practice. My hat goes off to them. They deserve our profound respect and gratitude. Today, during the current COVID-19 pandemic, the public is now acknowledging that. For me, I looked forward to relieving pain and restoring function to the entire upper limb, a subspecialty that seemed to be in the cards for me all along. I would soon begin the quest for a dedicated hand and upper extremity fellowship. Yet another hurdle was in front of me, one that required more applications, tenacity, and the uncertainty of where I would spend a year after my residency. Concurrently, there were more patients to care for… always.

SAVING the Sophia Loren of Physicists

In early 1993, a New York taxi inexplicably jumped the curb directly in front of the famed New York Hilton on the upper west side of Manhattan. He plowed into a long line of customers who were patiently waiting for some of his colleagues to take them to their desired destination that fateful evening. Because the taxi line was full, a multitude of bystanders were seriously injured, several of them fatally. One of the worst injuries was transported to Bellevue Hospital. As fate would have it, there was an international congress on optical physics at the hotel, and one of the participants was a young, beautiful scientist from Milan, Italy. She had sustained the full force of the taxi's impact, causing a severe open fracture of the tibia, just below her knee, in addition to something we term an "open book pelvis injury." Such injuries can be life threatening and this one was no exception. In an open book injury, the ring of the pelvis is interrupted and displaced, typically by two breaks in that anatomic construct. It renders the entire pelvis and abdomen highly unstable and often leads to associated internal injuries, whether the bladder, rectum, or aorta.

This young lady came in with labile blood pressure and diffuse injuries. Despite a concerted effort with fluid resuscitation in the trauma slot, the trauma team could not stabilize her. In an ironic twist, the chief resident at that time was engaged to a young lady I had dated during our early medical school days. At a subtle level, this was the stuff of "General Hospital" or "E.R." television shows. After all, most of us spend our time inexorably entwined in hospital life. It is not as exciting as Hollywood portrays, but it happens. Until then, there was the typical expected "tensions" between us, but this case was about to suppress them…fast. I was called down to the trauma berth, ala "4344", since the third year realized the complex nature of the case required a senior resident. After brief banter, my nemesis and I decided we needed to take her to surgery immediately. Her unstable pelvis was likely contributing to her hypotension and I informed him that I had to stabilize it with the application of a pelvic external fixator. The "ex-fix" is a large, stainless steel construct, resembling an erector set from childhood. It is attached to large, threaded pins that are inserted into the pelvic walls, two Schanz pins on each side.

After those pins are attached to clamps, the entire apparatus is manipulated to "close the book." This procedure not only stabilizes the patient's abdomen and pelvic viscera, but helps to control bleeding by decreasing the raw, oozing bone surfaces that are displaced from the fracture. As I rapidly attached the device, using the sterile hydraulic drills that are our reliable tools of the trade, we noticed that the pressure minimally stabilized. At this point, my now synergistic colleague decided to open the pelvis. "There must be a major bleeder," he uttered as he reached for the #10 scalpel and proceeded to open the pelvis via the classic Pfannenstiel incision. His prediction was an utter understatement: her pelvic floor was filled with blood that continued to well up, no matter how much suction we applied. To allow access, I had loosened the ex-fix temporarily and soon realized this was making the situation worse. There was no way to control the bleeding; we surmised we were losing the patient. We packed the pelvis and lower abdomen with multiple "laps" (surgical towels) and then retightened the fixator. Several minutes of intense discussion followed, a seeming eternity, before we made the mutual decision to "call in the cavalry".

Although interventional radiologists are not seen as surgeons (a fact little-known by the public), they often perform the most heroic procedures. If a vessel cannot be identified, clamped, or controlled from the outside, they can do it from within. It is the culmination of microcatheter technology, along with high-tech fluoroscopic imaging that often brings awe to even the most seasoned physician observer. The interventional suites were on a completely different floor. While we consulted with the radiology residents, anesthesia prepared the unstable patient for an even more unstable journey – out of the O.R., down the hall to the transport elevator bank, and then down to the radiology department. During that time, they had located the mythical chief of that division. He had been at Bellevue for decades and was rumored to be *the* highest paid civil service worker in all of New York State – more than the governor, the state district attorney, and even the hospital chief administrator of any city hospital.

This was the hospital's full-time chief of interventional radiology, Dr. Richard LeFleur, a "catheter cowboy" so to speak. He did not hesitate to come in and within 30 minutes from time of intra-op assessment, she was on *his* table, and he was ready to halt the bleeding via high tech intervention. He explained with clarity that the procedure to control hemorrhage could potentially also diminish the perfusion (blood supply) to her gluteal areas. She could essentially slough off her buttocks to save her life. For a Cuban red-blooded male, this was no minor matter. With the patient intubated and her husband back in Milano, we urged our colleague to move forward. He inserted a series of "micro-springs" that would lodge themselves in the origin of the deep circumflex iliac arteries – a major branch of the iliac arteries which bifurcate off the aorta itself. This was a risky but necessary procedure at this tense moment, else the patient would expire. Between several minutes and forever-and-a-day, the procedure was done. We noticed the patient's vitals had stabilized and we could finish the job at hand. I stabilized her lower leg with a ring-type hybrid external fixator. Another erector set: this time for the leg.

The patient not only survived, but while on the ward, we noticed that she did not have any significant adverse effects to the soft tissue and buttocks area, although we had our plastic surgeon colleagues on stand-by. As often happens with major trauma, one performs the needed tasks first, then asks questions later. Over subsequent days and weeks on the ward, I got to know the patient well and the impact of what we did took on even greater significance. I learned about her children, her husband, and her cherished career as a physicist. This vivacious, lovely, and brilliant scientist from Italy appeared to come out of a Fellini film, amid the denizens of the New York street life that surrounded her. These are the occasional long-term patients of the Bellevue wards, the ones we often call "citizens" – the more productive members of our society whose fate brought them to the hallowed halls of the oldest public hospital in the United States.

As much as it was a privilege to care for all patients on the Bellevue wards, it was an occasional patient such as this who did not seem to belong, but gradually began to fit in. We are all citizens of this earth, and the cruel hand of disease or major trauma relegate us to occupy the same place of humanity. It was a pleasure to witness the day "Dr. Italy- the Sophia Loren of physics," left the ward in a wheelchair, about to embark on a different journey of inpatient rehabilitation at an outside facility. Once she returned to Italy, she wrote me and recounted her recovery journey, now able to walk with her children and return to her scientific work. Caring for her and watching her recover day-by-day was an arduous but uplifting experience I will always cherish.

PLANES, TRAINS, AND AUTOMOBILES

During the fourth year of orthopedic residency, a surgeon also focuses on the specialty they might like to pursue. Increasingly, residents in many areas of medicine will pursue a fellowship, which means they will dedicate more time to honing their craft. Internal medicine residents may decide to pursue cardiology, gastroenterology, or perhaps infectious diseases, while others may elect to practice the broad spectrum of internal medicine.

In the past few years, orthopedic programs have reported that upwards of 95 percent of residents will pursue a subspecialty fellowship. While some may enter practice and do general orthopedics as a profession, the overwhelming majority will seek fellowship training. Why? Due to the explosion of knowledge, four years of orthopedic training will not suffice in many orthopedic specialty areas such as spine surgery, pediatric orthopedics, sports medicine (arthroscopy focused), or foot and ankle reconstruction. My initial interest in orthopedic oncology was related to my childhood experience of losing a close friend to a bone malignancy as well as my fascination for the magnitude of reconstructions that can now be done to save a leg or preserve shoulder function in large tumors.

However, lifelong decisions are often made from a collection of experiences, culminating in a gut decision or hunch. Amputating an adolescent's leg on Christmas Eve only reinforced my strong inclination to pursue surgery of the hand. While my earliest recollection of this calling was related to my beloved grandmother, the sentiment was reinforced when I performed microsurgery on the carotid artery of rabbits during my Cornell neurobiology research, and later when I saw the marked diversity of cases and pathology the microvascular hand surgeon managed during my training.

Much like the residency matching process, applications are submitted to the fellowship programs including USMLE board scores (licensing exams), letters of recommendation, C.V., research experience, results of the OITE (orthopedic in-training examination). In other words, it is the college application process all over again…this time on steroids. Aargh.

One barrier for me was the fact that on-site interviews are strongly suggested. I simply could not afford to fly to all the training programs I wanted to consider. The Mayo Clinic offered me an interview for a hand fellowship, which I declined. Although it is a prestigious program, I felt quite certain I did not want to be a full-time academician. I responded the same way to the famed Indiana Hand Center. During some engineering field visits, my dad had spent some brief time in Indianapolis. As a single Latino man from the northeast, he was certain his son would not be happy there during non-working hours. No insult to the Hoosiers, but I was not a fan of the Indy 500, nor did I care for the "vibrant" restaurant scene in this Midwestern city. Many factors come into play when making this type of career decision.

By then, I realized I would most likely establish my practice in the Miami area. However, the Miami fellowship did not have the breadth or scope I was seeking. Having spent a decade at a trauma center, I had dealt with my share of gunshot wounds, knifings, and IV drug-abuser hand infections. I wanted broad experience in community hand surgery, but I also had an interest in the entire upper extremity. Before it became fashionable, I was hoping to become proficient in shoulder and elbow surgery since those articulations place the hand in space. The upper limb functions as a unit; therefore, the ideal training encompassed the entire extremity. In 1994, there were only four upper limb touted fellowships. Turns out, I had good foresight: most hand fellow-ships today include upper limb training, despite the occasional protests of our shoulder/elbow and sports medicine colleagues. Again, competition persists.

One of those fellowships was at U.C. Davis in Sacramento. Since any in-terview agreement I entered implied that I had to pay for my own travel, lodging, and meals, I made careful, strategic decision. Lucky for me, I con-firmed an interview date for just prior to the 1993 AAOS Congress in late winter in San Francisco, which would allow me to kill three birds with one stone: have my interview, attend "the Academy" and visit friends I had made during my orthopedic rotation as a medical student almost five years prior.

The day of my flight, I arrived a bit late to the New York La Guardia Airport, thanks to a trauma case. I missed the bag check counter deadline and went directly to the gate with carry-on in hand. They allowed me to board and reassured me that ground crew standing nearby would get my bag on the plane. With a skeptical eye, I saw my lonely bag propped up against another passenger's suitcase and wondered if it would make it on the plane in time. Despite the ground crew's promise, when I arrived at San Francisco Interna-tional, my luggage was nowhere to be found on the carousel. Once it became eerily empty, I hoped against all logic it would somehow show up. After all, it contained my interview suit – and like many surgical interviews, mine was scheduled for 6:30 a.m. the next day. My interviewer and team had to be in the O.R. by 8 a.m. sharp.

As luck would have it, I then drove my rental car nearly 100 miles in the dead of night *sans* my suitcase. Keep in mind, this was well before Uber and even common cell phone usage. I grabbed my bulky map from the rent-a-car facility and began the long, lonely drive, worn out from my surgical schedule earlier that day. To my dismay, when I checked into my modest motel, I realized there was no way to get a suit or sports jacket the next morning in bustling Sacramento. I interviewed in jeans, a flannel shirt and cowboy boots.

I am not a "starstruck" kind of guy, but being a huge Olympic buff, I remember how disappointed I felt when I did not have the opportunity to meet Eric Heiden, one of the greatest winter Olympians ever. Since he was doing his training at this program, Heiden would have been my junior or-thopedic resident. Alas, it was not to be as he had to juggle other engagements as a famed athlete. A few days after my interview, I ran into the training pro-gram director in the hallway at the Moscone Convention Center in San Francisco, site of the orthopedic academy meeting. He greeted me with this reminder, "Hey Badia, aren't you the guy I interviewed a few days ago in jeans and cowboy boots?" Sometimes the best laid plans can work out for the better.

My most memorable interview experience, however, took place in the city where I decided to embark upon my hand and upper limb advanced training. Pittsburgh has long been recognized as a progressive healthcare city (along with technology and financial services), eclipsing its previous industrial reputation as the "Steel City." I was not familiar with any Midwestern city, let alone Pittsburgh, but do not tell folks from the "Burgh" that. They consider themselves northeasterners. Let us say that Pittsburgh is different in many good ways.

Alleghany General Hospital is a level one trauma center on the north side of the Alleghany river complete with helipad, outpatient surgery center, and a biomechanics lab in-house – all relevant features to a young surgeon seeking a broad experience within a tertiary care community hospital. While not as large or as well-known as the UPMC (Univ of Pittsburgh Medical Center) campus, Allegheny General Hospital's (AGH) hand and microvascular surgery reputation was stellar. The fellowship already had a rich history and allowed for a true private practice hand surgery exposure, coupled with major trauma center clinical challenges. The deeper appeal for me, however, was due to its division director and hand fellowship director, Dr. Joseph Imbriglia. Dr. Imbriglia had trained under the mythical Dr. Bob Carroll at Columbia Presbyterian – the man I met with my grandmother as an eight-year-old boy, some five years before Dr. Imbriglia would do his fellowship. While I am not one to suggest karma as an explanation for such serendipitous events, it seemed somehow fitting that I would now train with him.

My interview with Dr. Imbriglia was enjoyable and pragmatic, much like the program itself. Because I would engage with several colleagues that worked closely with him, it would be a broad fellowship experience, not an apprenticeship. In fact, I do not even recall a formal sit-down interview, but rather, being asked to join the department for the weekly hand surgery grand rounds – in essence a meeting of residents, A.G.H. hand surgeons, interested community surgeons, and the three current fellows. I recall sitting in the back in the rafters, so to speak, in a steep auditorium reminiscent of the old-time surgical teaching amphitheaters in turn-of-the-century realism paintings. Dressed in the typical interview suit, sticking out like a sore thumb, I tried to maintain a low profile while I listened with rapt attention to the main presentation and the clinical discussion of cases that came in that week to the hand service.

One of the cases pertained to a comminuted, intra-articular distal humerus Y-type fracture, or to put it in simpler terms, "a bad busted elbow." Dr. Imbriglia led this discussion on how to manage the injury and began querying mid-level residents, then fellows. At one point, he turned his whole body in my direction, facing backwards, and asked, "Hey Alex, how would you guys handle this fracture at Bellevue?" I looked around with a perplexed look on my face – he could not possibly mean me!

Since many people address me as "Alejandro," I thought perhaps he was talking to another guy named Alex. When I realized there was no one else in my vicinity, it hit me: Dr. Imbriglia was genuinely interested in my opinion. It was a dramatic departure from the stodginess and hierarchies I encountered in large New York City academic centers. I was taken aback.

With authentic interest and warmth, he fixed his gaze on me, his trademark bushy eyebrows raised in inquisitive expression. "Well, what approach would you take?" he repeated. In an instant, I felt comfortable and confident. I let loose with a detailed answer that began with a direct posterior approach, argued for olecranon osteotomy, and finished with a 90-90 plate construct with 3.5 reconstruction plates from the pelvic set…years before fracture specific plates would be developed. No sweat. I had done a bunch of these at Bellevue. The open, welcoming air in the conference hall just about crystallized my decision right there. After the conference, I met the other attendings including Drs. Butterbaugh, Hagberg, and Baratz, the guys I would learn from. Someone introduced me to the current fellows, whose brains I picked for a bit. Two of them, who remain friends to this day, followed instructions to give me the lay of the land, including a tour of the orthopedic ward, main hospital O.R.s, and the outpatient surgery center in the newer wing. They showed me the Singer Biomechanics Research lab, a favorite haunt of Dr. Baratz, who discussed basic science research possibilities with me. I felt very much at home and returned to New York with a hope that I would match in this program.

I continued my fourth-year residency confident that I had chosen the right path. I experienced the usual stress of selection and awaiting "the letter," but like most of my colleagues, I had grown accustomed to the competitive rat race. My confidence was rewarded in the spring when I matched at the

Allegheny General Hospital program in Pittsburgh, which enabled me to enter my final year of residency with my immediate and enticing future determined. I could enter my chief year with the ability to focus much of my attention to upper limb surgery yet realized that some areas of orthopedic care such as spine, would never be of primary importance to me. Still I did my best to embrace the opportunities. I tried to enjoy New York a bit more during my final year.

NEW LOVE, NEW CITY

The chief resident year is a culmination of thousands of hours of patient encounters, surgeries performed, and clinical pearls learned. Moreover, it is a time for further focus and narrowing down your vision for your professional life. It is also a period to harness leadership and organizational skills since the chief does exactly that: lead and oversee. Naturally, different surgeons have varying aptitudes in this area. Some may depend more on their junior residents while others may consult with the attending surgeons and professors for guidance. Regardless, the buck stops with you. This period of heightened responsibility is crucial for establishing independent thought as a clinician and surgeon because the time was fast approaching when you may not have another person to turn to when you are seeing patients, solo, in an office consultation. Peer wise, there would likely not be anybody with you in the operating room at 3 a.m. when you are called in to the community hospital to stabilize and repair that open comminuted (fragmented) elbow fracture or complete digit amputation. You will recall specific protocols, rely on some helpful tips, and simply get the job done. The chief year is the time to experience that independence and cultivate confidence and resolve.

The final year also represents a time of reflection as your decade of study and preparation comes to an end. The lengthy journey represents its own challenge. The fellowship year is determined to map out the location and subspecialty focus. It becomes a time to ponder a bit more on life and what aspirations one has for a professional future. Soon there will be no scrounging for money, perhaps some flexibility with time, and a chance to focus on oneself.

During my chief year, I was introduced to a medical resident at a networking event for Latin physicians. With few people who fit this category at that time at N.Y.U., I recall in vivid detail the moment I saw her. I could use an abundance of adjectives, but I will stay on point and simply say that after an extended courtship, she decided to join me in my fellowship year in Pittsburgh. I remember the exact moment she told me: she was applying lipstick and gazing at me through the mirror when she said something like, "I am thinking of applying for a geriatrics fellowship in Pittsburgh." *Wham.* The moments that followed seemed to unfold in slow motion. With a distorted facial expression and drawn out guttural voice like one used in a surreal, dream like film, I somehow uttered the word, *"Okkkkkkkkkkkkkk."* There, I said it. Up until then, my entire life – at least my educational process and surgical training – had been singularly focused on achieving the one professional goal of becoming a practicing surgeon. I had not allowed anyone to penetrate my exterior barrier and veer me off course. However, I now (albeit with trepidation) allowed myself to consider living with a young woman whom I fancied and respected. I had met several wonderful women along the way, some of them professionals and truly terrific people. But I was just not ready. The time had finally arrived for me to let my guard down and embark on several novel experiences at the same time. But first, I had to get through the chief resident year.

One of the most bizarre cases, replete with media frenzy, occurred halfway through my R5 year while on the Bellevue orthopedic service. An older, blind African American gentleman was brought into the trauma slot one late afternoon. He had sustained an open tibia fracture, routine for us, as well as a contralateral shoulder dislocation. I reduced his shoulder in the trauma slot, and promptly scheduled him for external fixator stabilization of his tibia. It goes that he was a well-known, almost iconic, figure in New York City lore since he had sold pencils outside of the Tiffany's storefront for the past 40 years, complete with seeing eye dog. That fateful afternoon, he was in his usual standing place when a taxi (yes, they can be dangerous as we have seen), jumped the curb, struck him, and took out his dog as well. It turns out that besides his owner's serious injuries, the dog reportedly lost an eye! So here was what sounded like dark humor, where an older sympathetic figure sustained a life altering injury and his seeing eye dog, a trusted companion, lost his own eyesight. Surgery on the homeless man went well and he was brought up to the orthopedic ward that night.

The next morning, the circus began. It seems this legendary figure inspired a human-interest story surrounding his dog and his unfortunate circumstances. He was on the front page of the New York Post, same paper that wrote about us "Sleepless Doctors," although with less genuine sympathy for the human patient than our canine protagonist. The story reported that his dog had been taken to the New York Animal Hospital, adjacent to the famed Hospital for Special Surgery, a competing orthopedic hospital with H.J.D. Having lost his eye, he was an inpatient since his master was downtown on our ward at Bellevue.

This cover story milked the collective pity of the New York metropolitan area as it chronicled the events of this lonesome figure and his trusted furry companion. You could almost hear the synchronous "Awwww" of the Big Apple as folks read about this mishap on the subway or street corners. As if one story was not enough, I believe he made the front page two more times, akin to a literary soap opera. At this point, it was rumored that the dog received many more sympathy cards and letters than his blind owner, and the speculation was whether a seeing eye dog can hold his job if partially blinded. I remember joking, in the O.R. of course, that perhaps we should pitch in and get him a seeing eye cat to stand by Fido! I do not recall the dog's name, but I am sure half of New York knew it back then. As the chief resident, I soon had to field some questions from inquiring parties, including the media, which culminated in a full-blown hospital press conference with the recovering patient, sans his dog, lined up for the photographers around a table with the Bellevue banner behind. While I participated, I cannot remember my comments. For that matter, I cannot even remember what the hospital administrators said behind the myriad of microphones. My participation in the event was brief because I was called away to do what I do as senior resident...put out fires up in the O.R.

Focusing on elective procedures is one of the perks of the chief year. If a spine case is booked, I might ask the R4 to do that with the spine attending. The chief generally does the bulk of the elective joint replacement cases on the Bellevue service, coming from the adult reconstruction clinics, but I also amassed considerable caseloads in hand and upper limb.

Running a surgical service in a city hospital is a singular experience in which one soon learns their strengths and weaknesses. I confirmed my proficiency in multi-tasking and utilizing limited time blocks to their fullest. However, I developed an awareness that I did not deal with bureaucracy well. I often relied on my junior residents to negotiate protocols and jump through logistical hoops. This was not a skill I would improve on in my future, try as

I may. On the flip side, I set the record for the most surgical cases the orthopedic department completed in a month, an achievement that depended upon developing a rapport with anesthesia but more so with the head O.R. nurse. I sometimes wonder if that role is held by the same person, or a clone, in nearly every large hospital O.R. They excel at saying, "No," but I soon realized that if you are true to your word and consistent in your actions, they begin to bend. For example, if I ask them to sneak in a wrist fracture to the schedule, I better stick to my promise that I can get it done in well under an hour. I also learned to not burn favors, or cry wolf. If something was not urgent, best to leave it that way. You never know when you will want to cash in that chip.

Organizing, delegating, managing, operating, and providing direct care outlines the job description for a surgical service chief. These skills would later serve me well in private practice. By year's end, around June in the residency training calendar, I began to reflect on many issues. I would soon depart the collective string of institutions: N.Y.U. Med, Bellevue, and Manhattan V.A., where I truly "became a surgeon." Now I fully understood what Dr. Nolen had written in his transformational memoir within that fabled place called Bellevue.

The end of my New York City training also heralded a departure from the entire metropolitan area and the greater northeast region of the United States, my adopted homeland where I am a citizen. I was to leave the vicinity where both my parents and many of my friends from undergraduate days lived, and leave behind my daily life, a.k.a. "grind," in the big city. Despite multiple changes there was one constant up to my last days of training: the monotonous routine of more studying and the requirement to jump through yet another hoop, the orthopedic boards.

Board certification remains a controversial area but there is little argument about adopting and maintaining standards for a profession that requires a significant amount of knowledge, with so much at stake. The ABOS (American Board of Orthopaedic Surgery) is the governing body that maintains the professional standards of the specialty, much like the 23 other specialty member boards that comprise the ABMS (American Board of Medical Specialties). Founded in 1936, the ABOS also administers the Orthopedic Board examination, which has been traditionally administered in two parts. The first part is done soon after the completion of the chief resident year, while the candidate is either commencing clinical practice, or more likely, beginning their fellowship training. That first part is a nine-hour rigorous exam, with a combination of clinical and basic science questions, including biomechanics. Many of the questions will pertain to entities the clinician has likely never seen, and basic science topics that were learned via rote memorization. This is not to disparage the exam, but most colleagues agree that practicing surgeons would not be able to pass this exam in later years unless they had weeks to months to fully prepare. For this reason, the exam is taken around that residency training period when the vital information is fresher in the mind. The timing of the exam also takes into consideration that the competing forces of maintaining a practice, patient care, and family duties make passing it simply unfathomable for practicing surgeons.

However, in the closing months of orthopedic residency, many surgeons focus on studying for the exam and must continue through the summer months until they complete it. Once a surgeon passes it, they must sit for part two – largely an oral examination – within five years to obtain "board certification." I will discuss the part two exam when I detail my initial year in clinical practice. An additional challenge to face.

As I bid farewell to so many familiar faces and places I encountered during my decade of preparation, I got ready for the next stage of training in a new city. I began to pack my humble belongings from my shoebox apartment, all the while studying for yet another exam. My then-girlfriend did the same. We combined our belongings and furniture in a 20-foot U-Haul truck as I picked her and her cat up in front of her building. With the cat sitting between us, we departed for our seven-hour drive to the "City of Bridges" ...and I never looked back.

Fellowship Year: Mastering the Hand and Upper Limb

The challenge of moving to a new city was overshadowed by the preparations needed to commence a fellowship and shortly thereafter, sit for an examination. I remember little other than being pleased with the area we selected to live in, as well as the apartment itself. In fact, it comprised the first floor and most of the second floor of an old, three-story wooden house, a typical northeastern dwelling in Shadyside area of the Burgh. We had selected it during a weekend trip to Pittsburgh some months prior to get situated for our year. I still recall with amazement the low monthly rental fee of $850 – I suspect you could not even rent a closet for that price in New York City during those years. Furthermore, the lovely home had three fireplaces, two of them fully functional, and both driveway and easy street parking. *Luxury.*

Although my girlfriend had also wanted to inquire about fellowships, she further procrastinated about the issue and did not work during that year, a tough pill to swallow for an internist, pun intended. I purchased my first car in nearly a decade, a convertible Chrysler Le Baron – wishful thinking for my Miami future, I suppose. For about six weeks, I enjoyed it quite a bit. The summer months in Pittsburgh were glorious and sunny…and coincided with my free time spent studying for the boards. Bummer.

With no internet at the time, I had no idea that Pittsburgh was one of the cloudiest cities in the U.S., even eclipsing Seattle in that department. I might have to delay my convertible deployment for my post-fellowship year but opted instead to put the top down and the heat on…unless it was raining, of course. It rained a lot in Steel City, too.

Once I began my fellowship, I could not have been happier. I had a direct commute, easy access into ONE facility, Alleghany General Hospital, and faced challenging clinical work with my co-fellows and the attending surgeons. How could I not enjoy it? This was quite a change from Manhattan where I walked almost everywhere and dealt with different hospitals, staff, and cultures. However, there was one challenging caveat: I was once again relegated to making $25,000 a year, just like my intern year five years prior. I had climbed to a whopping $40,000 a year as a chief resident, but the differentiator was my moonlighting, an opportunity I did not have in this new city. Yes, my expenses were markedly diminished, but I still had to return to a frugal lifestyle, plus I now had two mouths to feed. Frankly, it was all to be expected. In my mind, I knew no alternative so on I went. It felt like delayed adulthood: many friends were now well into their professional careers (including some medical specialties), building families, and setting roots. I was in my early 30s and still struggling financially.

My fellowship consisted of an every-third-night call, but it was humane. The orthopedic residents slept in the hospital, did the initial assessment, and called the hand fellow with anything complex or potentially surgical. When a patient showed up with two fingers in a Zip-loc bag, hopefully wrapped moist and on ice, I knew I would be up all night. Nevertheless, it was a much better lifestyle. You might call it a gentleman's fellowship. Sort of.

Besides covering the hospital incoming trauma, which included the entire western Pennsylvania region and northern West Virginia, I was once again immersed in the environment of private practice hand surgery, reliving days with Dr. Charlie Melone. However, despite some similar physical similarities, and both being excellent surgeons, they could not be more different. Yes, they were both short, Italian American men with strong personalities who graduated from northeastern medical schools around the same year. But that is where the similarities stopped. Charlie, as even the N.Y.U. residents affectionately called him, was a much more typical hand surgeon in manner and affect. He was detailed-oriented, with habits and methods that could almost be described as superstitious. In other words, he embodied the whimsical term used among other orthopedists, "hand weenie." While I feel he may have imparted some of this detail-oriented nature upon my psyche, he did not inspire me to become the (perhaps) overly practical hand surgeon I am today.

A demonstrative comparative anecdote illustrates the basic difference between them. I recall a rheumatoid hand surgery case wherein I assisted Dr. Melone. If memory serves me well, it was a metacarpophalangeal arthroplasty hand reconstruction. Dr. Melone was a master of this operation, the type of then-experimental surgery for which my grandmother had consulted, but never received, with Dr. Carroll in the early 70s. During that time of the Dr. Melone hand rotation, I would often finish the case as I had become well acquainted with his technique, but for some reason, he always scrubbed back in to apply the dressing. A precisely applied, compressive hand dressing/splint is a critical component of many hand procedures. Charlie was not going to leave this to chance. However, I remember he possessed certain idiosyncrasies. For example, the surgical towel we placed the hand on MUST be *blue*, not green. Lastly the one-inch paper tape we used as the final touch on the dressing must be on a specific blue plastic dispenser – no "pioneering" as he would say.

This was the antithesis of Joe. One of the first times I scrubbed with him, we too were applying a dressing but together when he asked for some tape. Not paper, silk, cloth, or surgical but ... tape. The nurse asked him, "Do you want one-inch or two-inch?" I still remember the reply, uttered with his frequent guttural and somewhat mocking laughter, "I don't care. Please just give me some tape." Ha-ha. Classic Joe. And as meticulous as I might be, THIS attitude was aligned with my sentiments: focus on the important things. Much of my professional character and stances would be shaped by Dr. Imbriglia.

Dr. Joe was a larger-than-life individual, charismatic but firm, pragmatic but entertaining. Much like my old swimming coach, Scarpato, he somehow managed to convey what truly matters, distilling some of the nonsense, or riff raff amid the challenges of providing care. His stance on "tape" was simply emblematic of his approach to medicine – concentrate on what's important, care about the patient, and do not be distracted by nonsense. It was not wrong or right – just a specific approach.

Out of all my years of training, the fellowship was the most enjoyable. Whether it was due to my excellent mentors, clinical facility, or overall work environment I am not sure, but I suspect it was something less obvious: for the first time in many years, I could truly focus on learning. I got sleep (usually), attended a gym with regularity, and did not have to deal with a lot of stress or bureaucracy. Consequently, I even managed to initiate *and* complete two different scientific studies in that one year. That was quite a feat given that one was a prospective clinical study, and the other a biomechanical study.

The biomechanical cadaveric study involved determining the amount of force required by application of an external fixator to reduce a distal radius fracture in a cadaver forearm/wrist specimen. Without getting too technical, I always felt that the standard treatment of distal radius (Colles' wrist fractures) was inefficient and even detrimental to the wrist joint. At worst, it was barbaric. Since my intern days, I remember going down to the emergency room, placing steel wire Chinese finger traps on two digits with the arm suspended vertically, then putting weight on the upper arm with elbow bent at 90 degrees. The idea was that with this traction, the end of the radius bone would disimpact itself and return to a more anatomical position.

Since many of the fractures are in soft, osteoporotic bone, the deformity would gradually recur once the weight (usually some sandbags/IV bags) is removed. Even more egregious, the collapse would recur while the patient was in her clunky, heavy plaster cast so the wrist would heal deformed, what we would call a malunion. These malunions could be painful and often lead to marked loss of wrist motion, strength, and overall hand function. The severe ones were taken to the operating room where a similar process was repeated, but then another "erector set," a distal radius external fixator, was applied externally across the wrist to maintain the reduction (restored position) of the radius bone.

To make matters worse, my prior professor Dr. Melone popularized a similar procedure in which two large, steel pins were incorporated into a heavy plaster molded cast to maintain the reduction traction. This was done for some years until the widespread incorporation of the fancy and expensive external fixators as the standard of care. I never bought either technique. Way too much stress was being applied indirectly to the bones via extrinsic ligaments of the wrist that can then cause a whole host of secondary problems. In some cases, the solution was worse than the potential malunion if benign neglect had been instituted, something that was done for nearly 200 years after Dr. Benjamin Colles famously remarked in 1814 that "All these patients do well despite some deformity of the wrist." I did not agree with that perspective either because in most cases, anatomy must be restored for optimal functional outcomes.

Given the conundrum of an indirect and problematic solution to a widely accepted surgery for this fracture, I decided to quantify the forces required to obtain that correction to prove my hypothesis. Furthermore, I could also provide some evidence to support the fact that Dr. Imbriglia, being a pragmatic thinker, was the one surgeon in his group who felt that these fractures should be stabilized and internally fixed. Most of his younger colleagues adhered to the standard treatment of external fixation application, which was a bit ironic. One of my other mentors – a major proponent of the external fixation method – oversaw my biomechanical study, which proved that the distraction forces were extreme and often resulted in capsular injury. This explained why many of these patients develop wrist stiffness and other complication such as sympathetic dystrophy (RSD now known as CRPS type 1). Therefore, I sided with Dr. Imbriglia and we routinely applied titanium or stainless-steel plates/screws – except this was to the dorsal (top) surface of the wrist to maintain the fracture in an anatomically reduced manner – and not indirectly. This early, somewhat unorthodox thinking epitomized how I came to view and manage many clinical problems. Dr. Imbriglia's forward thinking instilled a progressive approach to patient care in my psyche.

Early in my fellowship, I decided to further my understanding of fracture care by applying for an A.O. fellowship. A.O. is an abbreviation for a German phrase, "Arbeitegen Osteosynthesefragen", which loosely translates to "fix fracture." This progressive philosophy on fracture management originated in Switzerland and Germany in the late 1960s. They offered a competitive fellowship in a variety of centers focused on fracture care around the world, although most were in Western Europe. They informed me of their decision in early spring, then placed me in an appropriate training center. Considering my skeptical views on upper limb fracture management, I felt this would be a logical addition to my training.

Later, I would bring some of these progressive concepts of distal radius care to Miami, where I partnered with a colleague who largely changed the methodology of how this common wrist fracture is treated. Sadly, my contribution was not fully recognized during this revolution of distal radius fracture management, but I am keenly aware that the biomechanical findings my study brought to light was a major factor in rethinking how to address this injury. This was an early example to me of how physicians are often not good collaborators and the full synergy of efforts is either lacking or delayed for no good reason.

My other study was strictly clinical, but also stemmed from my misgivings of a well-accepted practice in the A.G.H. outpatient surgery center – the infiltration of local anesthesia into the field prior to wound closure. Often, after a major bone reconstruction was performed in the wrist, the surgeon, the fellows, and I were instructed to squirt in 5 to 10 cc of 2% lidocaine into the soft tissues under the skin. I thought, "This is fruitless. The pain stems from a deeper area and anything short of a nerve block is simply wishful thinking." I designed and wrote up the study to obtain I.R.B. (Institution Review Board) approval from the appropriate hospital committee, since it involved patients that might get a placebo. While this effort created some busy work, it also involved engaging the hospital statistician, obtaining buy-in from the recovery room nurses and anesthesia, and organizing the data I gleaned. While gaining I.R.B. approval was somewhat challenging, it dwarfs what scientists and clinicians must do currently to further our knowledge. Many I.R.B.s have become businesses, replete with arduous bureaucracy. I suspect I would not have performed this study in today's obstructionist climate. These often-senseless hurdles became amplified, and aware to the public during the viral pandemic. Some loosening of these absurd restrictions is one positive that may persist after the current crisis resolves.

Once my study results were compiled, they confirmed my suspicions that the additional introduction of lidocaine had no demonstrable effect on post-operative pain scores and patient/nursing comments as compared to no infiltration. Not surprisingly, while my study was locally hailed and later presented in a national hand surgery meeting, my colleagues continued the same practice even though most of them accepted my findings. I soon came to realize that medicine was often more of an art than science. The experience also epitomized physicians' resistance to change, foreshadowing what I would soon encounter many times in my career as I tried to introduce another perspective to my colleagues. It was not at all a matter of intelligence but rather open-mindedness, which explains why it is often difficult to introduce innovation in healthcare. I was just beginning to scratch the surface of Medicine's dogged adherence to the status quo.

The open environment fostered by my mentors during my fellowship facilitated critical thought. Just like the day of my interview when Dr. Imbriglia asked, "How would you treat this?", I was free to explore the field of hand surgery on many fronts. Oddly enough I do not have as much recollection about specific cases as I do from my Bellevue days, but maybe that is because this was a simple, broad exposure to community hand surgery. It was exactly what I was seeking, and my clinical confidence grew as I was exposed to the type of pathology I would see in a typical private practice. Little did I know that my practice would not be so typical in Miami, but I was certainly prepared.

Spring in Pittsburgh brought an acceptance letter to a major trauma hospital in Interlaken, Switzerland, near the base of a major ski resort and an outdoor sports mecca in the Swiss valley. Just when I was preparing myself to revisit open tibia fractures and pelvic trauma came the letter informing me of a change in venue. The AO fellowship directors became aware that I was pursuing hand surgery and decided to place me at an ambulatory center in Freiburg, Germany, smack in the middle of the "Schwarzwald," or Black Forest. My life was beginning to come into clear focus; however, I encountered yet another interruption or delay – something to which I was accustomed. In this case, it was my own doing.

Midway in my fellowship year, sometime after I submitted my A.O. fellowship application, I began to think about a future "job." Logical as it seems, this was a novel step for many of us who spent our late teens and entire third decade in life studying, training, and preparing for an actual paid profession. It seemed like an awkward yet welcome step. Like many occurrences during a person's life trajectory, my future aspirations had been taking shape during a long period of preparation, and now, reflection. I felt quite certain I did not want to stay in the Northeast. I grew up there and trained there but outside of my parents, I had limited roots in the region. My only sister had moved to the South to fulfill her vision of being a "Carolina girl." I on the other hand, am a big city person who loves the water, sun, and access to easy travel. Few cities on the East Coast could fulfill that criteria and besides, I had already envisioned where I would live during the cathartic water skiing moment I described earlier, when I announced I would someday "live in one of those waterfront houses near downtown Miami." Much like my profession, I soon embarked on pursuing a dream that started as a simple vision and prediction.

During my limited free time in Pittsburgh, I began to think about the job search. While I love academia and contributing to the collective body of knowledge in my own humble way, I was quite sure that I would not seek an academic position. Yes, I love to teach and enjoy the intellectual environment, but as this book clearly illustrates, I do not enjoy politics, bureaucracy, or jumping through hoops. I understand this is a necessary part of serving within a large organization; I just knew it was not for me. Therefore, I did not seek fellowships in Mayo, Hopkins, or Washington University. All offered excellent programs, but I was pursuing a different track, even though my research work during my fellowship showed me that I could contribute to those endeavors if I put my mind to it. That last comment is an understatement since private practice comes with major challenges – hence the title of this book on healthcare delivery. My goal was to continue learning and advancing our field's body of knowledge, but in a setting where I would be less encumbered and forced to jump through fewer hurdles. Little did I know what I was in for!

Certain of my decision to pursue a specialty private practice scenario, I began to speak with mentors, colleagues, and friends about possible opportunities available in specific geographies. I narrowed my search to the eastern side of the country to be close enough to my small, but tight-knit family. I investigated a variety of practice types in cities like Houston, New Orleans, and Fort Lauderdale. While I wanted good proximity to water, nightlife, and culture, I soon realized I really I wanted to satisfy a latent longing deep within: to remain close to my Latin roots and use my proficiency in Spanish to differentiate myself from my peers in a significant way. A doctor who could communicate in Spanish was important to many patients. And me.

What a huge advantage this could be in a private practice setting. Little did I know that I would later build a renowned international practice; back then I simply wanted to bond and communicate with patients in *their* native language. When one is in pain, stressed, and confused as to options, you want to inquire and converse in your native tongue. While my native tongue *is* English, I realized that communicating in Spanish could create a special bond among my fellow Latino population. This became clear during two separate incidents with my primary mentors in hand surgery.

One major foreshadowing occurred in Dr. Melone's lovely New York City office, where I performed the initial evaluation on an ophthalmology resident from Venezuela who was going to pursue training in the Big Apple. He presented with a complex fracture of the base of the thumb (a Rolando fracture), which he had sustained while throwing his opponent in a judo match the week prior. He caught his thumb in the gi (the two-piece white garment worn in martial arts) and was placed in a temporary splint until he could be seen by a hand surgeon. After Nelson uttered only a few words, I realized Spanish was likely his more comfortable language. As opposed to the typical scenario at the Bellevue clinics where I often heard, "Where is Badia? This lady speaks no English!" my patient encounters at the N.Y.U. faculty offices rarely offered me a chance to use my Spanish. It is a basic human desire to feel needed and relevant, and I relished the moment when a Hispanic patient could feel at ease and describe their clinical problem in their own language. Watching their facial expressions when I spoke to them in their native tongue with calm confidence was priceless.

This was the feeling I got from my Venezuelan patient who expressed his major concern that he might not have the thumb dexterity and motion to perform microsurgical procedures of the eye going forward. I instilled hope, explained the procedure in more technical language (in Spanish, of course), and presented the case to Dr. Melone. We subsequently performed the fracture pinning and Nelson did very well. Later, he went on to research and further training in a prestigious New York eye hospital, before relocating to Minnesota. To this day, we keep in touch and often refer each other patients. He, too, settled in Miami...for similar reasons, I imagine.

Today, I perform same procedure with sophisticated arthroscopic assistance, the type of surgery I have performed on many of his compatriots who fly to Miami from Venezuela. In the early 90s, that surgery was not even considered but the concept of a patient flying to another country to seek expert care, such as with Dr. Melone, appealed to me. It was pure medicine – and not an example of the patient's mother picking a doctor out of an insurance book, which is usually the case.

If my NYC private practice encounter with a Latino patient was somewhat rare, you can imagine how rare it was in Pittsburgh, long known for its strong

German, Polish, and Italian community. Twenty-five years later, the Hispanic community is still barely 3 percent of the population. It was quite a surprise when I encountered yet another Venezuelan patient (not just Latino), in Dr. Joe's office during hours. Sadly, this young man, a paraplegic, presented in a wheelchair. He had been shot in the back and also sustained severe bony injuries to his elbow as the bullet pierced his spine and entered his arm during a "routine" assault in Venezuela, an occurrence that is all too common in that increasingly violent nation. His lovely, supportive girlfriend accompanied him. Neither one spoke much English. After I translated for Dr. Imbriglia, we performed the surgery together a few days later. I could not have known then that my Venezuelan slang and idioms would be refined down the road. Regardless, I felt a special bond with this patient. Fast forward some years later. When this same patient showed up in my Miami office, it took me by surprise. I removed the hardware Dr. Imbriglia and I had placed back in Pittsburgh, more confident than ever that I had made the right choice by setting up my practice in the tropical yet urban environment of Miami-Dade County.

However, some interesting events led to my final choice of destination. As I mentioned, the small city of Fort Lauderdale had also been a contender after I spotted an ad in an orthopedic journal that a multi-specialty orthopedic group was seeking a hand surgeon. Not only did this location satisfy my requirements of surf, sun, and southeastern proximity, I knew the community well because my stepmother's parents had retired to a humble home in the residential heart of Fort Lauderdale. In my early teens, we often performed the typical Cuban mecca summer pilgrimage of driving from New Jersey to Miami and stopping just short in "Lauderdale." I had fond memories and assumed it was a somewhat Latino city since it was a few miles north of Miami.

The Fort Lauderdale orthopedic group I visited was in the penthouse space of a tall commercial building, complete with panoramic views of the aquamarine Atlantic Ocean. Strangely I did not get a sense of being fully at home. Although I enjoyed chatting with my colleagues and their staff, I was not convinced this was the right fit for me. I returned to Pittsburgh thinking that I could "make do," and that the proximity to Miami may suffice. The mutual chemistry was generally positive, therefore, they invited me back for a second interview to dig deeper into the practice opportunity and scout out the lifestyle options.

Between the two visits to Fort Lauderdale, I made a fateful phone call one afternoon. I had been looking at further job opportunities in J.B.J.S. (Journal of Bone and Joint Surgery) and noticed a small ad seeking an orthopedic partner in Miami. I called the number on the ad and easily managed to speak to the surgeon, Dr. Roberto Moya. A pleasant man, he informed me that although he was still practicing solo, he realized he was starting to get older and had a wonderful opportunity to bring in an associate. I reminded him I was completing training as a hand surgeon, with an interest in the entire upper limb, and inquired about the specifics. It seemed he suggested the need for me to do general orthopedics, but his next statement nearly floored me: in a calm tone, he stated that the position would pay $80,000 a year with some potential incentives we could discuss. At first, I thought I heard wrong since my colleagues inquiring about positions in the Northeast, Midwest and Western states were considering jobs starting at three-to-four times that salary.

In a succinct manner, I asked him to repeat the salary information, hoping that in my excitement over my first Miami inquiry, I simply misheard. He repeated the $80,000 dollar figure to start and I just about fell off my chair. As I fought to contain my surprise and even indignation, I reminded him I was in the middle of a coveted hand surgery fellowship following a Cornell/N.Y.U. education and N.Y.C. residency that included Bellevue Hospital. I mean, what would Dr. William Nolen say?? I sensed that the kindly Dr. Moya understood my surprise because he then told me about an industrious orthopedic hand surgeon who was also practicing in Miami. I assume he realized I was not about to start fixing hip fractures and managing back pain all over again. I recognized the name right away and informed him we had met in N.Y.C. some years ago. I thanked Dr. Moya for his time. A quarter-century later, I have not had any significant live conversations with him since that enlightening phone call. I would soon realize that Miami was no typical place by U.S. standards...but I am getting ahead of myself.

The Miami hand surgeon had been introduced to me by chance over six years prior, when we both stood in the operating room main corridor at the Hospital for Joint Diseases. We were not even seated in the surgeons' lounge when an H.J.D. ortho resident remarked, "Hey Alex, you should meet my fellow resident who is also Cuban...I think." He was standing at the scrub sink, five feet behind him, when he heard his name. He shut off the scrub sink, towel dried his large hands, and approached us. After his colleague made the introduction between us two token Cubans, he extended his hand, "Mucho gusto, Alex." We spoke at some length and I discovered that he too enjoyed conversing with a fellow Latino, although I was a lowly medical student that happened to be doing an anesthesia rotation there as a fourth-year clerkship. I told him I was applying within the orthopedic match, and that maybe we would encounter each other in the future. It was brief but monumental foreshadowing.

While I barely remember my second visit to the Fort Lauderdale orthopedic practice, one specific moment stands out in lucid detail. As I chatted with a possible future colleague near an X-ray box, staring out over the blue, tranquil ocean, I inquired if he ever had any Latino patients. "Sure, we have a couple," he replied. *Wham.* That was it for me. While I loved the location and the excellent opportunity to be one of the trailblazing hand surgeons in East Fort Lauderdale, and the potential for growth, I was not at all keen on being barely able to utilize my Spanish. Furthermore, after years spent amid non-ethnic colleagues, I yearned for a more diverse experience and to leverage some of my innate strengths. With perhaps adulterous guilt, I telephoned my old fleeting contact, the Miami Hand Surgeon. You see, I had a hunch that I would not be fully satisfied in joining the group to the north of Miami and had obtained his practice information in the meantime.

Days before I boarded a jet to the Fort Lauderdale Airport, I had spoken to this Miami surgeon, who suggested we meet. I promised to let him know. Keep in mind, in the days just before widespread cell phone usage, we were connected via "the service." It was our only option, unless we wanted one of those suitcase phones reserved for other Miami-based professions that also dealt with "pharmaceuticals." He returned my call some hours later at my hotel since he had been in surgery. No surprise there. In his usual gentle yet enthusiastic manner, he said, "Yes, yes, Alex. Come on by and we can talk. I am at Doctors Hospital recovery room." I told him I was probably an hour away, but he reassured me that was no issue since he still had lots of cases to do. Mind you, this was late on a Friday night and I would soon discover that these were elective cases. Further foreshadowing.

I threw on a suit and headed south down Interstate 95. By now, it was past 9 p.m. and I felt a sense of an illicit romantic rendezvous or perhaps another "Miami style" business meeting. It was at the tail end of the *Cocaine Cowboy* era, after all. Since neither G.P.S., nor Uber had been invented, I used a map from my hotel and relied on my decent sense of direction. I arrived in the quaint city of Coral Gables, the "Scottsdale" of Miami, and parked in front of a community hospital that bore no resemblance to Allegheny General, let alone Bellevue. Once inside, they directed me to the operating room entrance where a front desk nurse kindly ushered me into the recovery room area – complete with recovering patients and, unbelievably, others who were about to get an IV and pre-sedation. I thought, "This is certainly not the V.A. hospital. What time are they doing elective cases on Friday night?"

Yes, this was community private practice medicine. Suddenly, he stood up, noticing that a youngish man in an awkward suit was interrupting his surgical flow. He was writing post-op orders when he approached me, wearing dark purple scrubs, looking much like an overgrown Barney character. Reminiscent of our first meeting, he extended his hand with the words, "Mucho gusto, Alex," then invited me to sit down next to the recovery room clerk, where he began to tell me about his busy practice. I cannot recall if the conversation took place in English or Spanish, but I immediately felt a sense of comfort and camaraderie. I explained my situation, why I was in South Florida, and how I felt little excitement about the practice opportunity some miles north on I-95. After hearing me out, he shook my hand and thanked me again for making the trip. "We'll talk," he promised. No surprise, he was being called back into O.R. #2.

As I drove back in quiet reflection, I felt the culmination of years and years of study, *knowing* at last where I would end up and how I would practice. I should have strapped my seatbelt in a bit tighter, but I was soon back in Pittsburgh for my training finale. Not so fast. I recounted my experience with my live-in girlfriend, and we made plans to head to Miami to look for residential options (much as we had in Pittsburgh), while I cemented my agreement with the Miami hand surgeon for our association. He planned to pay me a modest salary with a major incentive: split profits with him 50-50 once I achieved a certain milestone within six months. It was my type of opportunity, capitalistic and merit-based, and not some hierarchy or scheme to enrichen my senior associate. A win-win. I had a sudden urge to call Dr. Moya.

Just prior to the Miami logistics seeking trip, I received positive news from the A.O. organization. They had indeed placed me in Frieburg, Germany, which meant I now had to work it into my plans, once again delaying my entry into "normal life." The opportunity offered no salary but instead a stipend to help me with living expenses while in Europe. "Delayed Gratification" was to be the name of my future boat in Miami, I concluded.

Of course, it also threw a wrench into my personal life. After honoring my lease, I would have to move out of Pittsburgh, then somehow head to Germany for my extended fellowship, delaying the establishment of a home base in Miami. On a subliminal level, I must have realized it would be a challenge for two people, particularly a fellow medical professional who had not worked in a year. While I bore zero responsibility for that, I sabotaged the relationship and she moved out with little fanfare…or notice. However, I did notice that the remaining boxes she left in the apartment for later recovery had a Miami address on them, although we did not see or even speak to each other for another eight years! A clean, but traumatic breakup indeed. My singular purpose overshadowed any personal path to building a family life, and I was determined to not be sidetracked or veered off course.

My final month in Pittsburgh was a bit challenging. This was a difficult breakup. Dr. Imbriglia jokingly remarked that I had to get off microsurgery call since my hands were trembling under the microscope. He was right. I tried to stay busy by completing my research projects with Dr. Baratz's guidance and to scrub in more with Dr. Buterbaugh, who did a lot of arthroscopic surgery, including athletic injury care, an early area of interest for me. Dr. Hagberg was generally our attending for the bigger trauma and reconstructive cases. He was interested in microsurgical reconstruction and late trauma management, including flaps. I barely operated with him in the closing months.

I packed up my rental home and secured another Ryder truck – this time a bit bigger, with a rear car dolly for my Le Baron – sans a cat. My two good friends, Dr. Luciano Stroia and his fiancée Mary Pat, came over at 5 a.m. to help me load the truck. I never forgot their kind gesture. Their friendship and support eased the final weeks of loneliness and transition to a new life. When I saw them decades later, I reminded them how grateful I was for that selfless gesture. That last week also included the A.G.H. gala where all graduating residents and fellows were sent off.

Prior to the gala, we participated in what would become my one and only disastrous golf outing: the fellows' tournament where we played with the attending surgeons. I had somewhat prepared for the event by going to the driving range a few times with either Mark Baratz or Mary Pat. Like many frustrated golfers, I soon understood the difficulty of a game that demanded steady practice. I was okay with that part, but when I discovered golf took upwards of five hours, I was out. For me, that time would be better spent on the water with a few Margaritas in hand, if not on a tennis court, or other more vigorous activity. It could be that I did not want to "get the bug," and become addicted to the preciseness required of putting a little ball in a cup hundreds of yards away. Such an activity can be a danger for a meticulous hand surgeon dealing with small objects. During the tournament, I struggled through the first eight holes before the sky suddenly opened, and in classic Pittsburgh fashion, the heavens relieved me of the ordeal. I arrived at the 19th hole early and a bit wet, with a chance to celebrate a stimulating and truly transformational year with terrific mentors.

As I drove away from Ivy street and turned onto Chestnut and the quaint shopping district of Shadyside, I reflected that this was indeed a turning point and the start of the rest of my personal and professional life. I drove straight down route 79, through the gorgeous Smoky Mountains, carefully selecting my limited bathroom/gasoline stops, as the truck rental agent warned me that I absolutely could not go in reverse given the car in tow. I pulled into Susana's neighborhood in Pineville, North Carolina, a lovely suburb of Charlotte and spent the night. We reminisced a bit about my professional journey but looked ahead to my European trip. This was to be more of a life experience, since my responsibilities would be minimal, other than to observe and learn different approaches to hand surgery and healthcare delivery. I had never had the opportunity to backpack through Europe, that soul-searching journey so many young students experience. During my school summers, I had worked multiple jobs and focused on milestones that would help me reach my goals. Now that I had accomplished them, this journey would allow me to reflect and transition to my new life of *being* a surgeon, not *becoming* one.

Two days after departing Pittsburgh, I arrived in Miami, where I put my furniture and belongings in one of those storage places whose existence I had always wondered about. Did people have that much "stuff?" Well, I had a condensed a lifetime of objects to stash and was now unencumbered to final-ize my European plans and travel itinerary. My step-cousin, David, helped me with that before taking me to see several apartments, including one I really loved in Brickell Key, a small, but convenient island right off the main com-mercial avenue of Miami's banking district. Although I did not have the resources to hold it, when I returned two months later, it had been placed back on the market. Meant to be.

I left for Europe with a combination of well-defined travel goals and the carefree spirit of a typical backpacker, who would typically be more than ten years my junior. Better late than never. I had purchased one of those famous Euro Passes, a collection of ten rail trips for one set fee. There was no distance limit on any of the legs which had to be within the four countries selected; therefore, I had to be strategic to avoid purchasing more tickets. My initial foray was pathetic as I burned one leg from the outset. I was not used to travelling, strange as that now seems, and my first rail trip was from Dusseldorf Airport to Freiburg station, my ultimate destination. I was quite tired from my overnight flight in coach, of course, and I recall falling asleep and waking up to see the imposing Cologne cathedral on my right, adjacent to the city train station.

I must have fallen back asleep because I later awakened to another spectacular cathedral, somewhat familiar looking, but this time on my left-hand side. Groggy-eyed, I collected my senses and soon realized it was the same station but from opposite perspective. I had slept through to the end of the train line at which point it changed direction – I was now back in the same place! I quickly collected my bags and wiggled my way out of the train car past entering passengers, so that the doors would not close and I might end up all the way back near Dusseldorf. I explained my dilemma to the unsympathetic station clerk in broken German, mixed with English, and ended up wasting an additional journey leg. The result? I arrived much later than I had planned with my mentor.

It was quite a start to my trip in a foreign land. The challenges continued as I arrived in Freiburg on a typical rainy day. Since it was a weekend, there was no easy way to reach Dr. Klaus Lowka, who probably wondered what happened to me some hours ago. I did see the universal symbol for Hospital from the elevated platform and walked with my bags to the distant location hoping to find help in locating him. Again, I spoke in broken German, this time to the small-town emergency room clerk, who found his home phone number and rang him. In characteristic fashion, Dr. Lowka promptly came back to fetch me and deliver me to my residence, which was in the Goethe Institute, adjacent to the ambulatory center he managed and saw patients in. The Goethe Institute is a German language and cultural immersion center for students of the language. I felt like I was a freshman at Cornell again, which was exactly a decade prior, but I was no college student anymore. It was a tiny austere room with a shared hallway bathroom and a hotplate in the corner. No TV or amenities. I made some close friends from Salamanca, Spain and Nairobi, Kenya whom I often went running with. It was clearly a different type of fellowship.

On Monday morning, I reported to the Zentrum fur Ambulante Diagnostik und Chirurgie, ready for a novel experience. I soon realized that Dr. Lowka and colleagues had built a truly state-of-the-art outpatient mini hospital only lacking overnight beds. It was my first exposure to the type of cost-effective and efficient orthopedic care that I would eventually advocate for in the U.S. Upon entering there was a diagnostic area, physician offices, and therapy center, and then directly downstairs, a robust outpatient surgery center with multiple O.R.s and a surgeons' lounge with coffee and strudel. No running between major hospitals and traveling afar to get to a medical office or speaking to the hand therapist by phone. This was a transformational time for me, and along with my recent Pittsburgh fellowship, it served as my most impactful professional experience. I soon focused on HOW Dr. Lowka practiced hand surgery – not so much the clinical details or treatment protocols. I learned how he used computers (well before the era of E.M.R.), maintained clinical data for future studies, and integrated care in one location from A-Z.

It would also show me the German system of healthcare, one I will comment on in the final chapter. As Americans, it is important for us to assess and evaluate other systems, particularly as our own system has become nearly unaffordable.

Lucky for me, my fellowship took place in August and September, which meant Dr. Lowka and probably half of Europe went away for a good part of late August on "holiday." I am grateful he had informed me ahead of time because I spent weeks before the fellowship confirming several visiting observerships with some of the brilliant European minds of hand surgery. The purpose was not only to observe their surgical techniques but to SEE how they managed their offices, scheduled surgery, and conducted follow-up visits. An additional benefit that was not apparent to me right away turned out to be the greatest gift of all: I learned how to create long lasting professional relationships and more importantly, deep friendships within my field. The latter would inspire me to continue travelling the world and gain perspectives, experiences, and rich memories that gave my soul another dimension, while promoting innovation and "outside the box" clinical thinking.

I began with a visit to Professor Ueli Buchler in Bern, Switzerland. While disappointed that I could only observe a few surgeries with him due to his summer schedule, I did get to participate in the Inselspital (University Hospital of Bern) Hand Surgery Department summer outing. This was no picnic and scrappy volleyball game but rather an excursion to go canyoning in nearby Interlaken, the outdoor adventure capital of Central Europe. Everyone participated in rappelling deep into a river gorge from an elevated highway edge, descending the canyon in wetsuit and helmets, and plunging into waterholes from massive boulders. There was no concern about breaking a nail or eating too many brownies. In fact, months later in the same location, nearly 20 canyoners where drowned when a flash flood occurred, sweeping the ecoadventurers away to their deaths.

Atlanta native Bob Lins (who was doing a more extended fellowship with Ueli) and I also made a lifelong close friendship with Dr. Phillipe Cuenod, his current fellow who hails from Geneva – the superior French part, he would often remind me. During the 96 Olympic games in Atlanta, I would crash in Bob's apartment. More recently, I spent 10 days with Phillipe in Koforidua, Ghana for a hand surgery medical mission in 2018. The downstream effects of this travelling fellowship remain to this day.

During one morning in the Inselspital, I heard someone call "Badia!!!" with Spanish intonation as I walked across the lobby on my hurried route to surgery. When I spun around, I saw none other than Jose Rodriguez, a talented New York Rican (mainland Puerto Rican) whom I had met through a girlfriend during my medical school days. Both he and his wife Iliana had studied at Harvard, and we had all met for dinner one evening. I did not see him again until the rigorous, and unorthodox, orthopedic residency interview at HSS, the Cornell-affiliated Hospital for Special Surgery. I recall the interview where Jose and I looked around, then back at each other and said, "Bro, there is no way they are going to take two Latinos in a residency class of only six trainees" It was he or I. Much deserving of the honor, Jose matched at HSS, and has gone on to a truly storied career, having served as Dr. Chit Ranawat's first partner as an arthroplasty (hip and joint replacement) surgeon.

I had not seen Jose since that fateful interview and it was truly a pleasure to get a taste of home and our Spanish culture, away from the Big Apple. So, what did we do? We planned our first trip to Paris together. I went first because I wanted to visit Dr. Francesco Brunelli at the famous Institut de la Main in the XVI arrondissement. Jose arrived the following day and we lit up the town, "doing the Louvre" in under 3 hours as if we were on surgical rounds on a massive service. We still chide each other over how our first trip to "The City of Lights" was not the romantic excursion we had envisioned ...but we had a blast.

The ramifications of these visits soon became crystal clear. My next one was focused on spending time with Dr. Riccardo Luccheti, a talented hand surgeon who was truly forging the path for wrist arthroscopy in Italy and even Europe itself. We had briefly met during a cadaveric wrist arthroscopy course in Chicago, at the renowned OLC (Orthopedic Learning Center) a lab adjacent to the AAOS headquarters (American Academy of Orthopedic Surgeons). The lab would later be a model and precursor to the now famed MARC Institute, the Miami Anatomic Research Center which I co-founded in 2005, which was the largest surgical teaching lab in the world at its initiation. Riccardo was a relatively young hand surgeon within the hand surgery division at the San Marino Hospital, the only clinical facility in the Republic of San Marino, third-smallest country in the world, after Vatican and Monaco. This was a history lesson unto itself.

Our visit started off in a strange way, one that was even more stressful than my entry into Frieburg. I had purchased one of those Sony handy cam "mini" video cameras (not so small by today's standards), an early precursor to the yet-to-be-invented smartphone. It was one way of chronicling my European experience. On occasion, I liked to video typical interactions with people in a clandestine manner. When the train conductor came to clip my ticket, I began to film my brief, pitiful exchange with him in my broken Italian, but with the camera partially concealed by my light jacket. He gave me some strange looks and moved on. We arrived in Rimini and as I exited the train car, I noticed he was hunched over a payphone and then looked back at me as he was speaking in his hurried Italian dialect.

Within minutes, two sharply uniformed officials accosted me. "Per favore viene con me," ordered the Carabinieri, the national police of Italy, often the butt of many jokes regarding their intellectual prowess. However, this was no time to mock or challenge their intelligence. They ushered me into a room, where they struggled to communicate the charge against me. After I explained my reason for coming to Rimini and gave them the phone number on my invitation letter, one of the policemen phone Dr. Luchetti. Within minutes, Riccardo arrived, looking part agitated but also chuckling. He then explained in English to me that the train conductor was in the country's national witness protection program. When he noticed I was secretly filming him, he thought I could be a member of La Cosa Nostra, the Sicilian Mafia. The office made me erase the filmed segment, although I tried to be slick and keep a small segment for posterity. Being an astute man, Riccardo noticed and became a little upset because I was already in hot water with the Italian police. After I obeyed orders, Riccardo took me to his apartment to meet his wife Maria and their young children, where Maria fed me a bowl of pasta with Funghi (mushrooms). Welcome to Italy.

We commuted every day from his childhood home near my hotel, which was on the famous Rimini Beach of the Adriatic Sea coast, a place I visited …once. It was fascinating to observe how Riccardo, like many European hand surgeons, juggled the demands of being in a public service system and attending to a private practice in the evening. To this day, Riccardo and I remain close friends, and have served as charter members of several specific themed hand surgical societies.

My last observership took place in Strasbourg, France with the indomitable Guy Foucher. Dr. Foucher was one of the most energetic people I have ever met, let alone a simply brilliant surgeon and unique thinker. His morning clinic consisted of seeing perhaps 35 patients between only two exam rooms linked by a large box on a lazy Susan type of construct, which allowed a rudimentary computer to be swiveled between both rooms. He documented every visit, and I do not think I have ever encountered a colleague who kept such detailed records. He was a decade ahead of any EMRs and would likely bristle at how the concept has been perverted. His image library was a veritable "Bibliotheque Nationale" of surgical Kodachrome slides. A reminder: this was the days before digital photos and PowerPoint presentations occupying a single slim laptop. Dr. Foucher devoted much time and space to this unique collection.

At lunchtime, he jumped on his bike and banged out 30+ Kilometers of hills outside the famous Clinique Orangerie. He always returned in time to change straightaway into the signature white European doctor garb – a la American ice cream man. We would see another 30 patients, perhaps perform two to three minor surgical procedures in his ambulatory suite, and then change again to head to the gym for a workout. Keep in mind, there was no time for a mid-day shower; hence the trip to the gym was a bit challenging for me when I joined him in his small European car sans AC on several occasions.

As often happens in these observerships, particularly in late summer, there was little elective surgery to observe and glean any clinical pearls. However, that was not my goal. I observed and learned how these men organized their thoughts, lives, and practices. I did find time to explore the cities, often alone.

On my third day with Dr. Foucher in clinic, I noticed a young, serious man assisting him, taking down dressings, and writing notes. A fit guy with short spiky hair and light eyes, he appeared to be a Frenchman. When I inquired about him, Guy replied, "Wala, you have not met Dr. Menvielle?" Sounded French to me.

"No," I said.

"Well, Fernando here is my fellow from Argentina."

"Whoa!" as my daughter would say when taken aback. *French is by far my worst romance language and I could have been conversing in Spanish with him all this time?* Fernando and I quickly bonded, and I joined him and his then wife for multiple gastronomic outings as a culinary threesome. I best remember the tart flambe' at *La Tete de Lard* in center Strasbourg. Fernando was the first of a long series of Argentine colleagues and friends I would begin to make after my first visit to the country as an invited speaker in 1998 and continuing to the present. He would much later become president of the prestigious Argentinian hand surgery society

Once I returned to Freiburg, I began to incorporate all the methodologies and practical wisdom into a mental framework about how I might practice medicine upon my return to the States. First and foremost, I finally got my "backpacker" experience and succumbed to the travel bug. From then on, I would forever seek to broaden horizons, make new friends, and add sights and sounds to my mental tapestry. This went far beyond surgery of the hand but was an integral part of life itself. You might have heard of a tombstone epithet that goes something like this:

"Here lies Juan. He wished he had spent more time at the office."

That was NOT going to be me, although many would judge me as a workaholic in future years. I know better. Onward to Miami, and the application of everything I had learned inside the O.R. – and out.

Chapter 3 – Entering Medical Practice: The Inside Story

"I will respect the hard-won scientific gains of those physicians in whose steps I walk, and gladly share such knowledge as is mine with those who are to follow."

I arrived in Miami the morning of October 1, 1995. I remember the exact date because I had been scheduled to start practice with my initial partner the following week. However, I was to begin days earlier, on Friday, October 6. The plan was to take a few days to move my furniture and belongings out of storage and into my apartment – the same one I had seen months prior, during my brief stay between Pittsburgh and Germany. Although October 6 also happened to be my mother's birthday, it took on a predictive significance for me.

That morning, my new partner phoned me and described a tragic case that required urgent attention. "Can you attend to it?" he asked. Mind you, I had no privileges at any hospital yet, and thanks to already typical inefficiencies of our system, I was not listed on any insurance network. In fact, I had not even set foot in the office. My partner requested that I go see a patient in Nassau Bahamas, where the hospital had asked for a hand surgeon to evaluate a patient. "Ah yes, the perks of having a junior partner," I surmised. My colleague informed me that the local hospital would handle all the arrangements, including transportation from the airport, courtesy of Dr. Thompson, Chief of Orthopedics. I thought to myself, "I haven't even started practice and already I'm seeing an international patient and performing a house call – abroad!"

Of course, I wondered if this would be a commonplace scenario in my new home. If that were the case, I would certainly hit the ground running. I packed a small bag, headed to the airport, and within 90 minutes, entered Dr. Thompson's car. A mild-mannered and affable surgeon, he explained that a terrible accident occurred, one that involved a premature infant in the neonatal ward. In routine fashion, a nurse had applied a cotton swab over an IV site that was discontinued and wound a cloth tape around the baby's hand to secure the compressive pad and preclude bleeding from the dorsal hand IV site. Hours passed before the tape/cotton ball was removed, revealing two ischemic (due to restricted blood supply) digits that had transitioned to a dry gangrene stage. The dressing had constricted the infant's delicate, micro digital arteries that perfuse the fingers. The family was naturally distraught and the hospital, while apologetic, wanted to bring in an expert to shed light on the issue and palliate the tense situation.

When I examined the child, I noticed that 2.5 radial digits (fingers) were already black and mummified. At that point, the incident was over a day old and it was up to me to somehow bring solace to the grieving family while assuaging the hospital leadership, which anticipated legal action. I could not bring myself to tell them I had just completed a second fellowship days prior and had not even set foot in my inaugural practice. This is a classic example of where medicine is more of an art than a science, and caring is more important than curing. With complete candor, I explained to the family that a baby's digital arteries are much more reactive than an adult's, particularly a delicate preemie, and that unfortunate incidents do happen. I could make no excuses other than reminding them that tiny IVs are always in use in this setting; a neonate's hands are very delicate; and although rare, the intersection of these facts can lead to tragedy as it did in their little girl. Throughout the conversation the sounds of profound weeping and desperate wailing punctuated my intended sympathetic, reassuring words. To offer some hope, I further explained that late reconstruction could be done, but it was no time to go into detail about ray resections versus toe-to-hand transfers, etc. It was not a time for science, simply compassion.

As I left, I experienced a strange mixture of sadness and relief. I knew I had given the family an opportunity to explore all avenues and receive answers to their questions, while giving the hospital team the sense that they did their best to placate a terrible situation. Such was my entry into the private practice of medicine.

Decades later, I would perform a complex reconstruction on his mother's elbow after a fracture, much like the one that Dr. Imbriglia grilled me on during my Pittsburgh fellowship interview. I would go on to see many Bahamian patients in future years but always harken back to this bizarre initiation to clinical practice.

The following Monday I drove my Chrysler Le Baron to the practice of my solo colleague, who had managed to build up a busy hand practice within four short years. While he had not specifically sought a partner, it seemed like ideal timing. He certainly could use the help I soon surmised. The small office was in Coral Gables, close to the University of Miami campus. The extent of my knowledge about U.M. was that Greg Louganis started his diving career there and Playboy praised its coeds and campus for being beautiful and fun. I remember thinking, "That would have been nice." A bit different than Cornell in upstate "sunny" New York State.

Both the office manager and the hand therapist – a personable and talented young Jamaican girl – greeted me warmly. As usual, the waiting room was packed, alerting me that my services would come in "handy," pun intended. Aside from these details, the commencement of my private practice was not very memorable outside of the Bahamas jaunt: it dealt with the usual scope of community hand issues. By contrast, the workload (as opposed to specific or notable cases) was truly unforgettable. Since it would take months for me to get on insurance plans, I began by helping him, which acclimated me to the flow and nuances of office practice.

To this day, I have no idea why it must take several months to become "credentialed" with an insurance plan and receive a provider number. It made no sense to me then, and it makes even less sense now, given the existence of the internet and almost immediate access to data and personal information. While writing this, I Googled "Alejandro Badia M.D. education." Guess what? It took exactly .72 seconds to come up with 13.7 million results. I do not expect insurance companies to credential doctors in seconds, but if they have the will and interest, there is no good reason why it cannot be done in days or weeks. It is symbolic of much that they do… or do not do.

The office manager submitted my credentials in a large manila envelope containing photocopies of every diploma, exam score, board application, and medical license data. In minutes to hours, the insurance company could have called my institutions to verify legitimacy and allow my credentials to be referred to a "committee" that could surely meet more than once every month. However, that would obligate them to pay me for taking care of their patients, right? Until I received my own validation, I saw patients under the guise of my partner, who signed off on any decisions along with the paperwork, billing materials, etc. It's an open secret in medicine that everybody does this to deal with a process in which the party holding the money wields the power. During accreditation delay, the insurance carrier keeps the money in their coffers that they can put to work via investments, the company portfolio, and kicking the can down the road…and we just accept it.

While my new associate and I saw patients – and boy did we see patients! – we discussed the structure of our new association. To my delight, his offer was more than fair. While his accountant would round out the details, it included a base salary with an incentive to divide the net revenue after I reached a certain collections milestone. Within six months, I attained it – an achievement that served us both well. I was not only willing, but happy to work hard, especially with an incentive to do so. My arrangement was much better than the ones accepted by many of my peers, and it was preferable to working for a healthcare system where payment is related to R.V.U.s (relative value units) and other complex formulas that can be slanted in the favor of the payer, not the payee. It allows for a lot of smoke and mirrors, so take heed my young colleagues coming out of training. It does *not* have to be that complicated but it is done intentionally. My first partner had the right philosophy. From that moment on, his ethic was ingrained in me. As a fellow professional, I do not think one's colleague should necessarily make money off another's clinical work output.

The next discussion we engaged in centered on naming the practice. You might have noticed that law and accounting practices tend to use the partners' last names...that is, until their businesses reach an impractical number of partners. Then it simply stops and forevermore, the professional practice remains as nondescriptive like "Doe, Smith, and Rodriguez." If a law firm specializes in speeding tickets, a better name for them would be "The Ticket Clinic." Ah yes, that has been done. Bingo. In a healthcare practice, a descriptive name becomes even more critical. *Hands- R-Us* etc.

Drawing from several well-known hand surgery associations across the nation – most notably, the Indiana Hand Center (yes, I'd declined an interview with them but they had an illustrious history and stellar reputation for clinical work and research) – I suggested "Miami Hand Center." Simple and descriptive. Having already agreed to take on another partner, Dr. Roger Khouri, who was the head of the microsurgery fellowship at the renowned Washington University in St. Louis Missouri, my colleague agreed with my choice of name. A year would pass before Roger joined us because he had arrangements to make, and an obligation to complete the current academic year, but his inclusion would truly make us a center. In an ironic twist, the Indiana Hand Center would much later return the favor. They are now the Indiana Hand to Shoulder Center. I first coined the term, "hand to shoulder" and perhaps should have registered the name as several friends suggested. The name arose from a conversation with an old fraternity brother, whose wife joined us and made this suggestion when hearing what I was seeking to describe. As for the Indy guys, I was not upset. After all, imitation is the best form of flattery.

However, Roger's arrival would not come soon enough. We plowed through a difficult year without him, and I realized that our practice was unusual in terms of workload and breadth. My colleague had made it a mission to truly dominate the Miami market in his field. Not only was he an excellent hand surgeon and workhorse, he had obtained contracts with virtually every insurance carrier in the area – a feat in and of itself. He worked closely with his accountant and his accountant's wife who ran a small, family-owned medical billing company. I soon surmised that our high volume was a result of incredibly generous insurance contracts that benefitted the carrier, not the clinician or our office. Being a young surgeon who wanted to accrue experience and caseloads, I did not mind it so much in the beginning.

However, when I noticed that some of our contracts were for only 60 percent of Medicare allowable – unconscionable for clinicians of our pedigree of training and expertise, my attitude shifted. We were hand surgeons, a specialty that is NOT replete with providers. Furthermore, we practiced in Miami, a city known for many foreign graduates – not necessarily with physicians trained in some of the country's best programs. While that may sound elitist, in any profession education and credentials carry weight. It is certainly up to the clinician to point that out and demand their worth. Something we really do not do enough of and it is now biting us in the butt.

In addition to a burdensome office practice, with hours that often ran into the night, we covered nearly every hospital in town, except the University program at Jackson. How did a typical scenario play out? I saw patients until 8 or 9 p.m. before getting a call about a fingertip crush injury at X hospital. On my way to that hospital, I often received another urgent call from Y Hospital. Whenever possible, my first case might get resolved as an E.R. procedure but the next case might be a severe wrist fracture or a rapidly advancing hand infection. I would call Y hospital from the X hospital emergency room to "Call the O.R. team in." This effort frequently required negotiations with the O.R. charge nurse and even the anesthesiologist about the urgency of the procedure. When I arrived at the second hospital, often near midnight, I might then be "bumped" because another surgeon booked a case that might have more urgency. I say "might" as sometimes these issues were highly subjective, for example a "hot bag," a gallbladder that the general surgeon feared could rupture. Since it made little sense to argue, I learned to make the most of the wait time. I met one of my best friends, Dr. Ignacio Rua, that way, in the OR lounge at Miami's Cedars Hospital, hoping to get another room so I could complete my case.

Long before smartphones came along, the O.R. lounges featured TVs that broadcast CNN or a sporting event, and a place where you could catch up with remote phone dictations. During my first years in practice, my colleagues and I depended on beepers to garner our messages and often sought a payphone if we were in a public area or a restaurant. That involved a search for the elusive quarter that neither I nor the restaurant proprietor seemed to have. Around 1996, I obtained my first cell phone, a Sony Ericsson with the small rubber antenna, which I thought was small. It was good for returning calls but not much else.

Within months, I realized I did not have much more of a life than when I was an intern. In fact, I was probably working more hours than I did as a senior resident – with additional responsibilities that private practice is known for: paperwork and administrative tasks. As residents, we did not always do the surgical dictation and we certainly knew *nothing* about coding and billing. Additional forms and questionnaires were never our responsibility. They added to the work burden, yet the effort was never remunerated. I remember thinking, "How can my mentors have never taught us what an I.C.D. 10 or C.P.T. code was?" I did not know the first thing about the nuances of workers' compensation and the commensurate paperwork since the doctor-patient relationship now had a third dimension: the employer. And the insurance company. And the defense attorney for the carrier. The work comp plaintiff attorney representing the "injured" worker. The claims adjustor. You get the picture.

All these people rely on our expertise, but it is often taken for granted. It becomes an art to learn how to get reimbursed for your time for some of these interactions. Many never will be. Besides the paperwork, charting, and dictations, the on-call burden was stifling and mostly comprised of hospital calls from an emergency room that needed my expertise. Usually. Still I often found myself relegated to speaking with the E.R. desk clerk because the E.R. doctor "was busy." *No kidding. I assumed he or she had their feet up on a desk while they read the National Enquirer!*

I countered, "I understand. I know busy. Do you think it would be too much trouble if they could simply present to me the clinical problem before

I jump out of bed at 3 a.m. and drive 20 minutes there?" Most of the time, they would answer. Eventually. They are often overworked too. There were weeks when I might cover eight or nine hospitals on an on-call evening. My partner was quite fair with the distribution, even though I was "the junior guy." As expected, however, I got the lion's share of the holiday calls. One of them that took place in my third month of practice would be memorable indeed.

A CUTTING-EDGE NEW YEAR

New Year's Eve, 1995 would be a special one in many ways – a celebration of a new year and a new life. It had been barely three months since I'd relocated to Miami, and thanks to a blind date arranged by my partner's wife (whom I suspected had an ulterior motive – removing the bon vivant, single "new doctor in town" status from her husband's office), I was dating a lovely young lady. Keep in mind, the phrase "blind date" in the mid-90s was most accurate. There were no smartphones, digital cameras, or dating sites that revealed a person's looks prior to meeting them in person (assuming they post recent photos…but that is another story!). While the concept of me having any free time to woo the ladies was laughable, I appreciated her introducing me to a beautiful, intelligent gal who was also a medical professional.

Because we did not know many people yet, we agreed to "crash" the New Year's Gala at the Biltmore Hotel, a feat we pulled off. One of my clearest recollections of the evening involves dancing next to Albita, a popular Cuban singer. Yes, I was on-call but there was no way was going to be a complete teetotaler on this most festive occasion. As someone who handles alcohol well, I had already handled several routine calls that had come my way that night: champagne bottle injuries, drunken falls, and hand fractures related to fights that broke out over women who might resemble my date. Although amplified on a holiday, these were all typical late-night incidents.

Well beyond midnight, we were still having fun as I bobbed and weaved my way out of running to any of the hospitals. By the time I arrived back at my one-bedroom apartment in Brickell Key, it was quite late. I do not even remember what time it was when I drifted off. First, my New Year's Day slumber was disturbed by a call from Hialeah Hospital emergency room, where a patient had shown up with a significant hand laceration. "Apply a dressing, give a gram of Ancef IV antibiotics, and I'll call the O.R. team a bit later," I responded in a groggy voice. No need to disrupt everyone's first of the year with a pre-8 a.m. call to come in.

I fell back to sleep, only to be roused again by the answering service. "Dr. Badia, they need you urgently at the Kendall Regional Hospital. Dr. Fondevila was asking for your associate." It indeed sounded concerning, so I phoned the hospital right away and asked for the emergency department.

"Doctor quien?" the voice on the other end greeted me in Spanish. Nearly one-third of all hospital E.R.'s in Miami answer the phone in Spanish, under the assumption that the doctor, patient, or family member on the other end speaks the language. Twenty-five years later, it still amazes me.

"Dr. Badia, I am the new hand surgeon in town," I replied. I tend to start with English until I run into real roadblocks. Then I succumb. As expected, the E.R. clerk told me that Dr. Fondevila, a prominent primary care physician and medical radio talk show host, was seeking my partner. I informed them that I was the junior associate and on my way to the hospital. Although tempted to grumble something like, "Of course, the new guy is on-call for New Year's Eve," I resisted. Gathering my senses, I washed my face, threw on my proverbial scrubs, and jumped in my Le Baron. No, I had not upgraded my automobile...yet.

These days Miami traffic is notorious for gridlock but back then it was modest. On weekend mornings, it was even calmer since Miami is not what you would call a "morning town," like San Diego or Boulder. It was eerily quiet as I sped – yes, *sped* – to the hospital, which was located many miles west, near the junction of the Dolphin Expressway, right off Florida's Turnpike. Because I had not been there before, I had to figure out where to park as I searched for the doctors' lot. Next, I rushed into the O.R. holding area, having requested that the E.R. personnel call in the O.R. team. It was evident that this would be a major case.

As I entered to collective sighs of relief from the staff, to my left I noticed an ashen individual with his left arm in a massive, blood-stained, and bulky dressing elevated by pillows. In the next moment, an anxious, frenetic doctor greeted me – the man I assumed to be the famous Dr. Mariano Fondevila. In a tone that assumed I knew who he was, he told me the patient's name, before inquiring about my partner again. I replied that I was the "new colleague," just a few months in practice and in Miami. To assuage his obvious concern, I put him at ease by describing my training and assured him I was accustomed to dealing with major trauma.

Next, I met the patient, Agustin Acosta, who despite being shaken and weak, thanked me for coming in. A true gentleman. I reassured him of the outcome before I even examined his arm, prompting him to reply, "My arm is completely lost and hanging by a thread. How can you save that?"

"Don't worry. My training will allow me to reattach and salvage your arm."

He replied that I perhaps came across as a bit arrogant and overconfident, considering the extreme situation – the near amputation of his arm. What he didn't know was that I had already reviewed the X-rays; noted the transection of the radius, with bone loss due to the wide kerf blade circular saw; and observed that his hand appeared well perfused (it had adequate blood flow). Thanks to his metal wristwatch, which stopped the forward progress of the blade, his ulnar was intact. I was trained to manage soft tissue injuries, including tendon and nerve. While it appears daunting to a patient or onlooker, it is akin to wondering how David Copperfield performs his illusions (something I still cannot fathom). When you know how, you just do. The trick is to inspire confidence in the patient and the O.R. team. I did not know it then, but Agustin would later recount the entire story in the documentary film, *Three Patients, A Doctor, A gesture of Gratitude*, shown during the DocFilm Festival in Miami.

While anesthesia and the O.R. circulating nurse whisked Agustin back to Room 2, I consulted again with Mariano, prepared my loupes, and began to scrub. I glanced at the arm as it was being prepped, devoid of the splint and dressing, noting that the saw had entered the radial side, likely taking out radial and median nerves, all the extensor tendons, and all flexors. In anticipation of having to take bone from the iliac crest (pelvis) to assuage the sectional loss of bone which could disrupt forearm and wrist function if not reconstructed with great care, I instructed the medical team to prep that area of the pelvis.

Barely four hours later, in a moment every surgeon cherishes, I approached Mariano to inform him of success. It is hard to describe the euphoria you feel when the task has been done to the best of your ability, you know a good outcome is nearly assured, and you can inform a patient's loved ones of the positive news they have been waiting for. Since I no longer deal with life and death, it is rare that I must confront the opposite situation. In general, my specialty enables me to provide good results for the patient. Although rare, dreadful outcomes tend to haunt me. Pleased with the news, Mariano wanted to know details – a natural reaction for a physician. I took ample time to explain the repairs, then informed him I had to be on my way to Hialeah Hospital, where another injured patient awaited my arrival.

The following week, I saw Agustin. I checked his wounds, reviewed his X-rays, and then placed him in a light, fiberglass short arm case. An astute man, he asked excellent questions in an obvious display that he grasped the significance of what had transpired. That was when I discovered that he, too, was a major radio personality who often interviewed Mariano on his morning show that scrutinized current events and informed much of the Latino (especially Cuban) community. Within days, he returned to work and, as you might imagine, began a running commentary on his medical progress. With pride, he shared who I was with his audience and described how I had "saved his arm" – quite a way to jumpstart my indoctrination into the Miami fabric and culture.

We became friends and he interviewed me multiple times on his radio program, and later, several local cable TV talk shows he hosted. These enjoyable experiences gave me my first sense of what patient education entails and how powerful it can be. My goal was not necessarily to advertise or develop a marketing plan, but rather, explain to listeners and viewers the key elements of various pathologies – whether the cause of carpal tunnel syndrome or how to treat shoulder pain. Via Agustin's fateful injury, I found myself explaining the difference between ligaments and tendons; microsurgery and arthroscopic surgery; and explaining why the process of choosing a specialist is critical. Did I mention I did all of it in Spanish? While I knew conversational Spanish, I had never lectured in my native tongue, not did I even know many anatomic terms in my other language.

Ironically, if not for my father I might not have retained any semblance of Spanish – something I yearned for when I moved to my new home. Although my mother had been a simultaneous interpreter and translator for almost four decades, in general she chose to speak English to my sister and me at home. A proud American, she had fully assimilated, perhaps to an extreme, but I could count on her for a masterful command of both languages. As if a professor of literature, she often quizzed us at home bilingually, giving me a solid foundation and proficiency to communicate in both languages when I developed an affinity for patient education.

As Agustin's progress continued, he reached a point where he developed more strength in his injured, non-dominant arm than his right hand. His commitment to rehab led to a newfound interest in weightlifting and fitness, and he became a changed man in many respects, much like me. One night over dinner at a local Italian restaurant to which he invited me, he reached for his glass of Cabernet with his left hand. As he held it high for a toast, he focused his gaze on me, awaiting comment. A clumsy silence followed while I anticipated an eloquent toast of gratitude…but no. Instead, as he stared at me intently, he remarked, "Alejandro, notice I can now fully abduct my thumb and wrap my hand around this wine goblet."

By the way, I was now known as Alejandro. Besides shaving off the trademark moustache I had worn throughout my decade in New York, upon my arrival in Miami, I insisted on using my birthname. "Well, Alejandro, don't you feel a heal," I thought to myself. In that moment, my patient was showing me that he had indeed recovered motor branch function of what was a completely transected median nerve. Mind you, this amazing recovery had taken almost a year, and I nearly missed its significance. Then again, I was distracted by the excellent vintage.

Agustin and I would enjoy many dinners together. I even welcomed the New Year with him and his family, eerily reliving another type of event. The close friendship we forged after meeting for the first time as doctor and patient was rooted in an indescribable bond that gives greater meaning to the practice of medicine.

As my practice grew, my partner and I worked well together. We had similar approaches to pathology but different styles of working. One Saturday morning, we did a series of elective cases. After the third carpal tunnel – or was it another trigger finger? – I announced that I would no longer be joining him Saturday morning surgery unless it was a trauma case. After all, it was a perfect winter day in sunny South Florida, a far cry from the cold and dreary climes of the greater New York metropolitan area where I was raised, and I preferred to spend it at the beach. I felt as if I had earned the right to shun the label of a workaholic and start to enjoy my weekends, especially if not on call. Part of my reason for moving to the area was to spend more time outdoors now that I could savor my freedom and growing financial independence in a tropical location. As he stood at the scrub sink, my partner then made the startling declaration that he had been diagnosed with a dreadful disease. Since he was on his way upstairs to begin treatment, he asked me to handle his next few surgeries, with the promise he would return later, which he did. It was admirable and unsurprising.

The fortuitous arrival of a new associate occurred as my colleague entered the graver stages of treatment. At last, Dr. Roger Khouri, a plastic and reconstructive hand surgeon, arrived in Miami to be our third partner. The three of us shared an amazing chemistry, and although we possessed starkly different strengths, we all had a firm commitment to excellent clinical care.

During a meeting one weekend for brunch at the Grand Bay Hotel in Coconut Grove, we agreed to focus on our strength and diversity as the only private practice hand surgery group in Florida. In addition, we included one other major element: academia. From that moment on, we wanted to be renowned as a driving force in academic hand surgery, nationally and internationally – a tall order considering the extreme amount of clinical work we were doing in the private practice environment. We covered almost a dozen hospitals and remained on just about every insurance network. It was an ambitious goal, but with Roger joining us, we were off to a fabulous start. Roger's experience as the Director of the Hand Surgery Fellowship at Washington University provided the perfect springboard. He had even brought a fellow with him from Bordeaux, France.

Add water in the form of our next fellow from South Korea, and later, Dr. Tony Connell from Perth Australia, and we had instant academia. Our founding partner had spent a year doing Ilizarov-type research with limb lengthening work/biomechanics in New York City, and I had developed research interests from my diverse projects in Pittsburgh. The simple premise? You do not need to be in an academic surgical department to do academia. That statement deserves repeating: You do NOT need to be in academia to pursue academics.

Within several years, we were presenting at almost every national, and even international meeting of hand surgery, orthopedics, and plastic surgery. We had also expanded our roles in microsurgery, while I developed an expertise in small joint arthroscopy. This was not a typical profile for a community practice group and there was certain pushback among some of the academic elites. One incident involving our own backyard department, the University of Miami, illustrated the extent of some of our colleagues' resistance to the concept. At a national hand surgery congress, we ran into the chief of the hand surgery division at UM, where Jackson Memorial is the teaching hospital. We expressed eager interest to participate in teaching residents and fellows, and our desire to collaborate on certain research projects, if interested. The response was classic academic snobbery, "Well, we just can't let anybody put the University of Miami logo on their letterhead."

As my partner steamed, I developed the laissez faire attitude I would come to fully embrace once I realized that egos and misplaced priorities often dominate the hand surgery sector (among many others). Forevermore, I would continue my clinical research and academic work unencumbered by university politics or the mandate to attend committee meetings. The same goes for our academic societies where the same speakers often present the same material, year after year. They are talented surgeons, but this is no way to foster innovation and encourage new ideas to be presented at a congress. This is not a criticism but an acceptance of reality. I felt secure in the knowledge that I was contributing to advances in our specialty that benefitted my fellow man and expanded my own knowledge. Medicine is a lifelong calling to learn and grow. Just as in many areas of life, I would not allow politics or sensitivities breach that noble objective.

Once our partner entered the most intense stage of treatment, Roger and I managed our hectic practice. It was incumbent upon us to ensure his patients received good follow-up care, and we tried not to bother him or his family while they dealt with a much greater and more personal challenge. We held the fort for a long time. I spent many nights under the microscope at hospitals like Baptist and Cedars Hospital (now the University of Miami Hospital), which reminds me of a very memorable case.

One lovely Saturday morning, as I was anchored on Biscayne Bay in my boat with my Venezuelan girlfriend (later to be my fiancée and wife), I received a disruptive call. It was from my answering service, relaying an urgent message from Port Charlotte, Florida on the Gulf Coast. As always, I promptly responded and spoke with an E.R. physician about a challenging situation, in what would turn out to be an exceptional case, and unique patient.

Joe Jacobik was a retired gentleman and proud family man who had been working in his garage on a circular wood saw when he suffered a terrible injury. While he was making the last of six Westminster Chime Clocks by hand, to be given to each of his beloved grandchildren, he somehow passed his left hand through the saw and amputated his four fingers, leaving only his thumb intact. The ambulance rushed him to the small, local community hospital, with his longtime wife by his side and his hand wrapped in a towel, bleeding profusely. When the E.R. doctor noticed two digits were missing, he instructed

Joe's wife to return to the garage to find them. There, she discovered two fingers almost buried in sawdust, rinsed them off, and placed them in a Ziploc bag.

Aside from the missing two fingers, the attending physician observed that Joe's remaining two fingers were hanging only by dorsal (top) skin. They were blue indicating lack of perfusion (blood flow). Realizing his hospital did not perform this type of complex surgery, the desperate E.R. doctor called Tampa General Hospital for a transfer. As he described the details of the case, he informed them that Joe was 73, with a cursory medical history that included a recent angioplasty procedure in which a coronary stent had been placed. Despite being asymptomatic and otherwise in good health, the hospital denied the transfer. The level one trauma center stated with firm conviction that an elderly gentleman with coronary disease was not a candidate for microvascular replantation surgery. Wow. Just like that.

To his credit, their refusal to accept the patient did not dissuade this committed physician and naturally, the patient's family. Somewhere along the way, he had heard about a "crazy group of hand surgeons" in the Miami area who might be worth a call. His intuition was correct. Within minutes of receiving the call, I pulled up anchor and navigated my way home. I gave them clear instructions to rinse the digits again in saline, place them in a bag, and put the bag on crushed ice, allowing no direct contact with the amputated fingers. This process slows the metabolic demands of the tissue and extends the window of opportunity to consider successful reattachment. My greater concern was for the two fingers that were still partially attached.

I contacted the Cedars hospital and discussed the case with the administrator on call, the O.R. charge nurse, and of course, anesthesia. I informed them the patient was already on his way by ambulance from Port Charlotte, a nearly three-hour drive. Because there was no need for air ambulance, we had time to ready the operating room and bring in the microsurgery team. I also took some brief time to rest and prepare myself for what would likely be an all-night affair. As often happened, this was yet another example of a typical disruption of my girlfriend's and my personal life. That evening, we had plans to entertain some friends at my home. I told her to proceed with the cocktail event, enjoy herself, and express my regrets to them. It does take a special person to engage in a committed relationship with a physician, especially in certain specialties. Alas, this was nothing new for us.

Around 6 p.m., I got the call that the patient had arrived at the Cedars E.R. I instructed them to transfer him to the O.R. holding area upstairs right away. Why had I chosen Cedars? A few key reasons: It was minutes away from my home on the Venetian Islands, and the quality of the operating microscope, enhanced by my familiarity with that brand and model. Oh yes, there was one more seemingly arbitrary and silly reason. I loved the adjustable O.R. stools in their surgical suite. While it may seem superfluous, I challenge you to sit up straight on a stool with no backing for eight, 10, or 14 hours. Much of the time, the surgeon stares into a microscope viewing eyepiece, which means comfort and steadiness are vital. What else was vital? Avoiding any thoughts of life stressors, such as the breakup of my Pittsburgh relationship, difficult insurance companies, or disturbing current events. Anything to minimize tremor and support the best outcome possible. Oh and no more coffee, chocolate, or sex before the procedure. Kind of like a pro athlete but not as well compensated, or revered. Until it is your kid's fingers...

The medical team promptly brought the patient into the O.R., and while anesthesia and nurses prepped him by placing monitors, intubating, washing the limb, and padding bony prominences, I dissected the amputated parts on a separate table, a mayo stand, to identify the relevant anatomy. Since it was a four-finger replant (two complete replants + two revascularizations), I reached out to Roger for help, and as always, he responded with enthusiasm. Remember, it was my weekend on call and his weekend off. But incidents like this happened countless times, and Roger knew he could count on me when the roles were reversed.

By the time my partner arrived, I had progressed a fair way into the surgery with the excellent help of my P.A. (physician assistant) at that time, Debbie, with whom I had been working for several years. This critical position was a second career for her. Debbie was a bit older than I and had run the full gamut in the retail buying field. In mid-life she sought something more meaningful and answered the call to go into medicine. In our healthcare system, the role of so-called "midlevel providers" is critical, a topic I shall explore more detail in a later chapter. Thanks to her proficiency as a microsurgical first assistant, I relied on Debbie to steady the vessel, cut the suture after a knot is tied, and dab the field of blood/saline. It requires a steady hand and steel resolve.

When Roger joined us, I had already stabilized the bone and fused the critical PIP joints (second joint from fingertip), because they blade had passed right through them. My patient would never be able to make a fist again, but it did not matter – he needed his fingers. He had been transferred to us be-cause he and his family recognized that he was willing to risk his life for the ability to maintain function in his Golden Years and finish his clockmaking. There was no doubt in mind. *Onward.* I had also repaired the flexor tendons, identified all the vessels and nerves, and tagged some of them in preparation for microsurgical anastomosis – a more challenging concept than readily ap-parent.

When a microsurgeon repairs a vessel, a series of micro-sutures are used to sew the walls together, bit by bit. In typical fashion, a suture is placed at each extreme to line up the vessel lumen (central canal), then multiple stitches are placed between those, in precise intervals, until the front wall is closed. The vessel is then turned so that the surgeon can complete the same process on the back wall, hoping they did not place previous stitches that may have en-compassed it, which would require removal and starting again. During this time, the micro assistant is irrigating drops of saline, occasionally with lido-caine (to paralyze the wall musculature of the vessel) to maintain its patency. It is an extremely meticulous, demanding, and pain-staking process: one stitch at a time, one vessel at a time.

Some say hitting a fastball in our national (U.S. and Cuba) pastime of base-ball stands among the most difficult technical feat in all of sports. Few athletes possess the hand-eye coordination to strike a small, round object hurtling toward them at almost 100-miles-per-hour, with a long, narrow wooden ob-ject. It is akin to microsurgery, which mandates training and practice in "the ole rat lab," where the aspiring surgeon repeats multiple anastomoses and connection types again and again. Of course, you are not reimbursed for time spent on this activity, suffice it to say. Some people possess a natural aptitude for this skill while others do not. They may acquire it with time and practice, but like a baseball player who can hit a speeding curveball or slider, others never will. Ever.

Those who master microsurgery may eventually receive renumeration for their honed skill in the form of an insurance reimbursement. Maybe. What is beyond dispute is that the most skilled and proficient physician who performs this task will never be paid as much as a major league hurler. Furthermore, a surgeon is not compensated in traditional fashion for his time spent on a task like saving our clockmaker's fingers. Time spent in the O.R. has no correla-tion to reimbursement. It is not an hourly equation like it is for our legal friends and countless other hourly professions. The insurance company pays according to code or codes that neglects to account for the time required, the intensity of the effort, and the necessary skill to accomplish it. There is no surgical version of a "free agent." Therefore, the surgeon does their best and hopes to be reimbursed for their evening spent working, reconstructing, and healing, so they can apply it to their overhead. Hopefully, they are fast and efficient, otherwise it is truly a thankless ordeal, other than the humanitarian aspect. However, being a do-gooder does not pay your bills and massive practice overhead. A harsh reality.

Medicine is one of the few, if only professions in which procedures are paid with little regard for expertise. This came to mind as I reflected upon my experience on the cardiac surgery service as an intern when often I spent enough time in the O.R. to nearly cry and noticed that some surgeons were extremely skilled and others…not so much. Some surgeons made themselves accessible to the patients, family, and me, and possessed excellent decision-making skills when faced with a complication or a clinical challenge. Yet Medicare does not pay exceptional surgeons any more than the mediocre ones.

Why?

It reminds me of an incident that occurred late one night back at Allegheny General Hospital when I saw a Japanese surgeon pace the O.R. halls one night in socks, cigarette in hand, obviously agitated and thinking out loud. At the time, the medical team and I were preparing for surgery on a patient who had shattered his elbow in a highway accident.

"Who is that?!" I asked one of the venerable E.R. nurses.

"He is the new neurosurgeon from Japan. A recent newspaper article extolled him as the 'Michael Jordan of Neurosurgery.' You didn't see it?"

When I revealed I had not read it, she informed me that he took cases nobody else would accept or even attempt. That night, he was already 18 hours into a delicate removal of a glioblastoma from the base of the brain. To avoid causing respiratory paralysis and death for his patient, who had traveled from afar with his hopeful, anguished family, the surgeon took frequent breaks.

"Wow," I thought. "Why isn't His Airness called the Dr. Neurosurgeon of basketball?"

Of course, Julius Erving was called "Dr. J." so perhaps there is some positive reference to my field. I once spoke to Michael Jordan at length. This would have been a good question for him as he was very pleasant, intelligent, and approachable. I am sure many high-level athletes are appreciative of their doctors who keep them "in the game". Others, not so much, as we will touch on later…

Silly, maybe, but you get the point. Here he is, one of the best brain surgeons in the world, taking on cases that many of his peers deem impossible, having trained for a decade, and he must rely on an insurance company to determine his worth. Furthermore, he is compared to an athlete whose job is to place a round ball into a circular ring surrounded by a net. A task many gladly do for free --- it is called recreation. No doubt the pros are very skilled but it is interesting to take a different view of it. For me, it made little sense then, and it makes little sense now.

This is not the case for all specialties, however. Aesthetic plastic surgeons often command their price base upon skill, reputation, and sadly, marketing. While I have no qualms with looking beautiful, I believe our society's values are a bit misplaced when a facelift or breast augmentation pays multiple times the amount that removing a malignant tumor or inserting a porcine aortic valve in a patient's heart does. These are further thoughts to ponder.

Back to our patient missing four potentially viable fingers. We reached the point where we were ready to perform multiple micro-anastamoses and readied the surgical microscope for a second surgeon. With Debbie's assistance, I had already performed several. We were well on our way to completing this taxing hand surgery. Roger sat down, and in his usual jovial, booming voice exclaimed, "Hey guy, you have half of this done!"

I replied, "Sure but we will work faster together. Let's get this guy off the table. He has a coronary stent ya know…"

An exceptional microsurgeon, Roger and I alternated repairs and completed the case in just under seven hours. Mind you, each digit requires the repair of at least one digital artery and to veins. If possible, you repair a second artery as insurance…sorry to use that word. Whether it is a replantation or a free flap tissue transfer, the challenge with microsurgery is that the tissue being reattached is dead. The microsurgeon brings it back to life via the introduction of blood flow to the detached part, then makes the necessary repairs to the veins – which are much more fragile and difficult to work with – and return it to the heart and lungs for oxygenation.

In what can only be described as a euphoric moment (though words cannot fully capture the feeling), we watched in sequence as each finger "pinked up." When faced with success like this after surgery, ALL members of the medical team often express quiet or solemn celebration: from the nurses who prepared the patient and the surgical techs who set up and manage the delicate tools, to the anesthesia team that keeps the patient alive. For any elderly man with coronary limitations undergoing a demanding surgery that required intubation for over eight hours, the latter presented a daunting challenge. Who was noticeably absent in the O.R. that exhilarating moment when we bore witness to clinical success? The hospital executive, insurance adjuster, and state regulator, although I believe they would have also relished this triumph for humanity, technical advances, and acquired skills. Surely the peripheral individuals in the healthcare equation must realize that we, the healers, deserve a major place at the table, if not a place at the head of the table, to debate healthcare challenges.

Post-surgery, the medical team continued to care for Joe. They brought him into the recovery room, hand elevated and still intubated, but stable, while I conducted the joyful task of informing his dear family of the wonderful outcome, although with a measure of restraint. Of course, they reacted with relief, gratitude, and elation, but now my next task was to educate and inform them of the potential pitfalls. Because the fingers remained well perfused, I did not have to "leach" any of them. Although it sounds Medieval and barbaric, the application of live medicinal leaches (Hirudo Medicinalis), is often a necessary part of achieving success after microsurgery when there is not enough egress of blood from the implanted part. Simply call 1-800-Leach-USA and our little friends will help us drain the blood from a congested part, while injecting anticoagulant (Hirudin) to help promote blood flow and avoid clotting – the enemy of microsurgery. The pharmacy often has leaches, but no calls were necessary in this case.

After an excellent post-op course, Joe was released a few days later and his family took him right to our Miami Hand Center for his post-surgical evaluation, mindful that he lived three hours away. Thanks to his charm and his uplifting story, Joe became somewhat of a celebrity while in the hospital. He even became the subject of an interview on CBS4, a local daily news channel. It was a welcome reprieve from the usual reporting of murders and heinous crimes – including health insurance fraud or another untimely "plastic surgery" death. Considering Miami is far and away the most prolific site of Medicare fraud, it behooves the city to report on the good things that transpire here and elsewhere.

Two weeks after surgery, Joe and his steadfast family drove back to Miami, where I removed the temporary pins that held his fingers attached and secured the PIP joint while bony fusion took place. Given the human-interest nature of the case, the news cameras were back on the scene, and we even allowed them into our outpatient center's operating room while I removed all eight pins and confirmed the success of the fusions. This would have been impossible in the hospital O.R. Why? Liability, I guess, that ugly word, but does the public not have the right to know what life and limb saving technology is out there? Yet, we focus on murderers and other "bad actors". A sad statement on our societal priorities, or perhaps the media's.

Next up in Joe's journey? Hand rehabilitation.

The media did follow the story in good taste, in alignment with Agustin Acosta's case, meaning they presented his ordeal through his eyes. Healthcare should not be a mystery. Patient education offers excellent benefits when the public understands the options that may be available to them. There is no better way to do this than through the patients themselves, not the person providing the care who is expected to know all. Now this type of education must extend to *how* the care is delivered, this time by the people providing that care – the doctors, mid-level nurses, and technicians. We are the *patients* of healthcare.

A model patient, Mr. Jacobik had a wonderful outcome. Psychologists long ago noted that patient optimism and full engagement with their treatment could yield almost near-miraculous results. For this reason, work-related injuries are often the most challenging to treat, due to bureaucratic and legal hurdles and secondary gain issues at play that must be discussed in an open forum if we are ever going to rein in healthcare costs. Joe envisioned the right type of secondary gain when he left my hand center, sans eight pins. He did his therapy, returned to A.D.L.s (activities of daily living) as soon as possible, and did what I fully expected – he completed the last Westchester Chime Clock for his remaining granddaughter. In a rare display nowadays, his family has kept in touch, sent me yearly Christmas cards with updates about Joe and occasionally, some photos, including him working on his table saw to finish the last wooden clock.

Ten years after the injury, his lovely daughter Tina called to tell me the news of his passing. She reminded me that Joe and his family remained eternally grateful that I could restore his function and allow him to live the rest of his life in a manner he deemed fit. Not through a nebulous, detached third-party as determined through either "authorization" or the clinical approval to perform the surgery. Thank you, Cedars O.R. team, the unknown Port Charlotte E.R. doctor, and Dr. Roger Khouri, in addition to my skilled mentors in microsurgical technique.

I often end a clinical lecture by presenting Joe's odyssey as an example of what can be done in medicine with cooperation, technology, and support at every level. I end with the last slide depicting the final wooden chime clock Joe constructed – standing alone, polished, and proud. Often, there is not a dry eye in the room.

Even in my first year, I came across many Joe and Agustin type of cases. The clinical cases a doctor encounters represent the tapestry they weave with the infrastructure they gradually create: a medical practice. I was fortunate to have co-founded the Miami Hand Center. It gave me the opportunity to work with a busy hand surgeon who shared the same aspirations of academia but did not have time to act upon them. From the start, I could contribute in ways that aligned with my strengths and I discovered latent talents I never knew I had. In a testament to my entrepreneurial nature, I came up with the name of the practice and even designed the first version of the logo, with my partner's enthusiastic approval. We were two rebels with a noble cause, who did things differently from the status quo.

We created a center where we could do it all for our patients: operate and do the rehab, because in hand surgery and certain other specialties, therapy is critical. In the hand, it is not about the pain, it is about the dexterity. The ability to make a fist. People take things like that for granted yet the use of your hand is ubiquitous and, for those who make their living working with their hands, there is an economic factor.

Our center featured something I used to call "the fishbowl," where you could walk down the hall of the patient exam rooms and look through the windows into the therapy unit. Quite often, I caught the gaze of one our therapists, who would gesture for me to come in, index finger flexing to and fro, like I was a grade-schooler in trouble. When I entered, she presented a patient who had reached a stumbling block. Together, we would discuss the problem, examine the patient together, and intervene. Try doing that with a therapist across town who is dealing with a problematic patient. Such commonsense solutions are an ongoing struggle with many insurance carriers and they *still* do not recognize the value, even above the economic, of this type of arrangement. In fact, many insurance companies penalize clinicians who have therapy within their facility, if you can believe that.

It's as if they are saying "Bad, bad doctor trying to profit off medical care. Let us dictate where the patient is sent, even though you have never met the therapist and they can't possibly understand the nuances of what you did for that patient." However, if the therapy center is owned by a businessman, that seems somehow okay. Simply amazing...

As I mentioned, one of our contracts was for 60 percent of Medicare – an absurd arrangement. While it had not been my decision to undervalue our services in that way, in later years many hand surgeons in my community complained to me that my partner and founding member of the practice undercut his colleagues with these insurance contracts. Regardless, my partner's decisions created a level of patient volume that was almost unheard of. It helped us become excellent surgeons. And, as has always been my philosophy, if you walk into a surgeon's near-empty waiting room, run the other way. If you are a patient, you need a medical doctor who deals with high volume and repetition in their practice.

The irony?

Patients will complain, yet most do not mind waiting an hour-and-a-half for the Dumbo ride at Disney World with their kid...they'll gripe a little bit, then accept that it's just the way it is. For some reason, they do not apply this same attitude toward their own healthcare. In fact, it still amazes me how many people grumble about it and even leave if they must wait too long. Sometimes, the inconvenience may be due to poor scheduling by our staff, whom we do not micromanage as a rule. However, it only takes two or three complex cases or some vociferous patients to upend the schedule. I will concede that my partners were not as cognizant as I about patient wait times. There is no question that people wait a long time to see their doctors. I am not justifying it but imagine this scenario: your waiting room is full while you provide the best care you can, one patient at a time. Then, the hospital calls you with a true emergency and you must leave right away. At the least, you need to answer the call and make some split-second decisions. It is very disruptive.

Therefore, the alternative is for the hospital E.R. patient to wait until the end of the night for the guy on call to run to that hospital. It is not ideal for the patient, E.R. physician or me, but that is what used to happen. It was not uncommon for us to see patients until about nine o'clock at night, then drive to the hospital to take care an open fingertip injury someone suffered when they, for example, put their finger in a car door, the blender or believe it or not, the lawnmower. These are ubiquitous scenarios in community hand surgery. I am not even talking about the horrendous fractures or soft tissue injuries like I described earlier. For every case like Agustin or poor Joe, there are 50 of these everyday injuries, every night. Back in those days, I could leave for the hospital at nine o'clock at night to see a patient but because hospitals don't work very fast, a case that took me about 20 to 30 minutes might consume three hours of my time. At midnight, I would be on my way to a second hospital that called me with another emergency as I previously recounted.

These experiences made us eager for our own operating rooms at the Miami Hand Center. Consider the difference: unless something was limb-threatening, the patient could be wrapped up in the E.R. and sent to us. Of course, the hospitals didn't like it too much because they wanted to capture the patient and proceed with the surgery – a vital source of income for any healthcare system, which brings me full circle back to crux of the matter, and the reason I started OrthoNOW®. To capture the patient from the get-go and manage their entire journey. More on that later.

Once we built our own operating rooms, the medical community soon learned that there was always somebody at the 'ole Miami Hand Center, till virtually whenever. Once our O.R.s became fully functional and ramped up, we sometimes ran around the clock. That is no joke. I would come in in the morning to do my elective surgeries and my partner and the anesthesiologist were still there. I knew the moment I walked in and saw either the anesthesiologist, or my partner Roger, sporting five o'clock shadows because they had been up all night. People received excellent care because we would say to an E.R. call, "Okay, ship them over." Once a patient arrived, the first question we asked was, "What time did you eat?" because we could fix them the same day. This was in 1998 when virtually nobody was doing that in Florida. The experience gave me a profound understanding for what makes sense when caring for patients – without any business training (I am still not proficient in reading a P&L statement). And that benefits both the clinician (or, to use the dreaded word, "provider," that has been ingrained in us) and the patient.

Here is the mind-blowing part: it is also excellent for the insurance companies, but they either do not see it or refuse to acknowledge it. One of the major problems with U.S. healthcare is that when people have a viable idea that saves the insurance companies money, the assumption is that they would pass the savings along to us, the consumers. But that is *not* happening. It is sad because we need good hospitals. We have reached the point where it is obvious; people know not every procedure requires a hospital stay. It started with ophthalmology and a lot of other areas. Patients realized, "I don't need to have a minor eye procedure or a colonoscopy in a big hospital."

Why?

Many of us are really convinced that the big insurance lobby and the big hospital lobby work together. I could support this with data but that is not the aim of this book. Some of the works providing that data are listed in my references. I want to convey what almost every clinician feels, particularly if they are trying to provide good, cost-effective care in the shadow of the local hospital system. It is a pity because we all recognize that we need good hospitals and tertiary care centers. However, there certainly is room in the sandbox for all of us. Medicine has advanced to the point where people now realize they do not have to be admitted to a hospital for a minor surgery. In fact, it is more cost effective and efficient to go to one ambulatory, stand-alone facility, where you can have everything done and be on your way. Yet despite the undeniable benefits, insurance companies have refused to drive this. Furthermore, they have not even encouraged it until recently.

The A.H.A. (American Hospital Association) has vehemently fought Medicare's (C.M.S.) proposal to expand the approved list of surgical procedures that can be done in independent A.S.C.s (Ambulatory Surgery Centers) despite ample data that many of these surgeries have superior outcomes in the outpatient scenario and lesser complications. The COVID-19 pandemic has simply underscored the need to avoid hospitals when dealing with non-life-threatening issues. Other issues such as M.R.S.A. (highly resistant bacteria), endemic to hospitals for many years, are now being highly considered. Now that C.M.S is finally accepting this data commercial insurance policies fall into line. Essentially, we have the government dictating efficiency and cost-effectiveness. Crazy concept huh? Most would agree this is not judicious. My previous V.A. hospital days alluded to the validity of the argument...or you can just inquire what the department of defense paid for the infamous screwdriver.

Despite multiple challenges, our surgery center soon became one of the busiest facilities in the entire county, even rivaling many small hospitals. In our peak year, we performed 4,700 surgeries, a measure of our patient volume but also O.R. efficiency, considering it was a two-room facility. We achieved this volume with a total of four surgeons (do the math), just prior to the addition of our fifth and final talented hand surgeon, Dr. Steve Alex.

Steve's addition led to some very welcome changes, particularly in terms of logistics and clinical work distribution. With five hand specialists, we could now focus on elective surgery every day of the week, both in office and in the adjacent surgery center. Each of us would have a hectic office day, along with priority to use all facilities, and the subsequent day would be surgical. Remaining days for each partner were often distributed by doing larger cases in the hospital, catching up with administrative or chartwork, and independent projects such as research. In some cases, this led to productive and truly landmark work in implant design and product development. But it also presented challenges in how we worked together and where we placed our focus.

I will reiterate we were quite an innovative group, not simply early adopters, and several of us began companies that would contribute to our unique specialty interests. Roger was the first to launch a company aligned with one of his other areas of expertise, breast reconstruction. Like many reconstructive plastic surgeons, Roger had an interest in breast surgery, but not the straightforward augmentation of simply inserting a silicone or saline bag implant. He had done extensive work on post-mastectomy and radiation patients yet sought to offer alternatives, including non-surgical solutions for women who were not comfortable with an implant.

He founded Biomecanica, which later became BRAVA and treated multiple patients. I supported my colleague as an early investor since non-operative breast enlargement seemed like an area anybody would believe in, right? Okay, I will refrain from making any crass any jokes. Regardless, these efforts demanded an abundance of time, energy, and capital for Roger, made possible by the newfound flexibility in our schedules. Yes, we still ran to many hospitals, but having our own surgery center for many elective cases freed us up to pursue projects, as most surgeons are not a fan of idle time. The same was true for my other partners.

Dr. Gonzalez-Hernandez founded a company called Toby Orthopedics, which focused on several products for upper extremity internal fixation – essentially, a more advanced plating technology for complex fractures and those with osteoporotic bone. Due to his physics background, he also devised a more efficient methodology for assisting flexor tendon repairs, a very technical area of hand surgery. Naturally, this consumed time and resources but was truly in our group's DNA. Some of the products were well aligned with a company that our senior partner had started some years prior; in fact, they were quite synergistic. This caused some issues that epitomized the difficulties physicians often confront with respect to collaboration – an extensive problem that contributes to the challenges we face in healthcare.

In my case, I later co-founded a company called American Hand Institute (A.H.I.). The goal was to forge innovation, in both methodology and instrumentation, in the burgeoning area of small joint arthroscopy, including the wrist. I had developed a particular interest in this after a pivotal course during my fellowship at the O.L.C. (Orthopedic Learning Center), where I not only met Dr. Luchetti, but other colleagues who would become renowned in the emerging discipline of wrist arthroscopy, such as Paco del Pinal from Spain.

Dick Berger from the Mayo Clinic had been part of that course faculty, a valued colleague who first demonstrated a technique he was starting to explore – arthroscopy of the thumb basal joint. For whatever reason, I saw it as having wide application and being a clear superior alternative to what most of us were doing: open complete resection of the entire trapezial bone, a technique I first learned with Dr. Melone, then later, Dr. Imbriglia and others. Much like wrist external fixation, I found it overly aggressive and almost brutal. That practical course led me to develop a profound interest in arthroscopy of that joint and even smaller ones in the hand. Consequently, I partnered with the few like-minded individuals who embraced these techniques: Drs. Tyson Cobb, Stacey Berner, and Steve Topper, to form A.H.I.

My interest was to develop a more ergonomic and specialized small joint arthroscope-camera unit specifically designed for these growing indications. This requires complex optical engineering and video camera technology that led me to attend Medica, a mega medical trade show in Germany, where an entire section was devoted to endoscopic technology. I soon learned how difficult it was to find others who share your vision; therefore, device development would not be my forte. It was a frustrating journey, fraught with hurdles that I was not willing to tackle, though our company did obtain two patents on related small joint instrumentation and implants.

Interestingly, there was another reason I developed this interest and focus on small joint arthroscopy. I was in the office seeing a patient with severe rheumatoid arthritis. While viewing the X-ray, my partner approached me with a puzzled look on his face. At the point, it was just the two of us, the other partners had not yet joined the practice. When I asked what he thought of my treatment plan, he retorted, "Don't you think I should be considered the expert on arthritis in this practice, Alex?"

Taken aback, I answered, "I think there is nothing wrong with both of us sharing this interest and besides, one of the reasons I became a hand surgeon is specifically because of this disease, rheumatoid arthritis." He suggested an alternative and advised that I should consider being "the expert" on arthroscopy. Not being a contrarian, I said "Okay," and promised to pursue that course. I had already developed an interest in it; there was no reason I could not continue my passion for treating arthritic conditions or any other entity that came my way clinically. I am grateful that he urged me into that area. I have since written multiple scientific articles and book chapters in the field of small joint arthroscopy. Many of our visiting fellows would remark to me that he often called the arthroscope, "the instrument of the devil," reminiscent of renowned shoulder surgeon, Charlie Rockwood's resistance to when shoulder arthroscopy appeared on the landscape. Disagreement and opposition often lead to progress. More on colleagues and collaboration in the next chapter.

Regardless, each of the surgeons at the Miami Hand Center had unique clinical interests. We enjoyed amazing synergy, since any clinical problem could have an internal second or third opinion. We also learned from each other; hence I can credit Roger for helping me refine my microsurgical skills as well as my decision-making capabilities. In turn, he thanks us for furthering his capabilities in addressing complex upper limb fractures, although he did not treat elbow or shoulder, not being an orthopedic surgeon by training. The teamwork benefitted our patients and us surgeons tremendously. Being a partner in the Miami Hand Center was a wonderful experience and a crucible of learning. We practiced together for over 12 years, but like many good things, it came to an end.

Chapter 4 – Cats, Colleagues and Collaboration

"I will remember that there is art to medicine as well as science, and that warmth, sympathy, and understanding may outweigh the surgeon's knife or the chemist's drug."

Our healthcare business colleagues, including practice administrators and investors, often use an interesting and familiar expression to describe the challenges of meeting with a group of physicians to decide policy: it is like herding cats. I encourage my peers to heed and embrace this commentary with humility. The expression, of course, refers to the failure of a collection of people to behave, or to be led, as a united whole. Anyone who has ever worked with a large group of physicians will grasp my meaning right away. Among orthopedic surgeons, however, the problem may be amplified.

Why do I bring this up? We, as a profession, must accept some blame for many of the developing problems in healthcare delivery. No, I am not suggesting that we caused the problem; au contraire, I am stating that we have had ample opportunities to manage the debacle and even reverse some of the disturbing trends. I speak from experience, having learned the hard way through the gradual and then, precipitous dissolution of the Miami Hand Center. Although it is painful to recount, past mistakes can be instructive, as Winston Churchill noted in a 1948 post-war speech to the House of Commons when he paraphrased philosopher Georg Santayan: "Those who fail to learn from history are doomed to repeat it."

With that in mind, I intend to share with you the lessons I learned from my mistakes, shed light on current issues, and humbly submit some ideas, along with contributions from other "providers." Many of the challenges and errors I have encountered represent a microcosm of our current healthcare mess in the United States and beyond. Let me be clear, the issue is not so much the quality of care, science, or clinical protocols but rather *how* that care is delivered to our patients.

As I described in the previous chapter, I was part of an amazing association of five incredibly talented, passionate, and hardworking physicians. The fact that our team disbanded provides a metaphor for many of the problems I see in the medical profession. We had accomplished just about everything we set out to do in our field, and in the realm of private practice and medical business. Throughout the duration, some of us began to innovate in the field of implant design and surgical methodologies, and even underwent paradigm shifts with respect to established treatment protocols. The changes in the way distal fractures are treated has become nearly folkloric among hand surgeons and general orthopedists, simply because this wrist fracture is THE most common adult fracture that requires surgical intervention. This is not a minor statement. In other words, the most prevalent bony injury that leads to surgery underwent a revolution in care – and this revolution was born out of our small, humble hand center in the southern portion of Miami-Dade County.

It is a well-known story among those who are close to me. Like my partners, I have lectured all around the world for reasons I have already discussed. In fact, I have lectured on all seven continents – yes, including Antarctica. It's not quite as sexy as being a member of the Seven Summits Club, but for me it's more rewarding, not to mention safer. These experiences have enabled me to "think outside of the box," since practicing surgery in a box does not allow for my professional growth or benefit my patients. In addition, the opportunity to present lectures around the globe has allowed me to transmit information, innovations, and knowledge extensively, and learn from others. I cast a wide net, something I continue to do to this day.

In the 90s, the distal radius fracture was treated in what now appears to be an impractical manner – indirect reduction (putting bone back in place) followed by securing that position with either a cast or cast incorporating pins (pins and plaster), and later an external fixator. I discussed these options in my comments on residency and fellowship training where I soon realized there must be a better way. Some colleagues in Europe (where A.O. foundation was founded) and less so at home, were promoting internal fixation as a better solution where the fracture was DIRECTLY reduced, not via external indirect means. I had confirmed my concerns via a biomechanical study while in Pittsburgh and received affirmation from my primary mentor, Joe Imbriglia.

When I settled in Miami, upon returning from my surgical experience in Europe, it quickly became apparent that the traditional technique was prevalent. I resisted this greatly, to the point where one of the distributors for a specific fixator became a bit nervous. After all, external fixators can be expensive because they require a multitude of metal parts and highly precise mechanisms. The problem is not the technology, which remains useful and relevant, but the indication in this case – the most common fracture encountered. I had placed well over a hundred tibial external fixators during my Bellevue trauma center days, but this was typically for open and complex fractures of the lower leg, not routine wrist fractures. I pivoted to applying titanium or stainless-steel plates for the distal radius of the wrist and could barely recall putting a fixator on any longer.

It was a radical shift in thinking. While many of my colleagues scattered around the world were already doing this, it was not commonplace in South Florida – a reality that fortified my attitude to seek and embrace superior surgical options and not always follow the status quo. To my good fortune, I chose to partner with a like-minded surgeon who was even better prepared to make this shift, with his background focus in mathematics and engineering. When I arrived back from Germany, we agreed to shift our wrist fracture care to plate internal fixation, further disrupting the pipeline of external fixation established within several orthopedic implant companies. Our decision led to significant economic consequences in the surgical supply side of various hospitals, well before we built our own center.

A brilliant, tangential thinker, my partner had already been dabbling in plate fixation for the wrist and agreed to phase out what I regarded as the antiquated, counterproductive practice of external fixation. However, his real brilliance was exemplified in a simple and perhaps, typical move. He took a contradictory approach to what was classic dogma in distal radius fracture surgery and placed the plate on the palmar (volar) side as opposed to the dorsal (top) part of the wrist. Doing that procedure was not at all revolutionary, as we often used it for specific fracture patterns (volar, Barton, etc.), but his indication *was* unorthodox.

I recall an afternoon where he came back from the O.R., at Mercy Hospital of Miami (if memory serves me well) and informed me with obvious excitement that he had placed a titanium plate on the palmar aspect of the wrist for a typical dorsally displaced fracture. In other words, he resisted the traditional dogma of using a dorsal plate for dorsal fracture, far and away the most common wrist injury pattern. I listened to his near heretical account with like-minded agreement because I understood his thinking. We could get into the biomechanical principles of applying plates on the tension side of the fracture, as in hip fractures, but that is well beyond the scope of this book. The almost Galilean principle here is that for change and consequent progress to occur, one must abandon certain conventions. Whether the sun moves around the earth, or plates should be applied to the dorsal aspect of a wrist fracture, accepted convention is not always accurate or preferable. I was proud of our alignment on this principle and was willing to embark on a journey of helping modify that doctrine.

At this point, however, my partner and I diverged. With his sound engineering background, he employed the help of two engineers to design a new titanium plate for volar application with some brilliant modifications of the emerging principle of locking plates (a topic beyond the scope of this book). The takeaway here is that ideas often emerge from collaboration. While I may not have thought of altering my plate placement when he did, he may have never moved away from external fixation if not for my work on refuting that approach. Furthermore, as with many novel approaches, innovators who are on the same wavelength often reach the same conclusion before another. With respect to staunch discipline of surgery, a radical change evokes challenges and requires a broader movement – not just the embrace of one or two clear-thinking visionaries. In fact, surgeons from Minnesota, Germany and elsewhere had already put into place the volar approach to both acute fracture management and late construction for malunion.

My partner's true innovation was designing a specific plate for this approach, and maybe even more importantly, educating surgeons on *how* to utilize this novel implant via hands-on courses. The pity was that he displaced me from his mission, despite the genesis in thinking that I described, and he might still even argue. I made a choice not to fully engage in the engineering process; therefore, I was not at all entitled to the eventual success of the commercial enterprise. My decision was based on several factors. I did not want to devote the time because I was already much busier with clinical practice than I cared to be, partly due to the insurance contracts I mentioned, and the practice philosophy. I was simply trying to toe the line and man the fort. However, as I stated after my fellowship experience traveling abroad, I do not consider myself a workaholic. Despite his initial kind invitation, I politely declined. Was there a subliminal factor at play? Maybe.

To use a cliché, past is prologue. Several of my partner's past actions and comments led me to realize he would not share much credit for this groundbreaking work. I chose not to devote the little free time I had to this enterprise, knowing I would only be a footnote figure in this orthopedic care revolution. I was fully aware of the value of my role in the evolution of that paradigm shift in fracture philosophy and did not need more. My only disappointment was his lack of acknowledgement of my contribution, which manifested in his purposeful avoidance of discussing our early change in thinking with our colleagues and peers.

In this respect, he was not unique. Failure to give credit where it is due is a common theme among our other colleagues who innovate. In a karmic twist, he had suffered a similar slight when a prominent surgeon in the field of limb lengthening published a mathematical equation devised by my partner. Imagine the frustration of someone else taking credit – in print – for something you yourself pioneered? It was not a monetary consideration, but rather a source of professional pride when your contribution to patient care via peer-reviewed literature, fails to assign appropriate or at least shared credit. Yet my partner did the same thing to me, resulting in the "line in the sand" that altered our professional relationship and our friendship, forever. And this was not even the first incident.

During our initial foray into changing how these common fractures are approached, I received a welcome invitation from Dr. Christophe Mathoulin from Institut de la Main, to present this concept at a Parisian conference devoted to wrist fracture treatment updates. On one of my many visits to Europe, I had visited my friend Francesco Brunelli at his innovative clinic that took a comprehensive approach to hand care. They had a surgical center within the ambulatory center where they evaluated patients – providing further insight as to how we would practice in Miami. In that setting, I met Christophe, who recognized the novel approach we were proposing for this fracture, largely because of my presentations at multiple international meetings. When he asked me to present at his meeting on the wrist, I agreed with unbridled enthusiasm. After all, the meeting focused on the wrist and is there anyone who does not love French cuisine?!

Exhilarated, I returned to Miami and shared the wonderful news with my associate with the suggestion that he could perhaps discuss biomechanics of the volar approach while I discussed a clinical case series, or vice versa. His response shocked me: "But Alex," he protested in his calm yet aggravating tone, "don't you think it should be I who attends the meeting and speaks on the subject?"

I could scarcely believe my ears. It was such a scalding and presumptuous response that I chose to be discreet and offer an unnoticeable reaction. For a moment, I was numb and dumbfounded. "But it was I who was invited, not you. I'm simply sharing the opportunity," I responded. "Fine, you go ahead."

Conflict avoidance is one of my faults. Yes, I wanted to go to Paris to speak about the wonderful advances we had proposed, but I was not about to get into a pissing match with a guy I had to work with day after day. I chose not to go. At that point, I preferred to use my valuable time to go boating. Right or wrong, that was my attitude.

The real damage, however, was in how my legacy would be perceived. I knew, as did many friends and close colleagues, that I was instrumental in this shift of treatment approach to the wrist. Understand, I have been fortunate in contributing to a variety of areas in my field, giving me not only a palpable sense of personal pride and validating my years of study, but also allowing me to be seen as a K.O.L. (key opinion leader) in these areas. These achievements have led to the accrual of strong orthopedic industry contacts and product development, opportunities to lecture across the globe, and the ability to direct patient care consequences as the more sophisticated patients can now seek treatment options from the palm of their hand. I have published extensively in most of these areas, which has traditionally been the vehicle for the transformation of surgical thought, in addition to society meetings and focused conferences. In this decade, we are seeing a shift to virtual and web-based education in many formats. However, some areas I have contributed in are highly specific and have nowhere near the impact that our simple shift in wrist fracture thinking represented in the late 90s.

In March of 2002, a monumental article entitled, "Volar Fixation for Dorsally Displaced Fracture of the Distal Radius: A Preliminary Report," was published in the Journal of Hand Surgery. The treatise introduced a novel concept to the most esteemed journal among our hand surgery colleagues worldwide. The date reflects that this was only a few years after we had adopted this methodology and was our presentation to the world of what we had already been discussing and even presenting at scientific meetings. The problem is that there were only two coauthors…and one of them was certainly not me. Even though we had developed and even promoted the concept together, to varying degrees. The second author, who happens to be a friend, was a highly respected wrist surgeon from Europe; however, he was not at all involved in the early development of the concept. Due to our personal relationship, it was difficult to discuss the issue with him. It was certainly not his doing. Despite my tendency to be non-confrontational, this was simply too much to overlook.

To clarify, our esteemed group of professionals at the Miami Hand Center, hellbent on being at the academic forefront of our specialty, had mutually agreed to list each other as co-authors on all papers, with rare exception of a specific technique foreign to the other partner. For example, none of us felt that we should co-author a breast paper that Dr. Khouri might pen. In my case, collaborative as I am, I even put Roger's name on articles involving techniques that he has never done and never plans to do. I assumed our gentlemen's agreement would be honored. When I confronted my partner, he claimed that the other coauthor did not want a third author on the paper. *Bullshit.* If the lead author brings forth a study, or a new concept, it is their prerogative to list the relevant coauthors, or at least the ones they feel beholden too. Of course, in his mind neither was the case, and this disrespectful attitude began to percolate and permeate through the group.

One might overlook a one-time slight, but when the same thing happened two years later, I had enough. What happened? My partner published a similar article, this time touting the technique for the treatment of wrist fractures in the elderly. By then, the other partners and I were using the plate manufactured by his company and supporting him philosophically and economically. I remember one week where I fixed 11 distal radius fractures using his wrist plates – yes, we were that busy. Aside from believing in the concept and preferring the implant (which had little competition at the time), I might stand to gain an economic benefit. The fast-growing company needed inventory, hence cash. Despite my previously mentioned issues with this partner, I invested with confidence and enthusiasm. I was happy to support him. Regardless, following this incident with the second article, I completely disengaged and forged my own path. To this day, I look back on my experience with Miami Hand Center with pride. All of us were excellent clinicians.

After that grave disappointment, I still published multiple papers. Even up until 2005, three years after the initial volar plate article, I published several articles in which I listed all my partners as coauthors. Several of them focused on small joint arthroscopy – techniques used solely by me within our group, unlike the volar plate. These methods were an anathema to my senior partner whom you will recall referred to the arthroscope as "the devil's instrument." No matter. One lesson I teach my children is that integrity is defined by your behavior when no one is looking.

In contrast to many groups, the rift at Miami Hand Center did not revolve around money. Rather, it developed in the realm of academia and in the breakdown of mutual respect. We maintained fairness in terms of distributed reimbursements with an "eat what you kill" model. Many physician groups deal with challenges with such an arrangement, because of discrepancies in human nature. Nobody likes it when someone else reaps the same rewards as them when they do not possess the same work ethic or simply choose not to work as hard certain months. Some of us who fled communism believed that individuals should dictate their own earning capability.

Although we shared the burden of overhead – including our therapists, surgery center staff, and front office staff – only one of us owned the real estate. In addition, each of us had separate "team managers," surgical schedulers, etc. With varying appetites for travel and attendance, those who chose to expand their knowledge in that way accepted its adverse effects on income. So long as you covered your emergencies and phone calls for the group during your on-call week, your schedule was your own responsibility. On the other hand, many physician groups pool their reimbursements and divide them equally after paying common overhead. While there is no right and wrong answer, that model would not have worked for Miami Hand Center.

As inconsideration began to mount in the group, it served as a warning to not only talk things over but as my mother's motto goes, to "deal generously." As I mentioned, Eduardo had started a company called Toby Orthopedics. He and our lead partner at some point had discussed a plate concept for fractures of the proximal humerus, the shoulder. Although I do not recall the details, they could not reach a mutual agreement about how to collaborate, rather than oppose each other on the design and who owned the intellectual property and development rights. Mind you, these are two renowned surgeons, brilliant designers and problem-solvers, and partners who shared the same office space, staff, and even patients. Yet, they could not agree on a simple design sketch. This event took place prior to Steve joining us. To resolve the issue amicably, the four of us went to dinner on two separate occasions, where Roger and I acted as mediators. Well…in my case that was irrelevant since I have always believed that $1+1 = 3$.

We each brought our own unique strengths and liabilities to the association. As I noted, early on I understood the concept of marketing and customer service in healthcare; however, my brain shut off during any discussion of P & L statements or insurance contracts. As we entered the internet age, I created a website, with scant contributions from my colleagues, respecting their preferences. I ensured that site represented us equally, portrayed our unique infrastructure, and became an access point for patients in the days long before physician websites were in vogue.

One afternoon, I happened to read an email exchange with a rheumatoid patient who was requesting a consultation for me, specifically. As I followed the trail, I soon realized that the message had been forwarded by our staff to my partner. No one ever showed me the patient inquiry. It was fortuitous that I saw this because it became the catalyst for me to decide to create my own webpage: www.drbadia.com. I continued to contribute to the group page despite the lack of interest from my colleagues, yet it dawned on me that my best efforts would be better suited to growing my own practice within the group. Until this incident, I had held the "musketeer" mentality close to my heart: One for all and all for one! However, the gradual erosion of that sentiment, further fueled by frequent disappointments, led to my questioning the viability of the group.

Bay State Blues

I am not the only one who has confronted difficulties in collaborating with colleagues. Robert Terrill, M.D. is an orthopedic, upper extremity surgeon who has been in practice for 30 years in the state of Massachusetts. He shares a real-life story about how one chairman's interference circumvented not only his career, but the career of another talented colleague.

"For the first 17 years of my practice, I worked at two different hospitals: The Trauma Center at the University of Massachusetts Medical Center and Memorial Hospital, which was sort of a community hospital. Then they merged and became a big entity. For the last 13 to 14 years, I have worked at another community hospital in Worcester. And so, I have witnessed a lot of the goings-on there. The ones that are external to me have been the development of large groups, including The UMass Memorial Medical Group, which, at least here in Worcester, is the 800-pound gorilla in the community. There is a multi-specialty private group called Reliant Medical Group, which is used to be called Fallon Clinic. And then there are small individual providers, a few small groups, at least in orthopedics.

"And what I have seen is doctors leaving private practice to work for the UMass group. I did not want to, but I was essentially pushed out by the Chairman of the Orthopedic Department without my knowledge, which was kind of interesting. His attitude was, 'You work for me, or you are not here.'

This occurred in 2003 when I was the Teacher of the Year of the Orthopedic Residency at UMass. And we were just getting bombarded with referrals from outlying hospitals and trauma centers for dubious reasons, like "Our hand surgeon on call does not take that insurance, they are in private practice" (they did not know how to respond when I told them I was, too), "Your hospital must accept any referrals," "I am not comfortable with this injury," etc. For various reasons, they were essentially, dumps. It was upwards of 50-to- 60 patients from a week on call. I had no extender, I saw every patient, and I had no partners or colleagues willing to share the load, which meant I had to shut things down for about two weeks, every six weeks to enable me to see and care for all the patients.

"That is why I told my chairman I could not continue to do it. 'Listen, I don't have a lot of other people to see patients from nine other hospitals,' I informed him. To which he replied, 'Well, too bad.' So, I really could not take call at UMass; I was taking call at the different hospitals. I was terminated in 2007 from my assistant professor position at UMass, and I just found out this spring that this chairman arranged to get it terminated without ever telling me. It is not what you are supposed to do for an academic appointment. I gave lectures around the world and across the United States.

"I remain on friendly terms with the hand surgeons there. I see their patients and they see my patients, so that is a collegial thing. But another hand surgeon at UMass did the same fellowship I did. And when he was given the opportunity for his dream job at Dartmouth Hitchcock Medical Center in Hanover, New Hampshire, where he did his residency, the chairman blocked him from going. Yeah, there is a little psychopathology as a backdrop in the practice of medicine."

A.R., R.C.M. AND THE PSYCHOLOGY OF LEAVING A MEDICAL PRACTICE

My psychiatric colleagues refer to it as "blocking" when one represses painful or self- damaging thoughts. I cannot recall the moment I decided to move away from my group, but the complexities of healthcare do not facilitate snap decisions. Yet once I made the move, the others followed. In one partner's case, it *was* sudden, like an embattled chef who rips off his apron, tosses his hat, and proclaims, "I'm blowing this taco stand!" (or Michelin 5-star restaurant du jour, etc.) In many professions, one simply seeks another position and begins to earn a new paycheck, following the two-week cycle of pay they collect from their previous job. It does not work this way in medicine. As a clinician in private practice, you have dependent patients who are scheduled for surgery, post-op visits, therapy, or late follow-up visits. You cannot rip them off like a Band-Aid, pardon the pun. Additionally, insurance companies tend to pay months later; hence the infamous A.R. (accounts receivable) can be quite substantial when a physician has reached his last straw with his associates. You cannot just pack up and leave. However, one of my partners did just that: he blew his stack, packed his medical books in a box, and marched out of the office, never to look back...until it was time to collect on his A.R. A.R. is such a complex and widely misunderstood process it even has its own fancy name and acronym about how to manage it: R.C.M. (revenue cycle management). Sounds like you need a PhD to understand it, and you probably do.

Leaving a medical practice on a whim is like leaving a live-in partner or spouse, where you soon realize you need to go back and get some of the clothes that were in the laundry bin; your toothbrush from the shower; and your favorite record collection strewn around the entertainment wall unit. Although I was tired of all the issues and the mounting general discontent within the group, I preferred to make my escape in a gradual, thoughtful manner. One by one, the initial partner had alienated all of us, and the monthly meetings often ended up being a discussion of what he wanted or decreed. I soon understood what the term "Banana Republic" really meant.

Another source of dissatisfaction for me with the group's overall lack of customer service. Lest you think I'm exaggerating, we had a "Wild West" reputation in the community, and although almost everybody respected us as surgeons and clinicians, including our direct competitors, we had a reputation for running a chaotic practice. It was not uncommon for our patients to wait four to five hours to see a doctor, and our staff soon bought into that culture. Among the clinicians, I tended to have much shorter waits, but when the practice adopts bad habits, they are difficult to overcome. Furthermore, over time I had developed a significant international practice, and these were not people accustomed to waiting long in their respective countries. After investing in the time and expense of flying in to see me, they would not tolerate long wait times.

I tried to influence our practice's culture and develop some protocols, but most often I met resistance – or worse, apathy.

My commitment to excellent customer service hinges on one simple fact: most patients do not understand my expertise, or lack thereof, for any specific pathology. Most of them do not ask where I trained or studied, or what papers I have written on the subject. What they do notice is how I care for them as a person and the way I focus on listening and taking their needs into consideration. The same is true for my staff and the environment, which must elicit a clean and calm aesthetic. It's an unfortunate fact that the medical profession is the only one in which almost all our reimbursement comes from a third party, not the person (patient) at the receiving end of the services; furthermore, our reimbursements are not commensurate with our level of expertise or client service. Cigna, for example, pays the top knee surgeon the same as the one with poor skills who uses antiquated techniques. I was not solely interested in treating patients who picked me out of an insurance book or were referred to me by their PCP (primary care provider). While I do not claim to be perfect, I knew I could not deliver the stellar level of service I envisioned within a group of five surgeons where that shared commitment to customer service is just not present.

Chapter 5 – Forging A New Path

"In nothing do men more nearly approach the gods than in giving health to men." – Cicero (106 B.C. – 43 B.C.)

In early 2006, I began to look for options outside the Miami Hand Center. I began by contemplating key elements: what type of practice I would build and where, along with my vision for the infrastructure, having developed a solid foundation working within a practice that was well ahead of our time. At one point, I served as Chief of the Hand Surgery division within the surgery department at Baptist Hospital, a well-respected "not-for-profit" hospital within the growing Baptist Health System. Although I had taken on many of my more substantial cases there and at several other hospitals, I had already determined that hospitals, designed for "sick" people, were woefully inefficient. My patients' problems were limited to the hand, elbow, or shoulder. In rare cases, they might have multiple comorbidities (illnesses), which required access to an I.C.U. (God forbid), or the type of surgery that called for close nurse monitoring, like a microvascular free flap, or replantation. Yet I soon realized that hospitals were for patients undergoing open heart surgery, neurosurgery, or even hip fracture fixation. Over time, my perspective on healthcare delivery changed, and I have the old Miami Hand Center to thank for that. We pushed the envelope and succeeded, proving the concept in real terms.

Because I did not want to regress in my methods of delivering upper limb care, I looked for a partner in outpatient surgery center development. The simplest solution was to pursue privileges in any of the locals A.S.C.s (ambulatory surgery centers) but there was one major issue: my office had to be nearby. Furthermore, I was accustomed to having a hand therapist adjacent to me, which assured optimal results for my patients, thanks to a strong association and direction interaction between the hand therapist and myself.

I discovered the issue came down to real estate. My previous experience taught me a valuable lesson; one I hope my colleagues reading this book will note. While leasing office space is like renting an apartment, it is worse. As you shop around, you will see that most apartments have the infrastructure you seek, and it is a simple matter of moving your existing furnishings and belongings. Not so with a medical practice. For example, some offices lack X-ray capabilities, or at least the ones you seek. As a hand surgeon, I only need one room with a stretcher or bed for minor procedures because I only examine the upper limb. For that reason, my exam rooms can be quite small with a table so I can sit across from the patient at eye level and focus on their upper limb. With any commercial space, the buildout is costly. Why invest that money in a property you do not own and cannot create equity in?

None of the options I looked at sufficed. Then, one morning in early 2006, I received a call from a commercial real estate agent who focuses on medical office space. He described a five-story building with an alleged focus on medical use that was still in the shell stage in the small city of Doral, in western Miami-Dade County, adjacent to the airport. At the time, all I knew about Doral was that it was the home of the Doral Resort (later to become Trump Doral) and La Covacha, a Latino outdoor nightclub. I thought, "I do not golf, and I do not have much time for salsa dancing anymore." However, Doral possessed one interesting draw that would prove to be a fateful decision in my career: the newly incorporated city was our chosen site for the DaVinci Center, soon to become the largest cadaveric surgical training lab in the world (at the time).

The DaVinci Center was the initial brainchild of an orthopedic implant distributor who often had visiting surgeons from abroad test arthroscopy systems on a cadaver knee set up in his warehouse. Realizing the opportunity for a much-needed business model, he invited an orthopedic device executive, two other surgeons, and me to explore the possibility. By coincidence, the five of us had recently selected a warehouse located in an industrial park in Doral, which was close to this potential office space. Being passionate about education and having just inaugurated a course on upper limb arthroscopy, I was enthusiastic about the project for which we had already engaged an architect for buildout. When discovered that the clinical space was barely one mile from the DaVinci Center's chosen location, I envisioned an orthopedic center that encompassed all the elements, including laboratory capabilities. The rest, as they say, is history.

On a hot sunny August afternoon in 2006, the day of my wedding, I was relaxing in the pool and catching some rays, when I received a call from my real estate attorney. He had evidently forgotten my exhortation not to disturb me on this specific day with any transaction issues or questions. We were negotiating a deal for me to buy the entire first floor of the Doral building, and the last thing I wanted was additional stress on this milestone occasion. My old buddy Roho, the Harvard neurologist as well as my best man, was keeping me company while I enjoyed those hours while my bride was busy dressing, knowing I could throw on my tux in a 20-minute ritual. My attorney's call symbolized the upcoming ordeal in confronting several new ventures at once. We enjoyed our wedding and honeymoon in Europe before I rolled up my sleeves to make major career and life changes. It is no cakewalk to be married to a surgeon, let alone a budding entrepreneur.

When people describe the real estate work as "cutthroat," they are not kidding. The negotiation process is a contact sport, even steel cage match level. I spent the months after my wedding balancing my busy surgical practice with making my exit from Miami Hand Center a reality. I needed a home. Commercial space is expensive under the best circumstances; little did I know, I would accrue mine just before the crash of 2008.

I paid a high per-foot price for a large footprint that included my medical office as well as an outpatient surgery center. Unlike many of my peers, I was doing this solo. While other surgeons were consolidating into mega groups, being hired by healthcare systems, or even retiring, I was building an empire and amassing debt. I am not sure where my absence of risk aversion came from, but like hitting a fastball, I visualized the entire process. Eventually, one hiccup worked in my favor. As we agreed on the real estate purchase, much to my surprise, the seller countered that the entire remaining first floor space was for sale. I was already in discussions with the broker over the smaller unit that would be my office. The deal in question involved my surgery center.

I replied that I did not need that much space, and for a solo buyer-clinician, I was already in over my head. Under the impression we had an agreement, I figured it would be no problem. He could find a buyer for the other one-quarter of ground floor space. His response? "All or nothing." That is when it hit me: the altruism and compassion inherent in healthcare does not often translate into business, let alone real estate. This guy and his partner had plans to build a mega diagnostics facility and soon realized they had way too much space for some M.R.I.s and C.T. scanners. They decided to flip the real estate and make serious money. For then, the transaction most likely equaled the running of imaging tests full tilt for two to three years at unpredictable net revenue. To add insult to injury, the commercial broker had doctored a document that was counter to the agreement I had in place with the building developer, and in truth, was flipping his space to me. We are talking Game of Thrones type shit. Consequently, I had to engage a litigation attorney, the second in a long series of attorneys I would "need" to simply heal my fellow man.

I spent much of 2007 in the arduous build-out process with a surgery center company I had met with the prior year, during a hand surgery meeting in Tucson Arizona. They were a pleasure to work with and oversaw the entire process from architectural design to staffing models, and then to buildout, which was fast. In fact, they moved at a more rapid rate than the contractor who built out my office and therapy spaces, the same one who was doing the buildout for our challenging cadaver training lab.

Because the developer had cut many corners on the building construction, as is typical in Miami, our surgery center buildout contractor had to improvise and often resolve basic structural issues, even with the building's cooling system. Furthermore, thanks to a lack of cooperation from other building owners, we often had to accomplish some tasks in a clandestine fashion to avoid a delay or shutdown while they aired their grievances. None of it made sense since it was no detriment to them. Many times, I felt like shaking them and saying, "Do you realize what we will be doing in these hallowed rooms? Relieving pain, restoring function, and maybe saving lives."

Although cynicism had never been part of my makeup, I imagined they would support the project if it were their relative or child in need of an operation. The project taught me how selfish neighbors can be, even in the health-care environment. I learned quickly about the concepts of priorities and work ethic, and real-life understanding of how things were done in my adopted city of Miami. As they say, it is indeed the capital of Latin America, with lesser resemblance to the northeast, where I grew up. The difference went beyond a warmer climate.

By now, the developer was long gone, which meant we had to deal with the "property manager," whom we paid as building unit owners. We still wrestle with the issue of groundwater seepage in our therapy center, which has led us to change the flooring twice. The property manager happens to be the builder of our therapy center, yet still does not help me. Although the building has sizeable reserves for capital improvement and repairs, somehow, they have informed me I am on my own, as of course, the insurance company negated coverage. I received this incredibly dry letter from the condo association lawyer, essentially saying NO. I did not even bother reading it as who really cares about that gobbledygook when the resultant action is what matters. Denying a claim is, after all, what they do best. Ironically, I had been the office condo association president since its inception, donating my time and energy for naught. Yet when I needed help, I did not get it, despite multiple attempts to remedy the issue. Once I realized there was little value in this figurehead role, I resigned from the board, even though I represent almost one-quarter of the entire building association dues. Yes, commercial real estate is a jungle. Oh, and we happen to be in the business of caring for people. Worlds apart...

My buildout struggles continued. I engaged a talented architect named Diana Boytell for my office, and the interior design, who worked closely with me to bring my vision home. When you spend nearly one-third of your life in a work environment, why not make it inviting to staff, visitors, and especially, patients? Somehow, this principle was ingrained in me. I understood that patients could not ascertain my surgical skills, or the astuteness of my clinical decision-making, nor did they even inquire about my education and residency. As the adage goes, patients want you to care for them if they know you care. And that care includes, the overall environment, its cleanliness and sense of tranquility, with a minimization of cold depersonalization. With that in mind, we built my waiting room to be warm, surrounded by wood on the walls and suspended ceiling slates, and the conspicuous absence of that one typical, impersonal feature of countless medical offices: the dreaded sliding window. I was determined to create a one-stop shopping facility where the entire patient journey could be completed under one roof.

My digital radiography experience at Miami Hand Center gave me insight as to its importance, and I leased the most state-of-the-art system, free of any cartridges (DR system) so that images would be transferred to the patient exam room within four seconds. The dealer told me that I was only the second facility in the entire county to have this unit, the first being none other than the ICE Krome detention facility, where immigration detainees are held. Nothing too good for our illegal immigrants the government must contend with.

As the shoulder and elbow component of my upper limb practice grew, I planned to install an in-office M.R.I. magnet, an emerging technology in the orthopedic space. This was a critical diagnostic piece for the upper limb. While it came with considerable cost, the convenience to patients would be enormous. Imagine a patient presenting with shoulder pain and receiving the customary X-rays and the definitive diagnosis all in one visit: wouldn't that be optimal for the treatment and recovery? Alas, the insurance industry does not value this capability. It is quite rare that we are permitted to offer this service to most domestic patients, and it is my international patients who utilize it the most. How ironic that affluent patients from emerging economies can travel to Miami and undergo the entire evaluation without interference, yet I cannot offer the same service to my domestic patients? In case you are wondering, the same applies to my Medicare population, who often have difficulty seeing me due to the travel logistics, and yet I cannot do a thorough evaluation without having to send them to an outside imaging facility. In addition to being foolhardy and inefficient, it is cruel.

Let me use a recent, but frequent example, to illustrate my point. A patient named Mrs. Gonzalez is in Room 1 with terrible shoulder pain, which I suspect is caused by an acute rotator cuff tear. However, my radiology tech is not permitted by Medicare to perform the study, simply escorting her to my open field magnet, just 20 feet away. Mrs. Gonzalez now has to secure an appointment for an M.R.I. across town, bother her children to miss half a day of work to drive her, and then schedule another appointment with me so I can *now* see the images and discuss the treatment plan. That means, she must make *three* appointments instead of one. And oh, for the second appointment my staff will bill Medicare, of course. I am not that charitable. Our system forces patients to complicate and prolong the patient journey to achieve a solution when some clinicians, like me, are willing to invest in the equipment needed to provide that care. It is no wonder other clinicians are not inclined to invest in infrastructure.

I am sure you are wondering why, and I wish I could give you an answer. It is kind of like when you were a kid and your mother told you, "Because you can't," without any further explanation. Now, there are bureaucratic hoops you can jump through to *try* to work with "the system" but even that is often of no avail. Some years ago, my staff took on the task of getting our M.R.I. machine "accredited" for which I had to assume the cost. There is an organization called the I.A.C. (Intersocietal Accreditation Commission) that certifies my magnet to be amenable to patient care and then eligible to submit billing charges to the respective insurance carrier. This is a process I will discuss further in a chapter detailing the opportunists in healthcare. The I.A.C. tagline is "Improving healthcare through accreditation®." I am trying to understand how. Tell that to Mrs. Gonzalez who still had to go elsewhere for her M.R.I. What was the outcome of our efforts? We still cannot bill C.M.S. So, I was willing to jump through that hoop, and of course, *pay* for the privilege. Shoot, I would wear a pink tutu if I thought it made a difference. What typically happens is that when C.M.S. sets policy, most commercial carriers will follow suit. Yes, private insurers allow Medicare, the government, to dictate the rules and senseless regulations. Is this a free market capitalistic economy? One wonders…

Since shoulder injuries are ubiquitous in the work environment, we often use our magnet for workers' compensation patients…that is, if the adjustor approves it. It is a random process and yet another topic I will delve into. Get the picture? Now, poor Mrs. Gonzalez will likely suffer from agonizing shoulder pain for at least another week since she must go to another facility and *then* come back to me. Just giving you a taste of our system as we move along.

Despite the hurdles, that is what I have in my center, all in one place. Each time I do a study, other than a plain X-ray, I have no idea if I will get reimbursed for the needed service. I also have fluoroscopy: it is like a live X-ray where you put the hand under, and it moves. It is valuable for checking for instability patterns of the wrist, assess healing of fractures or surgical interventions via multiple oblique views, and doing minor in-office procedures like a pin removal. With this expensive machine, I can often avoid the greater cost of a surgery center facility fee, anesthesia services, etc. We had this before in my prior hand center in yet another example of a component that put us ahead of our time. In fact, we had the first model mini-fluoro in the country, and as I mentioned, we were the second practice in the country to have digital X-ray.

The resistance to reimburse diagnostic tests stems from the fact that many clinicians tend to over order them. I believe we could solve this problem and lower healthcare costs in this country by implementing one major principle: the clinician who orders the study must be the person acting upon the result. Seems intuitive, right? Yet, most M.R.I.s are ordered by a doctor who is not the medical professional addressing the specific clinical issue. Consequently, they are likely not even sure what is the best test to diagnose a certain problem. Most times, they do *not* even look at the study, which is truly a problem. Instead, they simply read the report from the radiologist. If the M.R.I. comes back as "normal" that does not mean the patient does not have a problem, correct? For example, that person still has elbow pain, and their history and physical exam suggests a tennis elbow, or to put it in medical terms, lateral epicondylitis. Whereas, golfers' elbow, or medial epicondylitis, a similar pathology, occurs on the inner aspect of the elbow, location of the "funny bone" (ulnar nerve). The M.R.I. "report" dictates whether the patient will get referred to someone who truly *knows* how to treat the malady.

Although the M.R.I. did not offer any additional information, it added a lot of money to the healthcare cost, and the patient still needs treatment for the condition. As I mentioned, I have an in-office M.R.I. I could order elbow M.R.I.s all day long since tennis elbow is far and away the most common cause of routine elbow pain (having nothing to do with tennis, by the way). However, like most specialists, I abide by a code of ethics; I exercise responsibility when ordering tests, even if needed. Because I am an elbow specialist, I know the limitations of elbow M.R.I. for epicondylitis, a common ailment. As a resident in New York City, I dealt with it, yet when I learned to play tennis in my 50s, I experienced zero issues with my elbow (my shoulders are another matter). I simply do not need this specific test to clinically determine if an epicondylitis is present.

The converse problem is that the M.R.I. often comes back with a suggestion that there is a "tear" or disruption to the common flexor tendon origin in the elbow. Sounds dreadful, right? It is simply an M.R.I. finding of signal change, but the upset patient comes to my office, fearful that the tendon must be reattached or repaired somehow, which is not the case. This is an example of how the M.R.I. can be negative – or worse yield, an irrelevant finding that the primary care doctor of nurse practitioner in a general urgent care setting has uncovered because they ordered an unnecessary test. Good intentions are there but it is like asking me what specific test is needed for a patient with unremitting vertigo.

The elbow scenario is just one clinical malady. Imagine how much of this is happening in our healthcare system? The equivalent for a host of other orthopedic diagnoses, several unnecessary tests, and the testing that occurs in other sectors of medicine I am not qualified enough to comment on. I can picture my colleagues reading this and nodding in silent agreement, yet it is rarely discussed in a public forum. Yes, the so-called "experts" on healthcare policy – rarely the clinicians in the trenches – will debate the causes of our exorbitant U.S. healthcare spend ad nauseam but most of the time, they fail to discuss actual solutions in favor of knee-jerk policy.

Many will disagree with what I am saying here, but at least we are generating some dialogue, even if controversial. A multitude of studies have been done to document the overutilization of testing, which often leads to subsequent overtreatment, or inappropriate treatment across the board in our healthcare system. Similar studies have even demonstrated this in more so-cialized healthcare systems, such as the U.K., or our Canadian neighbor to the north.

I realized the significant divide among physicians when an article I wrote nearly a decade ago was recently picked up by a financial newsletter of all places, and then by Doximity, a sort of Facebook for doctors. The article, which made an argument for specialty walk-in centers, was first published in my local county medical society newsletter, followed by the state medical journal. As expected, I received little feedback at a time that predated social media, with its seamless ability to post, support, or vilify. Today, it is a different world; we see the stark contrast in COVID-19 awareness, compared to other pandemics in the past.

The recent reprinting elicited harsh criticism from my primary care col-leagues, and a bit less vocal support from specialists, particularly my orthopedic colleagues, who know exactly what I am referring to. I am making an argu-ment for the simple premise that the appropriate clinician ought to order the most apropos test that they will act upon to treat. I used the example that for many patients with wrist pain on the radial side (thumb side) the cause is DeQuervain's tenosynovitis. Yes, many astute primary care colleagues can make that diagnosis, but many others will order an unnecessary M.R.I. Fur-thermore, while they are often correct, there are other entities such as Wartenburg's syndrome, STT osteoarthritis, and early SLAC wrist arthritis which can lead to similar confusing symptoms and are missed, even with the most experienced clinicians.

How can a physician trained to treat a much wider variety of maladies be expected to sift through this differential diagnosis?

It is *not* possible. When I see a patient that presents with shoulder pain and realize the problem stems from a cervical etiology (cause), I consult with the spine specialist. Not just anyone, but a physician who deals with multiple cervical issues, aside from lumbar. I am an orthopedic surgeon, a specialist. Yet I will not work up the cervical pain as I will not be the one acting upon it and do not feel I am qualified to perform the most astute work-up. Even if I did, I may not know the best facility to perform that specific test. I simply do not do it every day, day in, and day out. Isn't it time we fully leverage the explosion of medical knowledge gained just in the last three decades since I finished my training? I know there will be ample, sound arguments against this thinking, but this is my goal: to generate controversy and bring the end-user, the patient - John Q. Public – into the dialogue.

In broad terms, two-thirds of physicians believe that almost one-third of medical care is unnecessary and wasteful, often starting with the ubiquitous ordering of tests. We can broach the issue of overmedication and unneeded procedures later. I want to stick to discussion of diagnostic imaging tests because this remains a huge issue that is hardly ever discussed among the public. To start with, be aware that at one point, there were more M.R.I. machines in Miami Dade county than the entire *country* of Canada. Curiously, many are owned by businessmen, not clinicians who take a different stance on revenue and appropriateness of the study. Recall that the commercial space I built out for my outpatient surgical center and rehab area was sold to me by two businessmen who were planning to erect a massive diagnostic facility. Will they police the necessity of the studies being ordered? That is doubtful because they are running a business. I mean no ill will; however, it is a fact that business professionals have no clinical knowledge to even assess the indications coming through their doors. In this case, the entrepreneurs owned multiple other centers and simply made a business decision, a smart one it seems, not pursue this venture.

Mind you, within a few years, a South American immigrant businessman had opened a small imaging center about 200 yards from our clinical center. The quality of the studies, at least pertaining to the upper limb, was simply atrocious. Of course, how would I be expected to do quality control in an information technology business? Yet a multitude of my upper limb patients present with their M.R.I. in hand (often via workers' compensation carriers) from this facility which I presumed must be excellent at obtaining the contracts. Although these studies are often useless, unnecessary, and poorly done, I must review them on a monitor adjacent to my own magnet which often sits idle.

Which is a more cost-effective approach? Letting the clinician decide which study is needed, if at all, and then having the M.R.I. done in potentially the same visit, in the same facility with the specialist looking at the images in real time, without necessarily depending on the radiologist's report; OR a non-specialist checking a box requesting the M.R.I., sending the patient on their way? It is an *everyday* issue and nobody is talking about it except in academic studies, like one by the A.C.R (American College of Radiology) which never filters down to the public. They present laudable data and make worthy conclusions, but specific examples, like the ones I presented best illustrate the problem to most layperson readers.

M.R.I.s of the hand offer another illustration of the point. Hand specialists will tell you that for the most part, they are unnecessary. The utility was much greater when a wrist specialist ordered a wrist M.R.I. versus the generalist, supporting the point I made prior, in a study by Chung et al at the University of Michigan. Conversely, for the shoulder, M.R.I.s are often critical except for scenarios where clear X-ray evidence is present for shoulder osteoarthritis, a much less prevalent condition.

Stretching the market and community need, but sensing opportunity, an Ecuadorian immigrant also opened yet another large, beautiful imaging facility behind my clinical center, in a newer commercial building. I only became aware of the center because he came in for a hand issue. As I see many patients from Ecuador in my practice, I tried to contact him to see how we might collaborate since, as mentioned, many insurance companies do not permit the studies to be done in our own magnet. I wanted to judge the quality of the images and tour the center. If it met my criteria, at least we could offer a convenient solution for some patients at my office and our walk-in orthopedic clinic. I reached out, to no avail, and within a year, I found out that the center closed. A pity. Immigrants are coming to our country to realize the American dream, but they walk into a hornet's nest when it comes to the complexities of healthcare. His failure to return my phone calls is a common issue. He chose to ignore the phone calls of a busy surgeon who could refer him "business". Amazing. The collaboration in our healthcare delivery system is simply not there. Of course, his focus was on his own "business," but healthcare takes a village and he paid the ultimate price for his uncooperative stance. The barriers are even more insurmountable when the owner of a clinic has no medical background and does not understand the ecosystem. More on that topic later.

The specialist will naturally influence what test is best suited for the specific clinical problem. I remember lecturing at a meeting in the Catalonia region of Spain, where a colleague from Barcelona was speaking on the utility of diagnostic ultrasound for differing hand pathologies. That was when people were just starting to talk about it. His reasoning made sense, and when I came back to the States, I researched the pricing and reimbursement potential for ultrasound. I realized I could quickly and more cost-effectively diagnose a variety of issues at the time of physical exam with this emerging modality in orthopedic space. I have now had an ultrasound machine for many years and the increasing use of this technique has driven down the cost – due to the emergence of smaller more cost-effective systems onto the market, including several that even connect with your smartphone. I was an early adopter, the drawback being that I purchased a SonoSite®, a hugely expensive machine that is really overkill for my clinical needs. While the market adjusts to clinical needs, it is actually optimal when clinicians drive that need, not just business interests. I now have an augmented reality headset, developed with McGinley Orthopedics®, that attaches to my ultrasound machine, allowing me to never look away from the patient, particularly when using it for guided injections. I fully absorb the cost, but if it makes me a better physician, I alone make the decision if it is worthwhile for my patients and my practice.

Therefore, the clinician specialist knows best in terms of necessary and appropriate tests. That person should be the one reviewing and acting upon every test they order. However, clinicians are not immune to over-ordering tests for various reasons including fear of malpractice liability, demands from the patient, and in lesser instances, profiting from those tests. We can and should work on addressing all areas, if perhaps we can improve fairness of compensation. It is obvious that the businessman who owns the facility is not driving costs down. He bought the facility for one reason only: to make money.

At around the time my new medical office was being completed, we finished our outpatient surgery center, The Surgery Center at Doral (S.C.D.). It was truly a state-of-the-art center with a three-room O.R. suite, spacious holding area and recovery rooms, and a simply gorgeous greeting area where friends and family could wait comfortably for their loved one undergoing the procedure. It was – and still is – the only Medicare-certified A.S.C. (ambulatory surgical center) in the city of Doral, or within at least a six-mile radius. Despite this fact there remains scant support from the community, and even the physicians who could benefit. The latter is often due to a combination of local medical politics, but more often, from typical physician adversity to perceived risk or even altering habit. The lack of community support is simply due to having to compete with "noise", the constant barrage in media and community education initiatives that are typically replete with big hospital information. When full page newspaper ads, billboards, and even municipal announcements bombard the public with hospital services, it is no wonder a smaller, yet more cost-effective and accessible option has difficulty competing. Oh, and we pay taxes. Another issue to take up later.

Our S.C.D.'s initial task, after jumping through bureaucratic and regulatory hoops, was to engage local surgeons who need facilities in which to perform their trade. Being a shiny new, beautiful, and convenient center, I thought that would be easy. Boy did I get a rapid, ongoing education about physician mentality, attitudes, and resistance.

Some years ago, I met with a cardiologist who was also an astute businessman. He had started a concierge health network, and soon was contracting directly with some major health insurance companies. I am not aware of his cardiac aptitude, but he was an innovative thinker and thought outside the usual healthcare delivery conventions. He told me "Alejandro, we are the 10 percent." I knew what he meant right away and never forgot it. Being open minded, fearless of failure, and willing to buck tradition are simply not typical physician traits. Now, as I admitted, hand me a legal contract or complex business plan, and I am lost. One must know their strengths and weaknesses and bring those more knowledgeable into their circle to fill those gaps. I soon found that this would be a decade long struggle. I always thought the adage, "Doctors make terrible businessmen" was a cliché, but I would soon learn why it is a cliché...because it is unequivocally true.

As the surgery center ramped up, I found myself representing over 80 percent of the case volume. This is no way to make a center successful. Firstly, no one surgeon could humanly fill a three-room center with procedures five days a week. I could only work so hard and of course, I had patient days where I needed to evaluate my patients with upper limb problems, most of them treated with non-operative methods.

Right before we launched, we had approached several clinicians with a ground-floor opportunity to invest and become charter medical staff at the new A.S.C. They included a podiatrist, a pain-management physician, and another orthopedist. Understand that by law, surgeons must buy into the center if they are to become partners and benefit financially from their own work and that of others. A law in almost every other state, it makes perfect sense. Well...no takers. There was alleged risk, therefore, nobody bought in. Of course, I soon realized it was also perceived as Badia's center and this is in line with a basic principle that nearly everybody in healthcare will affirm: doctors do not like the thought of other doctors profiting from them. Mind you, *most* will not take the risk of sustaining a mortgage, engaging another bank to build out an expensive facility such as an A.S.C., or weathering the early storm of business ramp up. I am not sure why I am not similarly risk-adverse, but it is a simple fact. Many say entrepreneurs are born, not made. Whatever the reason, I was willing to let others benefit from my initiative (and perhaps foolhardy venture), but there were no takers. Even when the opportunity is presented on a silver platter. The long path of medical education and surgical training takes its toll as the preceding chapters illustrated. I strapped in for a long and challenging journey.

None of the initial physicians we approached engaged us. While I have made many mistakes along my healthcare journey, developing, and investing in the facility where I perform almost all my operative procedures is a win-win. Why would I have an outside A.S.C. or even hospitals profit from my work? The fact that the facility fee represents much more than any surgeon's professional reimbursement underscores the reason that many specialists should be doing this. In fact, they have. It is a rare ophthalmologist or gastroenterologist who performs their procedure in a hospital facility, but rather a hospital affiliated or independent A.S.C. Why should this not be the case for many surgeons – for sure, orthopedists – while our cardiac surgery or neurosurgeon colleagues lament the fact that they *must* operate in the hospital setting? Due to the inherent mortal risk to the patient in these fields, they have no choice. I get an earful every time I run into my cardiothoracic colleague in our building's parking lot. He reminds me how lucky I am. I reply, "I know. I just wish many of my other colleagues would finally realize this."

While painstakingly slow, our A.S.C. volume increased, and our national partner soon announced a sale to a larger conglomerate which owned approximately 200 centers around the country. It was the typical move in healthcare. Terrific for the small center acquired, but not so good for competition and diversity in the marketplace. In our case, the national partner was offering a modest multiple to our E.B.I.T.D.A. (earnings before interest, taxes, depreciation, and amortization), even though we were nowhere near our potential. Furthermore, the model did not suit us, and cultures were not aligned. I did my due diligence and spoke to a colleague in the northeast whose center was purchased by the same company. He sheepishly volunteered "Us docs don't make much money." I asked, "How can that be?" I was well familiar with their center's robust volume, which was much higher than ours (still largely dependent on *moi*). Yet, all things considered, we did well. Obviously, their corporate partner was engaging in some fuzzy math.

Next, I spoke to my then anesthesiologist, and we agreed to partner up and approach a bank. Our reputable A.S.C. partner, Titan Health, agreed to let us buy our own center back from them at the same multiple that the "giant" was offering. Not knowing if the buyer would accept, I made it clear when meeting with "the suits" that I would be a troublesome partner, the red-headed stepchild, a thorn in their side. It was probably true, and Titan was permitted to proceed with the sale with notable exception of our Doral A.S.C. We reached an agreement that we, the doctors, could own our own center. Imagine that - a surgical center fully owned by the people who perform the actual surgery. It seems intuitive and expected, but I assure you that is not the case. It is a dichotomy that is symbolic of our healthcare system. We partnered with two skilled general surgeons, who were not ideal partners since their practice was hospital dependent for the most part, but the bank would not approve a loan to a sole surgeon center. We also allowed the anesthesiologist to buy in, foolish since the nature of their specialty does not bring patients to the center, but rather serves them. Logical insight but I would in fact continue to shoulder (no pun) the center for several more years. Partnering with other orthopedists would make sense but then again, getting surgeons to collaborate is a truly lofty and elusive goal.

The Birth of OrthoNOW® (Disruption of Orthopedic Care Delivery)

During the first year of operation, our A.S.C. went through some tumultuous changes, guided by our excellent partnership with Titan – well before they were sold to a larger player. However, not being based in Miami, they made some questionable decisions regarding staffing. For example, one of our early O.R. administrators had some bright ideas, but his failure to execute created some major problems. One of his innovative suggestions haunts me to this day. As we walked back from the Italian restaurant adjacent to the center, which we often used as our boardroom in the early days (yes, we did put on significant weight during that inaugural year), he posed a question. He asked, as he pointed to a row of dark windows on the second floor facing the restaurant, "Who owns the space above our A.S.C.?"

"I don't know, why?"

"Well, that might be a great place to put an urgent care center." Whammo. Much like my former girlfriend who signaled her agreement to move to Pittsburgh with me, his question often reverberates in my mind to this day. How might my life had been different if I had deflected her question, or brushed aside his comment by informing him that urgent care centers are saturated in the Miami market?

Alas, I did not. Whether due to my entrepreneurial spirit or foolhardiness, I engaged his question and agreed to research the commercial space. After all, it was not like I had already purchased more space than I could handle, right? Risk adversity is a trait I should have cultivated. Within months, I had made an offer on the large unit, from a practicing dentist who had grand plans to expand. Like my M.R.I. buddies, the husband-wife team wisely abandoned that idea and found a sucker in me, since I purchased it right around the time of the market crash. Who could have known? Well, some did.

I met an urgent care company, DoctorsNOW, at a medical meeting in the exhibitors' area, akin to my evolution with Titan, and they flew in to see my commercial space and discuss my joining their chain of centers. It was a franchise, a rare phenomenon in healthcare in those days, and it would help me get the center open. I knew nothing about urgent care, other than that it was still a growing concept with a noble goal – allow patients with less acute issues to avoid the E.R., right in line with my evolving thoughts on healthcare delivery. However, what I had in mind was fully focused on providing initial orthopedic care, not assessing sore throats, and administering flu shots. Furthermore, there were certain critical oversights that led to my failure.

For one, there was immense competition in the area, including a major healthcare system's reputable urgent care center. Secondly, my urgent care center was on the second floor, in a building not clearly visible from the main thoroughfare of my city of Doral. To their credit, they tried to dissuade me from doing the buildout on the second floor, rightly stating that a walk-in clinic needed more visibility and easy accessibility. They even suggested that I move my hand practice upstairs into that unit so I could put DoctorsNOW in my ground floor unit. *Blasphemy!* I had built a gorgeous, successful practice in an ideal space off the lobby. Besides, we were still barely visible due to building location. Despite my misgivings, I charged ahead with my optimistic and invincible spirit. Idiot.

The urgent care center failed miserably. We could not compete with similar local facilities; it did not generate orthopedic injuries that I envisioned could be taken downstairs for definitive management; and the excessive overhead was not commensurate with our limited insurance contracts. But I learned a lot. Having read a plethora of business books and entrepreneurs' handbooks,

I accepted the mantra that failure is part of every entrepreneur's journey. I soon learned that if I had not failed, I was not pursuing innovation. After his prolonged and dogged attempts to develop the lightbulb, Thomas Edison famously stated, "I haven't failed. I've just found ten thousand ways that don't work." That simple message kept me going.

On New Year's Eve 2009, I decide to close DoctorsNOW. As the first and only franchisee, I had to cut my losses, although it did go against the notorious contract obligation that typifies most franchises. It was nobody's fault. Granted, the parent company might have provided better oversight, or perhaps forbid me to open a less than ideal location due to my own ignorance. Unless terribly egregious, I am morally opposed to suing anybody. It comes back to the integrity stance I discussed prior. They did make some initial threats, but it soon became apparent that they were good people and similarly realized that there was no ill will or lack of effort. Besides, our society should sometimes embrace that most famous of wise maxims…*Shit happens*.

I wish I could say the same for many others. Lawsuits have become one of the pervasive stains on our great country and perhaps a product of extreme capitalism. Coming from a communist country, I am the most ardent supporter our system, but frivolous lawsuits are out of control. I would soon encounter many less ethical as they could not accept their own frailties or bad luck, as if somehow bringing a lawsuit would remedy that. The same happens in my profession, where both patient and clinician (notice I have avoided word "provider") seek the same positive outcome. Yet somewhere along the way, some patients, along with their avaricious attorneys, have equated a poor outcome with malice and ineptitude. We have plenty to discuss in this arena in terms of malpractice and tort reform but suffice it to say the same disgusting thing happens in business. Should I tell you how I really feel?

I began 2010 with an empty commercial space, complete with eight well equipped exam rooms, two waiting rooms, and a common administrative area. I now had one failure, colossal as it was, so only 9,999 to go according to a man much smarter than I, the prolific inventor, Edison. I chose a different approach and fine-tuned what I sought, the creation of a M.S.K. (musculoskeletal) focused walk-in center. I would now also engage more local help, with a fresh perspective on healthcare delivery. That help would come in the form of an intelligent young fellow Cornell alumnus via a chance meeting. During this time, my beloved sister and trusted confidante, Susana, would tell me that I should quit while I was ahead and focus on my best and most passionate vocation: surgery of the hand. She obviously had not met Thomas Edison....

Justin Irizarry and I literally met on a boat – mine. I had gone to a Cornell Zinck's club reunion (do not even go there) which occurs every year, nationally and internationally, one Thursday in October for the purpose of allowing Cornellians to socialize. If you must know, Theodore Zinck was a pub owner in Ithaca during the 1890s. You would have to know Cornell alums to understand.

Well, that day I happened to take my boat to this reunion which was held on a Miami River waterfront restaurant sports bar. The current Miami Cornell Club president, who was much younger than I, introduced me to a friend of his who had recently moved back to Miami after doing M&A (mergers and acquisition) work in Manhattan. Justin and I started speaking and I invited him on board for a cocktail that was certainly cheaper than the lounge's menu. I clearly remember the moment where I thought aloud how it might be interesting to join forces and truly disrupt orthopedic care as I showed him the layout of the boat's inside cabin. Justin had started his own consulting company, J. David Group, while I was deficient in many business principles and practices. But I had vision and quickly recognized that Justin was aghast at how poorly medicine was practiced from a business and systems point of view. It was a pivotal moment.

Justin and I spoke at intermittent intervals for months. He agreed with my decision to close DoctorsNOW, which I then decided to reopen as OrthoNOW®. That was the genesis. We soon married the clinical protocols needed, along with my experience as an independent clinic owner, with sound business principles. While I lacked the latter, Justin would literally learn the entire gamut of healthcare industry, inefficient as it was. I saw that as an advantage, although it presented certain challenges since logic and efficiency are sorely lacking in our healthcare gamut.

We would soon run through a gauntlet of so-called clinic administrators who made a series of blunders and miscalculations. Justin certainly didn't understand the nuts and bolts of running a medical practice, nor did I. Granted, it was ultimately our folly, but I remained myopic due to my busy surgical practice and the simple fact that nobody on our small team had run a boots-on-the-ground medical practice.

The inherent challenges of creating a new type of medical practice for orthopedic urgent care was further complicated by an array of conflicting recommendations by well-meaning individuals. DoctorsNOW had been staffed by a primary care physician and medical assistants who also had X-ray tech credentials. The little orthopedics they saw was often poorly managed. They simply did not have the training and background. It would be like asking me to see a patient with an eye disorder. Therefore, we turned to the growing specialty of orthopedic physician assistants, mid-level providers that did obtain expertise in post-grad training, along with real job experience. I should know their capability and availability since I was fortunate to have worked with only two talented ladies in this role during the span of my career. Between the periods of Debby and Kate's employment, I worked with two foreign-trained orthopedists who turned out to be problematic. Not every physician can take on the different yet vital role of physician assistant.

Our initial OrthoNOW® PAs were working out well until I received some truly some bad advice. We were having a hard time procuring many insurance contracts, as well as engaging referral sources, later to be told it was simply because we did not have a front-line physician. I argued that simply because a clinician has an M.D. or D.O. degree does not guarantee that they have the orthopedic knowledge base. After all, I could not ask a fully trained orthopedic surgeon to sit in a walk-in clinic and wait for patients with back pain or an ankle sprain to limp in. It was not a suitable role for their expertise, and surgical qualifications, particularly due to the well-suited skills of a trained ortho PA-C. It was also not an economically viable model. Orthopedic surgeons are paid at a certain level, and PAs quite another, but both are well-trained clinicians. No matter. If healthcare decisions were made smartly, and by the right people, we would not be at 20% of our national GDP.

In the earlier portion of this book, I guided the reader through my childhood, educational, and residency experiences. It is a long, arduous road, and that delayed compensation is commensurate with those years of high-level education and extensive post-graduate education/training. Physician assistants obtain their bachelor's degree, followed by two years of a master's degree and perhaps an additional year working closely with the specialty of their choice if they decide to pursue that track. It is a different course of study and sacrifice, albeit increasingly vital to our healthcare system, given the emerging physician shortages that are predicted, as well as a judicious alternative given the unsustainable increases in healthcare costs. Simply put, for many initial patient clinical presentations, the P.A. is trained to perfectly serve this role. But once again, the controlling elements of healthcare often make decisions that should be left up to the clinicians in the trenches.

My team was told that I should hire an M.D. or equivalent to obtain many contracts and even referrals from large employers or T.P.A.s (third party administrators). The latter is an oddly complex entity which acts as an inter-mediary between the people providing care and those paying for it, namely the insurance company. I will hazard to state that this is perhaps in the top five of utterly absurd concepts that the business forces in medicine created. I will be discussing the others in time but for now, understand that a T.P.A. is an organization that processes insurance claims and often certain aspects of employee benefit plans for a separate entity. The insurance company has out-sourced the administration of the claims processing which now adds another layer of cost and complexity to the system. We all know the insurance com-panies generate an obscene amount of money and over time, they transferred this essential task to someone else. It is as if I saw a patient, diagnosed them, and took them to surgery but then somebody else performed the procedure and I scrubbed back in to close the wound and put the dressing on. That somebody else plays a big role and ought to be compensated. But is it *needed*?

The intrusive T.P.A.s have indiscriminately decided that OrthoNOW® needed a "doctor" not a P.A., as much as we explained that the front-line clinician, regardless who it is, has the direct backing of a team of orthopedic surgeon subspecialists, something the existing myriad of general urgent care centers and occupational centers simply did not have. But, oh, they had a doc-tor ya know. How do I know? Well, I have been a hand surgeon for a quarter century in Miami and could barely recall an episode where those clinics di-rectly contacted me to discuss patient care, or even transfer for surgery. They simply write the Rx (prescription) and say, "Refer to hand surgeon" and now the hapless patient needs to wait for a desk worker to make that referral – an uneducated middleman, so to speak. For what purpose? To control costs? If the patient's finger is hanging by a thread, they just send it to the ER or call 911. Yes, they really call 911.

We jumped through that hoop, so to speak, and hired a "sports medicine" doctor I will call "Charlie." Ooh, sports medicine! Sounds great right? If he takes care of athletes, he must know what he is talking about. Well…Charlie was a family practice doctor who decided to do a one-year sports medicine fellowship. Please understand that the sports medicine term is widely used and unregulated. Chiropractors often call themselves sports medicine specialists, as do podiatrists and even primary care doctors who serve a younger, athletic population. Wonderful. They have that right and many are knowledgeable in their niche, whether spine, foot, etc. The problem is that an orthopedic urgent care clinic sees a wide range of acute and chronic M.S.K. conditions where the training and focus is the issue, not the title or label. Consequently, Charlie was adept at handling medical issues related to sports, such as dehydration or muscle cramping, but knew next to nothing about fracture care. I would say that it is not his fault; however, he had little interest in learning. The latter issue reflects a problem that you cannot simply teach or manage. Regardless, it should be me, the orthopedist and clinic owner, who makes the personnel decisions for the front lines – not the insurance company, not the T.P.A., and not the employer. This was yet another issue.

Charlie lasted a few years till I realized his limited knowledge was a true liability because it was harming patient care and, due to his title, costing me much more money than I could justify. When he came onboard, he did *nothing* to benefit our business model, despite the strong recommendations and some false promises. His employment did not positively affect our contracts, despite what our "consultants" stated, nor did referral sources even alter their patterns. The overly complex healthcare market simply could not adjust to such a positive disruptive innovation. We went back to employing knowledgeable and skilled orthopedic P.A.s and never looked back. So much for adjusting to "the system" when the system itself does not know what is best. Hence, the $4 trillion mess we are in.

But it is obvious the system does not reward, or even recognize, value. We discussed the issue that a clinician's level of training, expertise, and even clinical outcomes has no bearing on their compensation. Okay, you might make the argument that "the system" cannot easily discern these facts since they may be difficult to track. However, when an entire clinical facility is providing improved specialty care with convenience and for less cost, where is the paradox?

I don't claim to know the definitive answers but I will say this: if we could save money on what's being done now just by streamlining what we do and cutting out the fat, our healthcare costs would dramatically decrease. Statistics show there are only seven percent more physicians than there were in the 1980s despite the population increase. Yet there are *1,800* percent more administrators, representing all the barriers. All these people get salary and

154 · ALEJANDRO BADIA, M.D., F.A.C.S.

benefits. Think about where the money is going. We could achieve real reform through simplification. Yes, we need administrators and staff to run the show, but we do not need more chiefs than Indians…and the problem is getting worse.

When I started OrthoNOW® it was born out of sheer frustration of learning *how* my patients go to me, their subspecialty surgeon, at the end of the food chain. The concept made sense to nearly everybody we spoke to – friends, employers, fitness instructors, nursing home directors, teachers, and even insurance brokers. Yet we could not have a dialogue with the entire sector of the healthcare industry that pays for the care: the health insurance company.

Patients would ask us constantly, "Do you take my insurance?" The reality is, we would love to take their insurance, if only they would give us the opportunity to show them how we can better serve their clients (patients) while saving the insurance company money. It may seem intuitive, but government overregulation has erected formidable barriers to the achievement of that goal, something I will explore in Chapter 7. For now, our response to the insurance question is, "Yes, we take it. They just don't give it."

Some years ago, I read an interesting story about a Humana senior administrator who was featured in Hispanic Executive Magazine, the same magazine that had featured me twice. The well-written article detailed her corporate climb and business philosophy. Reading about her success despite some struggles and sharing the same Hispanic heritage, I felt a certain kinship with her. I took the initiative to send her a cordial email to congratulate her on her career and to send her one of the magazine articles entitled, *How OrthoNOW® eliminates the E.R. Middleman*. This straightforward piece explained my concept that patients who have orthopedic problems are better served by going to directly to an orthopedic doctor, much in the same way a woman who has a gynecological issue schedules an appointment with her OB/GYN – not her primary care doctor. So why are we not following the same principle when it comes to the musculoskeletal realm?

Well, by this point I would not be so naïve as to think anyone from the insurance industry would reach out to me and say, *Hey Alejandro, let's discuss how we can collaborate and save money for our patients and my company.* You would think that title of my article would catch her attention – especially when I took the time to write a pleasant email with a tone of collaboration. Yes, she did grant me the courtesy of a polite – if noncommittal – response. We shared some pleasantries but no substance before I decided to take a direct approach.

"Can we have a few minutes on the phone this week to discuss some ideas that may be of mutual interest?"

That is a clear request with a reasonable timeline, right? Wrong. Her answer read like something a Stepford Wives character might say. If I recall, her last email was a "Have a nice Thanksgiving," or something like that. We *never* spoke. Is it intentional? I believe it is.

Doesn't everybody in the 21st century – including health insurance executives – realize that hospital emergency rooms are exorbitantly expensive?

The magazine article was filled with accolades about the wonderful things this woman has done at Humana, yet she cannot be bothered to speak with one of the clinicians who wants to help her in her mission. I remind you my proposal would *save* her company money and better serve their clients. That is why I am convinced that their indifference is purposeful. Why rock the boat? There is an intentional veil between the health insurance industry and the people who provide the care. It is absurd.

Why do I suggest there is an intentional barrier? Because I know almost nobody in the health insurance industry, except for the same tired few who constantly receive awards at daytime business lunches and Chamber of Commerce meetings. I have attended many of these events with the "If I can't lick em, join em," approach. While there, I introduce myself, generate some banter, and launch into the value proposition I have for their company. Every time, I get the same glassy-eyed look before they move on to their next appetizer or glass of wine. I thought, "Is it my deodorant, or perhaps they don't want to speak about healthcare business at this business networking event?" Silly me.

These are my one-on-one experiences. However, the separation between "provider" and payor is institutionalized industry wide. Medical conferences are another example. I have rarely seen an insurance executive participating in a medical meeting, whether as an exhibitor or for the simple purpose of networking with the folks who provide the care they fund. Conversely, I have never attended or been invited to a health insurance convention where you would think the actual "providers" would participate. Yes, of course there are physicians present who either serve as medical officers or utilization review; however, I am not aware of any colleague in the trenches, who has been asked to attend, participate, or present. That should tell us something.

I want to be crystal clear and emphatic in stating that most of us in the medical community are not opposed to greater collaboration with our insurance colleagues. This book is not about statistics or figures but rather real life, daily anecdotes that illustrate the points I am making. I hope that there is disagreement, and this generates controversy, since any discussion is better than none. Many of us were shocked, baffled, and intrigued when former basketball star Dennis Rodman got married….in a dress. His publicist and PR team knew exactly what they were doing. We need to shock folks into a discussion "across the aisle" and finally work towards positive change. Our politician counterparts have become more polarized as of late, and recent challenges this country is facing, including COVID-19, demonstrate how this impacts all of us. It is no different in healthcare. How ironic that a medical crisis may now shock both sectors of society – government and healthcare – to compromise and pursue real progress. Hmm. Maybe I should put on that pink tutu after all.

Despite all the initial challenges (and there were many in creating a novel orthopedic care delivery model), we continued to move forward. This was not, as discussed, due to insurance acceptance, local colleague collaboration, or referral source engagement, such as local municipalities or large employers. It was patient driven. Plain and simple.

Some years after OrthoNOW® opened, we carefully looked at our data analytics and patient volume metrics and noticed a curious thing: over one-quarter of our patients were referred by "friends and family." This is almost unheard of in healthcare, particularly for acute and emergency issues. As our cofounder, Justin Irizarry, often declares. "Nobody in the history of the world has heard this comment from a patient, "Last night, I had a wonderful experience in the hospital emergency room." Of course, he is being facetious. In fact, I can relate a positive story that affected both my dad and later me, for a local emergency room.

In 2018, my dad experienced symptoms of shortness of breath that I soon realized went beyond his C.O.P.D. On one acute episode, I took him to the Mercy Hospital emergency room since his internist is on staff there. The excellent E.R. physicians worked him up expeditiously and soon alerted the interventional cardiologist that he needed a cardiac catheterization due to E.K.G. changes and other clinical signs. They placed a coronary stent the same day, and he experienced marked improvement. I thought to myself, "*This* is what an emergency room is for.*"

As we waited – and you DO wait in a hospital unless you are in the trauma slot, heaven forbid – I made many observations. I noticed an older Hispanic female awaiting consultation for hip fracture, which was diagnosed some hours earlier. She would need the orthopedic surgeon to either stabilize the proximal femur (hip) or perhaps replace the joint in what would be a hospital process since she probably had significant comorbidities as well. Near her, I noticed an adolescent with a swollen ankle or maybe knee – I do not recall exactly. The family was there, waiting for several hours, and I could see the stark difference: the elderly lady needed to be in that hospital emergency room, but not that young man. His diagnosis might not even be that obvious, as say a hip fracture on X-ray, and he should be splinted, iced, and sent on his way home, with the orthopedist clearly informed of the situation so that HE could do the appropriate work-up and initial treatment.

Now, if there was a walk-in clinic with orthopedic expertise available, and there was one – about 1.5 miles away – the patient would already be home, possibly with definitive treatment already completed. If the A.C.L. was torn, blood might have been drained from the knee under ultrasound guidance, and he would be getting on the O.R. schedule for definitive reconstruction if he and his family chose that route. *That* is the difference. As for the economics, I do not think I even need to point it out. But if you must ask…

There have been multiple studies and ample data comparing the cost of an emergency room to an urgent care visit. Cigna insurance published a 2016 study showing that the average E.R. visit costs $2,259 dollars while the average urgent care visit is just $176. Now, we are not exactly comparing apples to apples but that is just the point. We should have more complex care, cardiac or major long bone fracture, evaluated and likely admitted through an emergency room, whereas ankle sprains, low back pain, and hand fractures can be suitable for an urgent care center. Due to the severity of cases, the E.R. should cost much more but unfortunately, even minor pathology is billed at a much higher rate. This adversely affects not only the insurance company but also the patient in an era of high deductibles and copays. Often the patient is saddled with a shared payment percentage as well.

The issue does not end there. If cost alone would be the sole factor, perhaps we could focus on trying to have acute hospital care bill according to severity, nightmare recommendation given healthcare's complexity. Hence, an E.R. visit is usually…an E.R. visit. In addition, hospital diagnostics are much more expensive and the application of splints, etc. add more cost. Understand that hospital E.R.s do not apply casts as a rule, which means for many injuries, the patient incurs a second bill when presenting for definitive care at an orthopedist's office. That leads to the next major difference: quality of care and expertise. While E.R. physicians tend to be more adept at orthopedic assessment and care than most office-based primary care doctors, there are still many missed diagnoses and inappropriate care, due to the limited training in the musculoskeletal sector. In fact, a SOMOS study (Society of Military Orthopedic Surgeons) found that nearly 40 percent of hospital E.R. orthopedic conditions were discharged with inaccurate diagnoses and nearly three-quarters of those had significant impact on management. The problem is more dramatic in the general urgent care centers where many of the physicians or mid-level providers, do not have any orthopedic training. Recall my prowess for evaluating eye problems being a hand surgeon…Nada. Zilch. Zero.

A 2019 University of Maryland prospective study by Abzug et al, showed that 93 percent of splints applied to 275 pediatric fractures were improperly placed in either E.R. or general urgent care settings! I think soccer moms would be hysterical if they knew that over 90 percent of the time, their kids were not receiving optimal care. But we accept it. Fortunately, the most common complication was excessive edema (swelling) and in only 6 percent was there direct injury to skin and soft tissues. Regardless, we can all agree this is not acceptable. It stems from not seeing the right clinician at the right time. A basic concept. Until recently, there have been few alternatives and even less public education. I will discuss the issue of patient engagement and changing behavior in the last section.

For now, I will tell you that I experienced this firsthand since both my kids play soccer. In fact, my daughter plays for the Juventus Academy, an excellent program for kids who want to play above and beyond their school's team. I was amazed at how much resistance I met when simply informing the team administrators about the presence of an orthopedic walk-in center. I personally witnessed several minor injuries when accompanying my daughter to practice. The manager at the location near my home treated me like I was peddling soccer cleats, basically accepting the status quo- if a kid gets hurt, run to the hospital or the urgent care center. She was downright rude. Here I am, a caring physician, the right specialist for their paying client athletes, simply offering a better alternative. I guess I could have quoted the Abzug study- if she cared or would even listen. Their training field was close to our Biscayne location, even much closer than the hospital, to boot.

The Juvenutus Doral location was an even bigger program with nearly 1,800 kids practicing there every week. The organizer politely brushed me off each time I mentioned our easier option. As expected, the day there was an injury she called me, personally - as if I am a receptionist, triage nurse, or 911. When I answered, she went on and on about a kid's severe ankle sprain. I asked her why she had not taken eight seconds and downloaded the simple OrthoNOW® On my Way NOW™ app as I had kindly asked. Silence. I said, "Okay, hurry and you can send the kid and her mom to the flagship location which should still be open". Furthermore, she obviously did not understand that I do not treat ankles. I reminded her I am a hand surgeon and OrthoNOW® is what she needed. Understand this was my personal Friday night and I was out at dinner. She took my advice, and the following week she thanked me profusely. The kid was in and out in 45 minutes, including the application of a cam walking boot. Two weeks later, her own daughter had a similar injury and then yet another. So, three ankle sprains in two weeks on *one* girls' soccer team. What does it take to change behavior a little bit? The public is not completely without fault.

I experienced the same challenge and lack of engagement at my kids' own private school. I don't have to tell you what I pay for tuition but yet the school nurse had the audacity to tell me her phone "didn't have space" to download the simple app that would make her life easier, not to mention the parents and of course, the child in question. In fact, the only time the school administration even engaged me was to "scold me" for my mentioning to my own children that I had concerns about how one of their classmates was casted. Remember the Abzug study on pediatric splinting? I confided my concern to my son, all of 11, and he ran to tell the kid unbeknownst to me. Somehow it got to the parents who must have expressed outrage to the school headmaster. Shame on me, the only orthopedic surgeon parent at the school, who showed concern about a child. We even held an athletic physicals event since the students need this for kids, including mine, to participate in sports. We did this on site at the school, allowing parents to avoid this yearly headache, no pun. Well, two people showed up although we paid for the expert clinicians to be there for a block of time. Furthermore, my son's best friend's mother is the current president of the parent's association, seemingly designed to help make the school experience easier and more pleasant for all. I guess we needed to bring donuts to their meetings like one of the dentist's does apparently. The value our walk-in center brings was just not understood or appreciated. It is symbolic of our overall healthcare system ignorance. Until of course, it is needed, and then my cell phone starts ringing, or they run to the hospital. Again.

Despite many challenges, the OrthoNOW® model managed to succeed because it represents a commonsense solution, something often lacking in today's healthcare maze. It embodies the concept of "consumerization in healthcare". That term can mean many things but certainly implies that the "experiential factor" is important to many younger patients. A responsive digital experience is a key component, along with price transparency, and on-demand services. When COVID-19 hit, we were already prepared to provide telehealth consultations since we had already developed this option two years prior. This was a time when most clinics had only heard of telehealth yet had never engaged it. This focus on customer service, coupled with specialty expertise, explains why many of our referrals come from other patients, word-of-mouth, and reputation.

Given persistent obstacles to care, including the authorization process, over-regulation, and seemingly endless bureaucracy, many innovations in healthcare delivery have been thwarted. OrthoNOW® and similar models are not alone. Despite somewhat necessary hurdles in product or drug development such as the FDA, the actual delivery of care remains much more challenging. We get excited about a new drug, perhaps a COVID-19 vaccine or anti-hypertensive, but the value proposition is clear, and gaining market share simply relies upon educating the clinicians, followed by the patients who benefit. In healthcare delivery, it is much different. For starters, there is a "status-quo" factor and, as we have discussed, changing the behavior of the payor is a nearly insurmountable task.

This struggle is real…but it is not new. It was recognized several decades ago when it became apparent that we *must* radically change U.S. healthcare, or it could bankrupt the country. In a 2006 article in the Harvard Business Review entitled, "Why innovation in Health Care is So Hard" R. Herzingler succinctly identified the challenges. The stories, incidents, and anecdotes my colleagues and I share throughout these pages simply illustrate the challenge.

The author recognized that medical treatment has made dramatic advances in recent years, but the actual delivery of that care remains inefficient, often ineffective (such as the E.R. studies aforementioned) and consumer unfriendly. The last point is what today's consumers are most frustrated with and represents a major opportunity for disruption.

That disruption can be driven by, or thwarted, by six clear forces as outlined in the HBR analysis.

1. **Players** – Proponents and detractors within the system will help or hinder success of a true innovation. I will go into some detail here in Section II of the book

2. **Funding** – Healthcare remains virtually the only business where the person receiving the service is likely not paying for it. Seeking capital for innovation in actual care delivery is tied to this omnipresent obstacle.

3. **Policy** – Most of the rules and regulations are not made by the people who deliver care. Patient safety and HIPAA are good examples and the latter is now being finally ratcheted down due to COVID-19 and common sense.

4. **Technology** – Innovations in this area can improve direct care as well as facilitate delivery. The OrthoNOW® On my Way NOW™ app is prime example as are remote monitors for everything from cardiac rhythms to blood sugar levels.

5. **Customers** – Increased engagement, awareness and demands for "experiential" care goes above and beyond what the term "patient" signified.

6. **Accountability** – Consumer (patient) demands that a product or service be of high quality, while cost-effective and safe." Patient safety" is a somewhat redundant term, but the market is now highly vigilant.

While navigating these forces, my specific, yet broad innovation for orthopedic healthcare delivery somehow persisted. When discussing patient care, I believe one really needs to start with the clinicians as we have harped upon. Their expertise is paramount, followed by accessibility. The barriers on our local level have been considerable. We have discussed the insurance obstacles, which we will expand upon later, since the one paying for the service must embrace innovation and understand how it benefits them, above and beyond the entire ecosystem.

The referral sources are also vital. If large entities, such as a municipality or major employer insist upon that mode of care, the payors may fall in line. This has been a surprising challenge for us given that most large organizations gripe about their healthcare costs. Soccer teams, as mentioned, and large employers with industrial injuries should have the sense to embrace a more logical, and direct, solution. The fact that they do not demonstrates how utterly screwed up and convoluted the system actually is.

The OrthoNOW® headquarters is in Doral, Florida, and the flagship center remains in that small, dynamic city. The city was founded in 2003, only 3 years before I purchased the entire first floor of what was to be the first independent medical arts building in the area. I was fortunate in getting to know the entire city council, very devoted public servants who had a passion for transparency in government, no small feat for Miami-Dade county, a county with a storied history for corruption and back room dealings that are better tolerated within our South American neighbors, but not the good ole U.S. of A. The reader might enjoy exploring this history via books such as *Cuba Confidential* (Ann Louise Barach), *Sins of South Beach* (former mayor Alex Daoud) and *Miami* (Joan Didion).

I remember my real first encounter with Doral City Hall. It was before I embarked on my clinical orthopedic center, but rather leading up to the establishment of the renowned MARC Center, then named the DaVinci Center. As previously discussed, this was the brainchild of Charles Bourland, an orthopedic medical device distributor, who asked several surgeons to get involved in the project. When I heard "cadaver lab," I suggested we present this to the city leadership to get their blessing. We easily obtained a direct meeting with Mayor Bermudez, who was a major force behind the city's incorporation and is currently Mayor once again – stepping up to oust the previous mayor who had tarnished the city's progress and reputation.

Mayor Bermudez entered the city conference room with clear charisma, positive energy, and a Guayabera shirt, often the official garb of Latino politicians. He carefully listened to our proposal to build what would then be the largest, and most technologically advanced surgical teaching lab in the world. He understood the benefits to the city, including the frequent influx of surgeons, industry colleagues and their families who would then stay in our hotels, dine in local restaurants, and shop in nearby shopping malls, popular with international visitors looking for great deals. The advantages were obvious, but this was quite a different business. I looked the mayor in the eye and solemnly remarked, "Mr. Mayor, we simply thought that you should understand that we are bringing lots of dead bodies to your city". He paused, reflected, and understood the value proposition as well as the importance to the wider surgical and scientific community.

I do wish the sentiment extended to our innovative walk-in center, likely hindered by all the above barriers to healthcare innovation. While I could discuss facts and patient statistics, the story is best told via some anecdotes that reflect the challenge we have had in furthering our goal in providing optimal orthopedic care.

At the time of my new hand surgery office opening, the Doral Business Council (D.B.C.) was the dominant business chamber and networking force in the area. The Badia Hand to Shoulder Center (B.H.S.) was barely open when the current president of that organization kindly called upon me. Granted, these organizations sustain themselves with dues-paying company members, but I also felt they had genuine interest to welcome one of the first medical players in this growing city. Keep in mind that Doral has about 50,000 residents, but nearly 150,000 people come to work in the city every day, as it is home to some of the Fortune 500 companies that established headquarters here. Doral also boasts that it is one of the top 50 American cities to live in, third best place to retire in, and the fastest growing city in Florida. It was also named best city in Florida for business start-ups and 51st out of 100 top US cities to launch a business. While I recognize the accolades, this has not necessarily been our experience and we continue to face many challenges.

Many community leaders, along with active members of the D.B.C., kindly attended our ribbon cutting ceremony with Mayor Bermudez in mid-2008. It was an exciting time and my focus on a welcoming, but high-tech environment, for hand & upper limb patient care was evident. The guests marveled at the digital X-ray machine, M.R.I. suite, and Surgery Center at Doral O.R. suites directly across the expansive building lobby, as well as the therapy center, then called Integra, down the opposite hall.

I attended nearly every monthly meeting of the D.B.C., almost always in scrubs since it was always on a Tuesday. This was my set O.R. day where I ran three rooms of non-stop procedures, maximizing efficiency and delivering patient care in a very different manner than when I waited endlessly in hospital O.R. lounges, begging staff to bring my next patient into the room. A familiar and painful scenario to my surgeon readers.

I would substantially delay my O.R. start time by attending the morning breakfast meetings of the Doral Business Council at the nearby Intercontinental Hotel. Although I was deferring my "cut skin" time, I thought it was important to network with the business leaders and community, networking in my scrubs and white lab coat to maximize time. Most of the time, I was the only physician in the room. An hour later, after a poignant Pledge of Allegiance, reminiscent of my school days, the keynote speaker took to the podium. I would listen for a little bit and then leave. Regrettably, I could never stay till the end.

I thought I was laying a solid foundation in the community, and frankly, I did. No regrets, but I will confess I did not get the type of real engagement and actual results our team was hoping for. We were completely disrupting the patient journey for any orthopedic issue, with dramatic impact on patient care, particularly acute traumatic injury. If you are an employer, this has a major impact on your bottom line. My naivety clearly demonstrated that I was then unaware of the barriers to entry I would later experience from the business community and most civic bodies. Several anecdotes, from literally hundreds, tell the story in the small city of Doral. You can extrapolate what this might mean for the other 2.55 million citizens of our county, let alone adjacent ones.

Like many business leaders, I usually received relative receptiveness and modest engagement when discussing how an OrthoNOW® concept could help their employees, families, and the wider community. Granted, healthcare is complex enough, so I often had to explain the difference in care when an injured person walks into a hospital or a general urgent care, versus a focused orthopedic immediate care facility. After all, *that* was my purpose in attending these breakfast meetings, besides the yummy fruit platter and hot coffee. We were all there to network and explain how we might benefit from engaging each other's businesses. Keep in mind I was not selling insurance, real estate, or men's suits. You now understand the difference in our value proposition via the literature I presented and elaboration regarding this relatively novel method of providing care. However, the average layperson is not so clear on this, unless of course they suddenly remember the protracted, arduous experience of bringing **their** injured kid, or a parent, to the local hospital E.R.

While statistics matter, my charge in this book is to present real-life examples from the trenches, to illustrate these points. I do not have an M.B.A., nor written an analysis documenting the inefficiencies and cost, but I do have the real-world experience that only a "provider" can put forth. The D.B.C., then the cornerstone of the business community in Doral, was led by a slate of officers, leaders in local business community and a governing board. The initial chairman brought me into the organization, for which I am grateful. A later chairman, a managing director of a local major hotel, would recommend my current international patient coordinator, a vital role in my hand surgery practice, apart from our orthopedic care center. These were not only valuable business relationships, but many of them became trusted friends.

The challenge remained, however, to truly engage local businesses in understanding the value OrthoNOW® could bring to them, not so much my specific hand surgery practice, which is certainly not a "walk-in center." The next step would be formal contracts for care or at least companywide awareness of the local, convenient option that was available to their employees. That never happened and it was not for lack of trying by our business development team, marketing staff, and even me, a busy surgeon.

One Monday morning, I saw a young lady who worked for one of those membership retail clubs, who presented with a significant fingertip amputation. She caught her finger in a steel freezer door when checking inventory. I can imagine your visceral response to that imagery; I am glad I got your attention. Imagine the fear, panic, and pain during those moments as blood gushed from the raw tip and exposed the bone. I imagine a paper towel or nearby rag was quickly wrapped around the tip and now what? If I recall, someone called 911, and the patient was ushered to the nearest emergency room, even though she could ambulate and did not have chest pain. You get the point. Now, I am not so naïve to think that an acute and traumatic injury like this will not first think about "running to the emergency room" and I understand that everyone around her is also panicked.

She started the usual "doctor shuffle," which can be particularly grueling for the patient, and the employer who (hopefully) values her. She was seen in the E.R. where yes, diagnosis of fingertip amputation was made. Bravo. Then it was noted that she is a "workers' comp" patient, meaning it was a work-related injury which completely upends the patient journey. Granted, if this was a hand amputation, there would be near zero discussion on this fact and I, or a colleague on hand surgery call, would come in and hopefully succeed in performing microvascular hand replantation, ala my earlier friend Agustin. But that does not happen.

A fingertip injury is a routine injury (of course, not to the patient), but the system cannot accommodate everyone as they may like. In a large teaching center, like my beloved Bellevue, we have an army of surgical residents who would be happy to tackle that issue, immediately, so long as they can get O.R. time or sometimes knock off the procedure on an E.R. gurney with digital block anesthesia. In community practice, the hand surgeon on call and others may be in surgery elsewhere in the hospital or at another institution. Obviously, they cannot just "break scrub" and go running. That means, the discussion with the astute E.R. physician is simply to confirm that IV antibiotics were administered, X-ray discussed, and appropriate dressing applied. That likely occurred that day, but since the injury happened at work, the work comp insurance adjustor contracted with that wholesale warehouse center, now directs the care. The problem is that it does not go straight to a hand surgeon like me or even to an OrthoNOW® type facility where the logistics would *immediately*, in real time, plug the Orthopedic clinician to the hand surgeon via something novel called, uh, a smartphone. Yes, healthcare ranks 5ᵗʰ of 7 major economic sectors in terms of consumer ranking for ease of communication and digitalization. Government was last. *Surprise.*

What happens? The patient is sent to what most workers call "work comp." An occupational healthcare center, or occasionally a general urgent care that accepts and works with workers' compensation, a state-run program that sets premiums and benefits for all work-related claims within their respective state. Those states, including Florida, may permit private insurance companies to handle their work comp policies. Now it gets complicated. We have a state government agency delegating care to a private insurance carrier who in turn – you guessed it – turfs it off to our T.P.A. friends.

Aaargh.

What happened to our friend with the bleeding finger stump, now well stabilized with a fingertip amputation and appropriate dressing? Besides keeping her hand elevated so she does not bleed all over her driver's upholstery, she needs to go the pharmacy and fill prescriptions for oral antibiotics and pain medication. She likely will do that, certainly because of the opioid Rx (more on that later).

Next, she must go to the "work comp" center (there are at least four within the two mile radius of our OrthoNOW® specialty center) for an assessment with the workers' comp doctor, usually an hourly paid general physician or mid-level provider. What does that entail? They "assess" it is, in fact, an amputation all right. In a finger, which means we need a hand surgeon. Back to square one. That center, by the way, *never* calls me, even though I have been practicing hand surgery for a quarter century in Miami. They fill out the silly E.M.R. template notes where only the last sentences spell out the problem, a fingertip amputation, and they document "refer to hand surgeon." Now, the same adjustor (or maybe a different one) gets this and must find the accepting surgeon in yet another phase of the process, which amounts to more lost time. The occupational health center generated a four-to-five-page note of mostly *gobbledygook*, since the only relevant information is the description of fingertip (rarely accurate), and the treatment plan they send to someone like me. You cannot make this stuff up.

I saw the patient about four or five days later. As a medical professional who understands definitive treatment, I explained how a minor outpatient procedure, whether an Atasoy V-Y flap versus reverse flow homodigital island flap, could restore her fingertip...and likely get her back to work within a week or two, after some hand therapy to manage the wound and subsequent scar and desensitize the finger. And that hand therapist is across the hall from me, not across town. Where was the minor surgery done? Down the hall from my office in the three-room A.S.C. O.R. that we discussed earlier? When?? Within an hour of me seeing her since the first question my knowledgeable hand P.A. posed to her was – "What time did you eat?" then alerted the anesthesia and O.R. team. I took care of her as soon as the team finished fixing an ankle fracture in another room.

The patient was out of our building, a one-stop shopping orthopedic center, within a few hours. Pulp reconstructed, hand elevated, medication dispensed on site, so she did not need to wait in line at Walgreen's, and problem resolved. Sure, the services were billed, but we did something. The previous two facilities and well-meaning clinicians also sent their bills. Now you understand why healthcare is so expensive. And cumbersome.

How is this appalling, but commonplace, story relevant to the Doral Business Council? Well, the chairman of the D.B.C. at time of her injury had already been to visit our center in a demonstration of great interest and personal consideration for me. Like most everybody, he loved the facility but most importantly, its concept and mission. After his visit, I had visited the wholesale warehouse and asked to speak to the H.R. director, who took little interest but heard me out. Mind you, a busy surgeon is taking time to visit a major employer and explain that their boss understands the value of what we offer as a clinical facility, barely half a mile away. How can we work together to provide better care for *your* workers? I mean I care that much. In fact, I believe I even saw the steel door that might have injured their employee since we met in a back room adjacent to the storage freezers. Apathy was the operative word.

Several months after that meeting (where nothing constructive resulted), the injured worker was in my exam room with the mangled fingertip telling her story. I typically utter to my staff, "It's like Groundhog Day. Over and over."

I believe that was the inciting event, or one of, when I decided to stop attending that organization's breakfast meetings. I'll get my own bagel and coffee in my surgery center back area, and start my schedule on time so that I can finish earlier and have time to spend with my kids before they go to sleep on a school night. Frustrating issue, right, especially if you are the young worker who lost a fingertip and her supervisor who is scrambling to find a temporary replacement.

The same sequence of events has occurred with many of the other civic societies and chamber organizations. The president of one of the larger business associations in Miami was a patient of mine years ago. At the time, he was president of a major wellness related organization and sustained a significant shoulder injury. He had an upcoming long distance cycling event and we made a fun bet that he would help create a strong synergy between both our companies for mutual benefit, if I was able to get his shoulder to recover well enough to ride the 100 miles. He did the event, his shoulder did wonderfully, and yet we never followed up on our gentleman's agreement. He once served a role of influence for multiple companies yet had no sincere sense of how we could work together, even though we would save member organizations more money than they would bring us. That is the ironic fact with healthcare. I thought the point of these business networking events was to find better solutions to then do business more effectively. Guess I needed flashier business cards....

We have had similar direct discussions with multiple large companies in the South Florida area with the same result: initial interest followed by inaction. It likely stems from the fact that healthcare delivery is *so* complex that the benefiting parties are not even clear what the problem is, yet they realize they are paying too much. The CEO of a major cruise line shook his head when I asked if healthcare costs were an issue for them. "We spend 100 million dollars a year for healthcare-related issues," he groaned. I told him we had a simple system that could make a major dent in that and he referred me to the appropriate person but never followed up. After a nice lunch, two in-person meetings and multiple emails, zero initiatives were attempted. No pilot programs. A bit late now as our type of healthcare is now irrelevant. A microscopic virus has halted that industry.

A major airline, of which I am a proud upper echelon frequent flyer member, did take the time to fly to Miami from their headquarters in Texas. Their risk management team, a crew medical coordinator, and their in-house legal counsel came. It seems that one of their Miami-based risk managers inadvertently copied me on an email that read, "The OrthoNOW® thing is this clinic that some Dr. Badia has been hawking."

Can you imagine?!

I am the hand surgeon concerned about how *their* employees are receiving their work-related related injury care, not to mention the costs they are accruing. Some mid-level employee referred to my laudable efforts in this manner, as if I were peddling snake oil. Or compound creams. Or cannabis products. More on the latter much later. It would be interesting if I gave specific details regarding the jet engine mechanic who finally got to me nearly a week after multiple open fracture/nailbed injuries sustained at work, his definitive care being delayed by the typical, in fact routine, hurdles. Well...I would be slapped with HIPAA violations, as if being a concerned physician and human being was a crime. That overreaching legislation has had its share of unintended consequences and costs. Now, during the COVID-19 crisis, we are realizing the absurdity of it and using more commonsense measures to avoid interference with care. This, too, needs to be discussed as a contributor to our healthcare debacle.

Multiple attempts with dozens of large employers have been met with resistance, indifference, and even a touch of hostility. For what? Trying to save the company healthcare dollars while providing more streamlined, cost-effective care to the very people who perform their assigned tasks? This can only represent a system-wide ignorance as to how care is delivered.

As expected, municipalities and public organizations are even more challenging due to the inherent red-tape and prolonged timelines. In a meeting with a mayor and former county mayor, OrthoNOW® was asked to quantify what the estimated savings could be to local government. They are both intelligent men, grasped the concept readily, and the younger politician went so far as to visit our center. We compiled the data within weeks and prepared the report. To this day, nearly five years later, we have never been able to show this data to the people who requested it. This is disturbing. I am a local taxpayer and I would like to know that our leaders have vetted out processes that could save us money. The layers of decision-making are so dense that it goes nowhere even though there is some interest. Obviously not enough.

Poor collaboration and resistance to change does not, however, stop with large complex organizations such as corporations, civic groups, municipalities and even sports teams. The one place where healthcare could immediately benefit from greater interaction and cooperation is among the "providers" themselves. Yes, us clinicians.

A fellow orthopedic surgeon recently quipped to me that once you get more than 10 surgeons in a room, it is near impossible to agree on anything and you are less likely to achieve any definitive change. This is a major issue. Not only are we dealing with strong minded, highly driven individuals, but a lingering sense of competition that never fades. I tell my colleagues that the race started during organic chemistry and never let up. It is time to work together, not against each other. MCAT scores were long ago submitted and most of us have achieved our goals.

I learned this the hard way when franchising the OrthoNOW® model. Our objective was to package the program so busy colleagues of mine could simply replicate the model by inserting our turnkey methodology into their existing practice models. I would have probably done better by pretending that I was another healthcare businessman, not a fellow surgeon colleague who devised our system with a team to resolve the shortcomings of orthopedic care delivery. The same problems they have. All liked it, yet almost none of them engaged despite hours of conversation, ZOOM call presentations, and follow-up meetings, often on-site – either at our center or their offices.

The stories are too numerous to tell but a very recent one certainly highlighted the issue. I had met an orthopedic surgeon on a recent destination type conference to Antarctica where the social program was as stimulating as the academia. A small group of the faculty and participants got to know each other quite well and one of my talks was on the emerging sector of orthopedic urgent care. The surgeon asked me about it, as well as a unique medical device that I had been utilizing in surgery. His hospital O.R. acquired the device and he was thrilled and thankful that I had connected him with the founder, a surgeon in the same sparsely populated state of Wyoming.

He also was interested in OrthoNOW® due to its potential to solve some issues his group was having with acquiring patients and streamlining care and efficiencies. By that point, we were a licensing program, not a franchise, because it gives the licensee much more flexibility to engaging with only the offerings that interested them; furthermore, it did not obligate them to a long term commitment. Our onboarding team explained the process and he told us with noticeable enthusiasm that he was already bringing this up to colleagues and administration. The dialogue ended some weeks later. At the start of the COVID-19 pandemic, our V.P. of operations received a web link announcing that this group of orthopedic surgeons was opening an orthopedic urgent care.

No cordial follow-up by the interested surgeon, no explanation of why they preferred to "go it alone." What is clear is that many of our principles were divulged during the discovery process and of course, that information would certainly help them if they decided to proceed alone. They will experience many of the pitfalls and mistakes that any new business will encounter, but they evidently did not value the experience we brought, having made many past mistakes ourselves, and the process guidance that is inherent in our joining forces. I expressed my grave disappointment and pointed out the lack of courtesy in not simply informing me through ONE simple email, even though we had invested considerable time in addressing their questions. After all, he reached out when he needed help and we responded right away. Weeks went by and I received an email informing me that he passed along my one email to his attorney as my threats would no longer be tolerated. Plural: *threats*. Integrity is a difficult quality to impart. I guess he does not realize that if you wield a scalpel in South Florida, you better not be afraid of lawyers. Now a rodeo bull in Gillette, Wyoming? Definitely.

When I told my colleague, another foot and ankle surgeon, Dr. Greg Caban, about this incident, he remarked that he always remembers something that one of his surgeon mentors told him during residency, "We eat our own." What a short but powerful statement. Greg further added that physicians are the worst in collaborating and hold back the profession. He felt the current state of healthcare, post A.C.A. (affordable care act) is our own fault because the A.M.A. (American Medical Association) allowed it to happen. His comments were interesting, considering that I have spoken to many clinicians, mostly fellow physicians, about the goals of this book and asked many to contribute their thoughts and anecdotes as it was apparent that we agreed upon this fact – physicians hurt their own cause.

Many colleagues agree with Dr. Caban's stance regarding the A.M.A. The largest physician organization in the United States, it was founded in 1847 with the mission "To promote the art and science of medicine and the betterment of public health." Their noble cause resulted in many positive accomplishments over decades, including the war on cigarette smoking, the promotion of liability tort reform, and the creation of a National Opioid Task Force. These initiatives ultimately benefit the patients we serve, our primary common goal. However, the A.M.A. has dealt with criticisms surrounding the protection the profession from the many outside factors that continue to erode it, and consequently, healthcare. In 2010, The A.M.A. offered "qualified support" for the Patient Protection and Affordable Care Act, colloquially known as Obamacare. The benefits and pitfalls of this major act are well beyond the scope of this book, but one thing is clear: healthcare costs have continued to rise, and both "providers and patients" remain increasingly dissatisfied with U.S. healthcare delivery.

Lack of physician collaboration is largely at fault and even my request for comment from a leader within organized medicine was met with resistance and perhaps apathy. A trusted friend and colleague, past president of the A.M.A., declined my request to contribute to this book, which is solely intended to give the public insight as to our healthcare challenges and present some hope.

My own forays into organized medicine have been largely met with frustration and the sense that we were not making real progress. I occupied the District 2 seat within our own DCMA (Dade County Medical Association) for a three-year term during which time we met one evening a month as a board, as well as the additional meeting, depending upon committee or task force responsibilities. The group was comprised of committed and caring individuals, who took time away from family, self, and the ever-present patient care responsibilities. I remember many a night where I would delay my surgery start time to comply with my charge and watch when my colleagues would drive to make rounds at a hospital after the meeting concluded. While we achieved some key goals, including Florida state-wide passage of Amendment 3 to limit excessive medical liability compensation, we were often met with apathy and certainly limited financial support by our community colleagues. The fact is, physicians are busy, often day and night, and have not seen a compelling reason to lend support to most initiatives that protect patients and preserve our ability to treat them. A pity as it only hurts us and the patients we serve.

In 2004, 63 percent of patient voters approved Florida Amendment 3, which allowed for commonsense measures to rein in runaway jury awards and plaintiff lawyer compensation. If a patient was indeed harmed due to a legitimate act of malpractice, should they not receive the lion's share of the judgement? As expected, the trial lawyers poured money into the coffers to oppose the vote by a factor of 3-to-1 compared to supporters including the Florida Medical Association, multiple hospitals, and healthcare systems, and the A.M.A., thank goodness. The fact that state voters supported the initiative, despite poor physician backing, underscores the fact that true healthcare reform will largely come from the populace, not the insurance industry, government, healthcare systems, or, sadly enough, physicians. The term "consumerization of healthcare" will take on greater importance.

I continue to face major resistance from well-meaning colleagues who must have a subliminal aversion to simple collaboration. I first noted this when our beloved Miami Hand Center disbanded and the disgruntled partners could not even agree to take the model elsewhere, away from our initial partner who sabotaged it. Fortunately, all five of us have continued to do well – regrettably *despite* increased costs and the pain of starting anew. When I built the new center at Doral, amid considerable expense and effort as I have discussed, I was completely open to looking beyond and splitting the pie evenly. While I admit I have many faults, I am a proponent of the adage, "All ships rise in a tide," and would always prefer to have a smaller piece of a bigger pie. Despite taking all the risk, I was willing to consider completely equal partnerships in the surgery center. We could not move forward, however, paralyzed by individual concerns and ego, and the initiative faded away despite maintaining our friendship and good professional rapport.

The odyssey of the Surgery Center at Doral was discussed as I had to move on from the failed attempts at rejuvenating a hand surgery consortium. The A.S.C. finally achieved success, despite many struggles, and now continues to move forward. Nevertheless, we continue to face hurdles while we seek to increase patient volume and bring in more surgeon users. OrthoNOW® was almost solely designed to create a more facile patient journey that may end at the surgery center, if clinically necessary. This is a logical and economically viable – if not seemingly apparent – goal. The acceptance and support for

OrthoNOW® has been lukewarm at best by my colleagues and even the business forces behind the surgery center. If anybody would "get it", you think it would be them.

In our efforts to tie together our clinical center, an orthopedic ecosystem if you will, our V.P. of Operations had the brilliant idea of branding an all-inclusive orthopedic center, tied to the Doral name, our home. DoralDOC (Doral Orthopedic Center or D.O.C.) represented a comprehensive integration of every step of the tumultuous and inefficient patient journey and simplified the care of nearly any orthopedic malady. This includes initial patient evaluation via either the walk-in center (OrthoNOW®), or the individual orthopedist's office, many of which are now on-site. Diagnostics could be done at the same site on the same day (in most cases), with nearly every imaging modality. If surgical intervention is warranted, S.C.D. is down the hall and can now accommodate almost any type of surgery including total joint replacements, long bone fracture fixation, and even complex spine surgery – all outpatient. Comprehensive rehab services are down the hall, another concept that was met with indifference.

The website includes every surgeon's individual website and contact info, coupled with direct links to surgery center, walk-in facility, and rehabilitation. What is not to like? I am not sure, other than because a fellow clinician came up with the idea and took the risk to build it. I went so far as to offer to be excluded from the site's listing, since my esteemed hand colleagues would be portrayed, and the goal was over-arching. No matter. We remain in the prolonged and somewhat arduous process of achieving acceptance, which has revealed the depth of my stubbornness, and perhaps naivety.

Indeed, a multitude of forces and entities must collaborate to truly transform healthcare delivery to the seamless, cost-effective, and high-quality commodity that patients desire and deserve. Ironically, it is those patients who will ultimately drive that change since the referral sources, employers, payors and yes, even the "providers" themselves will not bring that change. My anecdotes and examples bear witness to that. I have heard similar grumblings from colleagues around the country who too tried to bring positive, but disruptive change in healthcare delivery. Until that change happens, physicians continue to strive for better patient care via lifelong learning and education. If only we could channel some of that energy and intellect into changing *how* that medical care is delivered.

Chapter 6 – There is No End:
The Ongoing Education of a Doctor

*"I will not be ashamed to say, "I know not," nor will I fail
to call in my colleagues when the skills of another are
needed for a patient's recovery."*

In the medical profession, the lifelong process of learning is unique. While university academicians in all fields can boast that their job is centered around teaching and learning, it should be considered an implicit part of their occupation. They ARE scholars. However, for most physicians in private practice or working within a healthcare system whose primary mission is to provide care, this is not the case.

Except for the atypical medical school professor in a research and clinical teaching position, most physicians cannot claim that research or academic pursuits are paramount in their job description. Yet, we attend conferences. *Do we ever.* There are local community medical meetings, specialty societies, regional meetings, national conferences, and international congresses ALL pertaining to one discipline. Then there might be the same myriad of meetings focused on a subspecialty. This stands apart from meetings of organized medicine to advocate for our profession care for our patients through national organizations including the AMA, the American College of Surgeons, etc. and state, county, and local societies.

In my case alone, I attend several meetings a year for orthopedic surgery, but then more for hand surgery, and then some additional ones for specific areas such as arthroscopy or trauma. Granted, this is largely a personal decision. I not only enjoy the academic exchange but have reaped the benefits in my own practice of hand surgery because I can provide my patients with a wider range of treatment options, since I also travel internationally. However, make no mistake: this is my own investment of my time and money. Like most of my colleagues, I receive no reimbursement for time spent "working," unlike other fields where a business trip is part of work description and comes with a nice expense account.

The issue is not about compensation but rather opportunity cost, something rarely discussed among the lay public. When you telephone your doctor and the staff tells you he is at a conference, it is to ultimately benefit you, the patient, and the fact that he cannot see you means lost revenue to his practice. Furthermore, the receptionist may say "he is away" or even on vacation, when the truth is that the prime focus of travel is the learning event, with perhaps a few days of R&R tacked on. Many physicians do this despite its significant impact to the bottom line. Why? Medicine is a calling, and physicians' continued investment in knowledge ought to be recognized.

Many years ago, it was not uncommon that a company whose device you use would invite you to a specific conference, or even pay some of your expenses to a national congress. Some may call that an inducement, but it seems in almost every other profession it is just part of doing business. After all, there is a communal component. We humans are social creatures and as you must have gathered by now, physicians are often too busy to socialize. Therefore, most of my colleagues don't think it is wrong when a company that wants to get your attention asks you to read some scientific or product literature, and invites you to lunch or dinner in order to discuss *their* products. Yes, they could do that during the day; however, ask any pharmaceutical rep or device distributor how easy it is to speak to a busy clinician during normal working hours. Regardless, we often do, for no remuneration.

Scheduling an educational meeting outside the busy clinical environment is a logical solution. Away from work concerns, the physician or health practitioner can concentrate on what the company representative is saying. It should not be a crime to have a conversation like that over dinner…or should the doctor pay for the meal? Should they "Go Dutch" like two teenagers who do not want to feel obligated to each other? This does sort of border on the ridiculous and reflects the extent to which society has become overly politically correct. Decades ago, none of these activities raised any red flags. The fact that they do now only contributes to the increasing stress that physicians are under.

The bottom line: if a doctor uses a specific drug or titanium implant solely because some company rep threw a steak and glass of wine down their throat, we indeed have much bigger problems in medicine. I think most physicians are both critical and ethical enough to make the right decisions for their patients without a "nanny state" breathing down our necks and wagging their index finger. It would be interesting to have the same standards applied to our politicians at every level. Come to think of it, the $10,000 monthly "lobbying fee" to induce my city leaders to consider a better healthcare delivery option for the populace likely suffers from the same issue. I will elaborate on this in the government chapter. Interesting how that somehow seems acceptable.

Nevertheless, the Sunshine Act was released in 2013 and became yet another onerous component of the ACA (Affordable Care Act), namely section 6002, which states that companies covered by any federal health program must report any consulting fees, food, entertainment, travel, honoraria or "transfers of value". Dr. Lynch, a prominent spine surgeon, echoed what many physicians felt when he stated during a Chicago orthopedic and spine conference, "The transparency is noble, and it enables patients to look at their doctor and make individual assessments, but a secondary thing is the government is trying to wrestle some control into this, trying to rein physicians in a little bit." We all took notice and most of us are, to be quite honest, resentful.

The real irony is that most medical educational conferences or even orthopedic industry dinner events are often "bare bones", pun intended. I speak to friends in the financial, banking, or real estate world, and it is a different reality. I do not pass judgement because there is nothing wrong with entertainment being interspersed with doing business. In the aftermath of the 2008 financial crisis, the financial industry underwent major regulation, and with good reason. Their activities extended far beyond lavish dinner parties or even the shocking cocaine scene at the beginning of the film, *The Wolf of Wall Street*. I stand my ground in assuring the public that most physicians are ethical, although there are bad apples in any bushel. We do not have to punish the entire profession for a few deplorable actors.

The over-regulation and penetration of micro-surveillance even affected educational events put on by well-meaning individuals or small groups. In 2005, I initiated a yearly hand surgery conference that was focused on an area that I feel was neglected in our field – upper limb arthroscopy and arthroplasty (joint replacement). Many conferences and specialty-specific workshops focused on fracture management techniques, microsurgery, and nerve surgery. As mentioned, I had developed a specific interest in small joint arthroscopy. I realized that larger orthopedic conferences did not give this discipline the attention it merited.

We held the inaugural Miami Hand Course at the Marriot Brickell, a hotel that is no longer in existence. The didactic conference was attended by many surgeons and therapists from abroad, while the faculty consisted of a stellar group of surgeons who self-funded their trip to Miami to teach the participants. Think about that for a moment. Surgeons, many in the late stages of their career, supported me and our educational mission by jumping on a plane, staying at the hotel, and sacrificing time away from their professional practice and family. Frankly, I was not surprised. These were colleagues, friends, and mentors who understood what I was trying to accomplish and supported the noble goal of the meeting. This is, however, often surprising to those outside the medical profession.

To defray the cost to participants, we charged some exhibitors a modest fee to set up a display table with their products. Most interesting was the shared exchange of knowledge in this subset of hand surgery. A key part of the course was a cadaver demonstration of a few select techniques by the faculty, transmitted to large screens in the ballroom to illustrate the methods and encourage discussion.

The following year, we moved the course to a hotel in Coral Gables since the downtown hotel was being levelled for yet another high-rise development on the water. This, too, was a monumental success. The course paid for itself and attracted even larger numbers of colleagues, many from Latin America and Europe. We even provided simultaneous translation, including a laudable performance by my own mother, Maria Voltmer, owner of Maria's Interpreting and Translating Service. I paid for Mom's flight and provided accommodations for her at my home. Thanks Mom.

Why should a course like this undergo such intense scrutiny? Well, in later years, as the grumblings of a "Sunshine Act" became an enshrined law, many orthopedic companies wanted to mitigate their risk. After all, my meeting was not meant to attract a huge audience, nor did it have wide-reaching influence. Consequently, each year, it became more difficult to attract exhibitors, as if we were doing something wrong or clandestine. Fortunately, the course content and reputation expanded in such a significant way that many companies did want to participate, which allowed us to finally fund the faculty's travel expenses. Furthermore, the course was further revered with the addition of a "hands-on" component on day two at the renowned DaVinci Center for participants. Quite amazing that we had to worry about the ramifications of a scientific and educational endeavor that would ultimately benefit patients. Some years later, to add salt to the wound, the company Intuitive Surgical threatened to sue the surgical training lab, claiming "confusion" over the name, which was shared by their now famous surgical robot. It seems that a wealthy company could somehow lay claim to the name of one of history's most revered inventors, artists, and anatomists. Something tells me Leonardo would not be amused. We were not interested in a legal fight or hassle. The DaVinci center was solely interested in cadaveric education and learning. So sad that some would interfere with that lofty goal, solely over a name used the world over.

As more years went by, I realized that most of the companies supporting us could least afford it. The billion-dollar players stood more to lose, a ludicrous and shameful concept. To reiterate, I see no wrong in combining a social networking event with education, as many of the techniques discussed were further elaborated upon over a mojito and a cigar rolled by a Cuban legend roller. After all, this is Miami, and many colleagues looked forward to this event where they could meet some of the most illustrious names in our field while listening to a live Cuban jazz ensemble.

One year, our course director informed me that Stryker, a billion-dollar orthopedic device company, would not support the course because the conference social was being held at "The Jungle" as stated in our conference announcement flyer. "The Jungle" is my home's nickname, and I figured if I kept conference costs down by opening my home to colleagues and industry, more participants could attend. I suppose the corporation's "compliance army" imagined that participants and faculty alike would be swinging from tropical tree limb vines or emulating our Wall Street counterparts. We cannot have that now, can we?

So, what happened? I stopped organizing and hosting the course, though I did not let go easily.

Congratulations bean counters.

Having devoted a huge portion of my time and significant energy to this important course objective, I wanted its maintenance to be seamless. To keep growing it and share the workload, I engaged our professional hand surgery organizations. Yet even the prestigious American Society for Surgery of the Hand (ASSH) made me jump through hoops when I inquired about their interest and willingness to adopt the course. If one lone surgeon could grow it, painstakingly, over the course of ten years, imagine what a large professional organization could do with an extensive database and resources, including capital and manpower?

I argued that the course took place in the winter months in tropical Miami, and included a well-organized, hands-on cadaver lab, which I knew was a big draw for my colleagues. The society also claimed to have an interest in attracting a broader international presence and membership. Due to my passion for travel and networking with colleagues, the course was comprised of nearly 80 percent international participants. No matter. They never gave me the courtesy of a response, despite completing some extensive paperwork. I am not sure why. The same happened with the hand association (AAHS), a smaller and more pragmatic practice focused organization, and even EWAS, a tremendous society focused on helping teach hand surgeons wrist arthroscopy in multiple countries. This was a large component of our Miami Hand Course. There was, and remains, no American city that holds these esteemed courses, despite my noble and unselfish intent. Sadly, politics is omnipresent, even in medical education.

Regardless, it was a rewarding task to help disseminate specific techniques to my colleagues, among world-class faculty and key opinion leaders. However, it was an exhausting effort that gained little support from surgical societies, as mentioned, and occupied countless hours during the six-month period leading up to the course. Susan Rylander, my sister and executive assistant, devoted innumerable hours to conference logistics, which often pulled her away from other vital tasks. Still, we immersed ourselves in the effort with gusto and passion. It is truly a pity that over-regulation and concern for inconsequential details would stymie a busy professional from trying to share knowledge and promote the exchanges of ideas between colleagues. I have no regrets that I ran this course for a decade; however, it is a telling sign when our overly intrusive system dissuades the teaching and learning, that would benefit the greater public.

The ongoing education of a physician involves not only conferences and travel to meetings, but the never-ending duty to read, read, read and "keep up with the literature." Most physicians will subscribe to several peer-reviewed journals, which are essentially publications that share medical and scientific knowledge shared by colleagues. Under the direction of a journal editor-in-chief and assistant editors, a review board thoroughly vets the papers. It is a painstaking process to get published but the reader can be assured that frivolous articles will rarely make it through the gatekeepers.

Staying abreast of journals alone is a Herculean task, but there are also books, online articles, and throw-away journals which, as described, contain valuable information that does not typically join the long-term body of knowledge. Deciding what is important, relevant, or even worth reading is a task unto itself usually due to several conflicting duties (including writing this book)

I recently stepped down from my long-standing commitment of serving on a hand surgery journal review board due to being pulled in multiple directions, primarily the entrepreneurial endeavor of impacting orthopedic care delivery. After reading and reviewing hundreds of technique-type articles of hand surgery, I felt a twinge of guilt when I resigned. For physicians, the pursuit of knowledge is in our DNA. Most of us feel obligated to contribute to mankind's body of knowledge, even if restricted to one narrow field of medicine.

An alarming fact I only recently learned from a colleague who lives in Spain is that the medical publishing industry exploits a physician's sense of duty, dedication to knowledge, and altruism. His sobering account opened my eyes to another injustice in the medical profession.

THE BIG BUSINESS OF MEDICAL JOURNALS
Dr. Juan Manuel Rios-Ruh
Chief Executive Officer en Aware Health Communication

I attended medical school in Venezuela. Afterward I migrated to Spain, where I did most of my specialized training. I did my orthopedic surgery residency in Valencia, followed by a foot and ankle fellowship in Barcelona. Since then, I have been pretty much involved in medical education. I founded our medical education platform with some colleagues that focuses on orthopedic surgery. It has been an interesting experience because it has allowed me to see a different side about medical education – the positive side of scientific and medical education, but also the darker side, along with where the medical professional is trending relative to the industry.

In Europe, we have a major (and relatively new) problem. It's frowned upon for a medical doctor who provides medical education – for example, a lecture at a conference or a meeting – to charge for their time or expertise, *even if they spend the entire day teaching younger residents or younger fellows*. It is not illegal, it is not unethical, but it is discouraged. The prevailing attitude is, "No, no, doctors shouldn't charge for going to a meeting and giving a lecture. They shouldn't charge for teaching younger residents or younger fellows."

Think about that: here we are in the 21st century, where you can find a course on a social media platform like Instagram about how to take a great selfie. The guy who presents the course can charge you $500 Euros per day… and that is fine. He must charge for his time and expertise in selfies, after all. But if you are a doctor who takes a day, several days, or a week or more away from your private practice or from the hospital where you are on staff (after you obtain permission) to travel abroad to give a lecture, you're supposed to do it all for FREE. If a doctor is willing to sacrifice their time and money, they should be paid at least as much as someone who is teaching an online selfie course.

For example, here in Spain, the National Society of Orthopedic Surgeons hosts a national meeting. When you calculate how much income they receive, from the cost of the tickets to the pharmaceutical contributions, it amounts to about two-to-three million Euros in profit for this event. Remember, doctors attend to hear the lectures from doctors. That is the *only* thing that draws us there. We want to hear key opinion leaders discuss their work. I have been invited a couple of times as a key opinion leader. Guess what? Not only did they require me to pay for a ticket to present a lecture they invited me to make, I had to pay for all my expenses – airfare, food, hotel, etc. I compare it to going to a Metallica concert and asking the band to pay for your ticket.

As physicians, we face a difficult situation, which is part of the same problem that stems from the practice of taking advantage of our altruism. Yet there are middlemen who declare, 'Okay, this is a business. We can make money from this.' These people are not doctors. They are not providing value, nor are they giving the lectures. They the people in the middle who take these profits while asking the doctors to speak for free and pay for all the expenses they incur to do it. You could be the key opinion leader who takes an hour of his time to educate and entertain the attendees, and you must pay not only to get *into* the event, but for everything else. It always surprises me that we medical doctors fall for it. Yet another aspect of moral injury.

Speaking of middlemen, there is another facet of this "middleman enrichment" that astounds me, and that is the immense business that has grown from medical journals. I am amazed that doctors have allowed it to go on for so long, but it has been investigated in Europe. For anyone who does not know how these publications function, allow me to explain. On their own and for free, medical doctors develop articles, which they want to get published. These doctors invest a huge amount of time and money on these articles – sometimes having to pay for translation, statistics, and other things. After that investment of their own money and time, they send it to the medical journal. Now, that journal does not have to spend a dime on editors because they have volunteer doctors to edit the articles. Yes, these doctors edit the articles for *free*. From there, if the journal decides they are good enough, they publish them.

Here is the rub: they charge anyone who wants to read an article a minimum of $60. They will inform the author how many people have read or cited their article, but neither the author, nor the editor receive a cent of that money. It is a perfect business for these medical publishers because they keep all the profits for themselves. For example, Elsevier, a Dutch publishing and analytics company specializing in scientific, technical, and medical content, made a profit of $9.8 billion U.S. in 2018. That is a lot of money. Elsevier enjoys a profit margin of 36 percent. To put that into perspective, other magazines like Time, which pays for authors and editors, have a profit margin of about 10 or 11 percent. I am sure Time and other publications would love to know how Elsevier got these guys writing and editing for free!

However, the European University Association noticed that this was an unfair deal and released a report entitled, *The Lack of Transparency and Competition in the Academic Publishing Market in Europe and Beyond*, in which they expressed their concerns "about possible irregularities concerning pricing and market conditions in the research publishing sector." The report states, "The bulk of the editorial burden (peer review) - checking the validity and evaluating the research – is done by working researchers (also often employed on public funds) on a volunteer basis. The publishers then sell the product back – at a high price – to government-funded institutions and university libraries to be read by researchers – who, in a collective sense, created the product in the first place."

Researchers are often employed on public funds on a volunteer basis. The publishers then sell the product back at an astronomical price to government-funded institutions and university libraries to be read by researchers. It does not make any sense. We are investing as countries, not only as individuals, a huge amount of money in vain to these editorials to let their scientists have access to these research – which the *researchers themselves* have done. These medical publishers have the perfect business going...on that runs completely on free labor.

Although the unfairness of it all has garnered the attention of government officials, it is likely an untouchable problem. Why? Five companies own more than 70 percent of all scientific publications. They not only take advantage of doctors' altruism; they hold the scientific research in their hands. They have the power to decide which ones will be published because there are so few of them. It is dangerous. It can be an advantage in some areas, but a disadvantage in other areas of medicine that they have no interest in publishing. It is an unfair practice and explains why the problem goes beyond the money. In fact, in 2017, The Guardian published an article entitled, Is the staggering profitable business of scientific publishing bad for science?

I hope this opens other people's eyes to the big business of medical journals, which exploits doctors' scientific production and altruism. As with other aspects of medicine, once again we physicians are eliminated from the decision-making and the revenue.

SECTION II

THE ECONOMICS OF HEALTHCARE

Chapter 7 – Government Interference and The Politics of Medicine

*"I will respect the privacy of my patients, for their problems
are not disclosed to me that the world may know.
Most especially must I tread with care in matters of life
and death. If it is given me to save a life, all thanks.
But it may also be within my power to take a life;
this awesome responsibility must be faced with great
humbleness and awareness of my own frailty.
Above all, I must not play at God."*

The role of government remains a hotly debated issue throughout history, but few will disagree that defense of its citizens and enforcement of its laws are applicable, unless you are a true libertarian anarchist. However, many would argue that government should also safeguard the health of those less fortunate, and the proverbial safety net is in place for even the most anti-socialist systems. This mission is not only moral but has a profound economic consequence as a society cannot be productive if many of its citizens are ill or infirm.

I have always told government officials that hand surgery, specifically, should be well developed and supported, because the majority of industrial injuries naturally involve the hand, and that a person can only go back to being productive if the sustained trauma is appropriately managed. There is a huge cost of not providing appropriate and timely hand care, but also a major benefit when that investment is made in future productivity for that patient and society beyond.

The recognized father of our specialty, Dr. Sterling Bunnell, was asked by the U.S. military to set up a series of hand centers to manage the profound injuries sustained while in action during W.W. II. It was estimated that nearly 90,000 injuries would be sustained to the upper limb during that conflict, one-quarter of them to the hand. Government realized this required more focused care than had been done in the past by general surgeons, orthopedists, and plastic surgeons. Hence, the field of hand surgery was largely borne out of a public-private partnership as then directed by the U.S. Army Surgeon General and private hand surgeon, Dr. Bunnell.

The argument is not whether government should have a role in healthcare for its citizens, but rather how obtrusive it should be. And given its size and inefficiencies, is government an ideal steward? For example, any clinician who has worked in the behemoth V.A. (Veterans Administration) system can attest to its frequent ineptitude.

My intention is not to debate "Medicare for All" or even argue for or against a one-payor system. I simply want to point out how government has increased the cost of care in many cases, from the city and county level, up to the federal level. In the final chapter, we will present some positive arguments for alternate systems of care, but it will be evident that the private sector is always involved and greater collaboration, as I urge in this book, is needed. It is not who provides care, or even who pays for it, but rather *how* that care is delivered. The last discussion continues to elude us.

You may recall the heated debates in 2009-2010 that preceded the passage of the Affordable Care Act by the Obama administration, legislation that added to the burdensome healthcare system in the U.S. It's important to note, however, that even though opponents of this bill decried it as socialized medicine, healthcare in the United States had already been socialized in many respects several decades earlier with the passage of The Medicare and Medicaid Act of 1965.

In fact, the concept of government involvement in medicine dates as far back as 1912, when Teddy Roosevelt ran for President of the United States and included health insurance in his platform. Then, in 1945, President Harry S. Truman urged the United States Congress to create a national health insurance fund that was open to all Americans. Truman's plan would provide health coverage to individuals and pay for expenses like doctor visits, hospital visits, laboratory services, dental care, and nursing services. Despite his passion and tenacity on the issue, he failed to convince Congress to pass such a bill. His successor, President John F. Kennedy, followed in Truman's footsteps by pushing for a national healthcare program for seniors after a national study concluded that 56 percent of Americans over the age of 65 were not covered by insurance.

However, it was not until 1966 – after President Lyndon B Johnson signed The Medicare and Medicaid Act of 1965 – that Americans started receiving Medicare health coverage when Medicare's hospital and medical insurance benefits first took effect. Harry Truman and his wife, Bess, were the first two Medicare beneficiaries.

How did the medical community react to it? According to A.J. DiGiovanni, M.D., retired general and vascular surgeon, "When they passed The Medicare Act of 1965, it created a tremendous inflationary spiral. I remember, the fee structures we got were excellent. Everybody who saw that payment scale was pleased, and I must admit I was amazed. But that was the selling point that got us into this. And then after that, government control impacted that program so that the fees did not match the general inflation that took place. It created a downward spiral. Medicare was a come-on to induce physicians to accept government-sponsored insurance and an appeal to our instincts about returns, which were fair in the beginning. However, as time went by the Medicare fee structure was not commensurate with inflation."

It should also be noted that Medicare, and certainly Medicaid, was designed as a lower reimbursement program to care for our well-deserving elderly and the less fortunate, as a civilized society should. However, as often happens with well-intended laws, the private sector insurance industry began to base its rates off the Center for Medicare and Medicaid Services. They started to reimburse doctors for medical charges using a multiple of the standard C.M.S. charge for individual services, which is not sustainable. Consequently, practitioners and hospitals had to bill at three- to- seven times that figure just to stay afloat – not that any private medical practice expects to receive that. I call it "monopoly money." If I got paid what I bill, my God I would be a multi-millionaire. We must bill this way because the insurance companies only pay us a percentage of our billed charges; therefore, they must be higher. Insurance companies never pay us for the actual value of a service provided. I know of NO OTHER profession like that.

The Health Maintenance Organization Act of 1973

With such a confusing, and increasingly expensive, system, the government stepped in during the 70s and passed a bipartisan bill to curb medical inflation. The term H.M.O. (Health Maintenance Organization) was first coined by Dr. Paul Ellwood, a pediatric neurologist who felt that economic factors in healthcare took priority over the need of patients.

This act provided federal funds to initiate or expand a Health Maintenance Organization (H.M.O.); It also required employers with 25 or more employees to offer federally approved H.M.O. options if they offered traditional fee-for-service health insurance to their employees. However, it did not require employers to offer health insurance. The government program gave H.M.O.'s greater penetration into the employer-based market, a strangling issue for businesses ever since.

Interestingly, The Dual Choice provision expired in 1995 although it had already opened the doors for the H.M.O. industry. This development perhaps represented the major turning point in U.S. Healthcare because it allowed businessmen not clinicians, to engage in providing care indirectly, while garnering wild profits. It is no coincidence that some of the wealthiest people in Miami made their fortunes in healthcare. They will admit that they know not one stitch – pun intended – about delivering care (more on that later). For now, it should be clear that the United States government opened the door to permit non-practitioners to further escalate the cost of healthcare in this country.

The staggering amount of money that local healthcare businessmen make on simply buying, and selling, Medicare patient lives, in the so-called Medicare "Advantage" plans is staggering and frankly embarrassing to me as not only a clinician, but a taxpayer. The collective patient pools are peddled like cattle with huge multiples on the sale. This despite our ongoing national challenges with healthcare costs. Somehow these healthcare plans for seniors seem to have the money to place full page newspaper ads in every issue of our only daily, and billboards dot the south Florida landscape as if we need to announce and advertise a plan that simply flips your Medicare benefits to an astute businessman. Naturally, they do. More enrollees mean more dollars. Providing more cost-effective care would also yield benefits, but that is not low hanging fruit. For now, expect expensive bus wraps of a smiling Magic Johnson. Yes, our healthcare dollars are partly in the hands of a charismatic ex-professional basketball player. Is anybody paying attention in Washington?

Dr. A.J. DiGiovanni M.D. on the Problems with H.M.O.'s

I must admit I was in an H.M.O. After discussing the issue at length with my colleagues and friends, we all decided to accept it. However, it was not long before the insurance companies developed the restrictive type of overseeing about the kind of a treatment we could offer to our patients. H.M.O.'s became less and less desirable than their original entry into medicine seemed to indicate. I never liked the idea of being in that type of organization, but it was almost a necessity. As a surgeon, you were captured in a way, if you wanted to survive and continue to practice medicine.

One incident from decades ago involving an elderly gentleman on an HMO stands out in my mind. After evaluating him, I determined he needed a hernia repair, yet his insurance company refused his application. When I spoke to a physician at the insurance company about it, he informed me, "Well, we don't believe it's something we should allow at this time."

"Wait a minute," I replied. "Are you a surgeon? Do you know about hernias?"

"No, I'm not," he admitted.

"Well, what do you do?"

"I'm an internist."

"What do you know about hernia treatment?" I pressed him.

"I learned something from friends of mine."

"What do you mean, 'friends of mine,' off the curb? You're ridiculous to use that kind of information as standard for surgical practice."

I don't remember what insurance company it was, but it angered me that this representative – an internist with no firsthand knowledge or experience with hernias – had the authority to evaluate whether hernia surgery was appropriate for my patient or not. It was wrong for the insurance company to use that as a standard for making decisions about the appropriate care and treatment of patients. After much wrangling, I won the case and received authorization to operate on my patient. But it was ridiculous to be forced to go through a process like that, especially when it was being evaluated by someone who did not have the background to make these evaluations on a sound basis.

HIPAA

The French philosopher Voltaire famously stated, "Common sense is not so common." Nowhere is this axiom truer than in the healthcare industry, thanks in large part to government interference. HIPAA (Health Insurance Portability and Accountability Act of 1996) is a classic example of the lack of common sense in medicine.

According to HHS.gov, "The Health Insurance Portability and Accountability Act of 1996 (HIPAA) required the Secretary of the U.S. Department of Health and Human Services (HHS) to develop regulations protecting the privacy and security of certain health information.[1] To fulfill this requirement, HHS published what are commonly known as the HIPAA Privacy Rule and the HIPAA Security Rule. The Privacy Rule, or *Standards for Privacy of Individually Identifiable Health Information*, establishes national standards for the protection of certain health information. The *Security Standards for the Protection of Electronic Protected Health Information* (the Security Rule) establish a national set of security standards for protecting certain health information that is held or transferred in electronic form. The Security Rule operationalizes the protections contained in the Privacy Rule by addressing the technical and non-technical safeguards that organizations called "covered entities" must put in place to secure individuals' "electronic protected health information" (e-PHI). Within HHS, the Office for Civil Rights (OCR) has responsibility for enforcing the Privacy and Security Rules with voluntary compliance activities and civil money penalties."

Now consider the costs of HIPAA, as revealed by Medical Economics.com:

"At the time of implementation, the Department of Human and Health Services (HHS) estimated that HIPAA would initially cost healthcare systems approximately $113 million with subsequent maintenance costs of $14.5 million per year. The actual costs of HIPAA compliance are estimated at closer to $8.3 billion a year, with each physician on average spending $35,000 annually for health information technology upkeep. The true costs, however, are unknown and buried under layers of purportedly necessary bureaucracy. These costs do not account for the added stress inflicted upon healthcare clinicians and patients struggling to allow each other access to important and necessary healthcare information."

Think about that: $8.3 billion spent on HIPAA. Then consider that before its passage, doctors, nurses, pharmacists, and other medical professionals respected patient privacy. We did not need a government agency to tell us to do the right thing. I have never walked into a pharmacy and heard the pharmacist yell out, "Hey Joe, your HIV prescription is ready!" It just does not happen. But like many unnecessary government programs, HIPAA has inflated costs and created another barrier to the efficient care and treatment of patients.

As doctors, we are forced into it. As much as I try to streamline it, there is only so much I can do. I've asked my staff, "Guys, can we condense all this paperwork? I understand you need legal stuff; I get that." Our society is driven by legal issues, which is sad. In the case of HIPAA, it makes no sense, yet I assure my staff that I'll jump through the hoops if they can get everything we need to comply on one paper with one signature at the bottom. We have become lemmings, the little rodents that blindly follow each other's march into the sea. But our compliance has enriched others and spawned a cottage industry (which I will explore in further detail in an upcoming chapter), as evidenced by the example below of a recent email I received.

Recognize and lock down your HIPAA compliance risk areas.

According to AMA and Accenture, 83% of physicians have been victims of a cyberattack. Such an alarming statistic serves as a reminder that HIPAA compliance programs and breach reporting should remain up to date, impermeable, and above reproach.

AAPC's **HIPAA Medical Reference Guide** was created to safeguard the compliance of your medical practice by equipping you with the knowledge you need to secure the frontlines and back doors to your patients' protected health information.

Our nationally recognized HIPAA compliance experts lay out best practices and guide you step-by-step through the do's and don'ts of compliance. This comprehensive guide shows you how to recognize and lock down your risk areas, including how to:

- Evaluate your vulnerabilities and guard against cyber threats
- Assess, analyze, and manage your EHR
- Plan for emergency management
- Properly dispose of PHI
- Ensure your BAAs are HIPAA compliant
- Prepare for community-wide disasters

The HIPAA Medical Reference Guide will also provide official guidance on cybersecurity, highlight new technologies to boost your practice IT, and discuss CMS interoperability. Take advantage of numerous toolkits to facilitate breach reporting, analyze your practice's risk assessment, beef up your cybersecurity, and boost your e-health vernacular.

The **HIPAA Reference Guide** also includes helpful features like:

- Answers to commonly asked HIPAA compliance questions
- Secure measures to add to your compliance checklist
- Quick reference to related rules and regulations
- Dedicated section for notes in the margins to keep important details at your fingertips

Affordable Care Act of 2010

Intended to slow the rise of healthcare costs, the Affordable Care Act was enacted in March 2010. Sometimes referred to as "Obamacare," this comprehensive healthcare law has three primary goals, according to Healthcare.gov:

1. Make affordable health insurance available to more people. The law provides consumers with subsidies ("premium tax credits") that lower costs for households with incomes between 100% and 400% of the federal poverty level.

2. Expand the Medicaid program to cover all adults with income below 138% of the federal poverty level. (Not all states have expanded their Medicaid programs.)

3. Support innovative medical care delivery methods designed to lower the costs of health care generally.

While assured that "if you like your doctor, you can keep your doctor," and "if you like your plan, you can keep your plan," according to The Balance.com, three-to-five million people lost their employment-based health insurance. Thirty million people who had private health insurance plans found their policies canceled multiple times because they did not cover the ACA's 10 essential benefits. The ACA requires services that many people do not need, such as maternity care. For many Americans, the law resulted in higher insurance premiums and less coverage.

Some of the pros of the Affordable Care Act is that it provides insurance for millions and offers free preventive care, which means patients receive treatment before they need expensive emergency room services. Some of the 10 essential health benefits include treatment for mental health, addiction, and chronic diseases. Proponents of the law often pointed to England's National Health System or Canada's socialized healthcare system as models we should emulate in the United States.

Instead, this famous legislation, along with the government programs that preceded it, have further accelerated, and expanded the medical profession's bureaucratic inefficiencies. One example is electronic medical records (E.M.R.). When the United States Supreme Court upheld the Affordable Care Act's constitutionality on June 28, 2012, it paved the way for a mandate to take effect in 2014 that required E.M.R. for all practitioners, adding yet another barrier to the efficient delivery of care.

According to a South Florida pediatrician who wishes to remain anonymous, "E.M.R. has transformed our workday. By its nature, pediatrics is 'touchy-feely' because you are dealing with someone's child. With E.M.R., I fall behind because I must make eye contact and show empathy when I am dealing with a parent and their child, who is my patient. I can't spend that time typing on my computer, which means I spend another two hours later writing down what they said and documenting the visit."

One of my former partners from the Miami Hand Center, Dr. Roger Khouri, M.D., F.A.C.S. concurs, "Medicine is getting to be more and more frustrating for physicians. We spend more and more time doing paperwork and on computers than on the patients, especially in the hospitals, which both Dr. Badia and I, being a little too old for this, have learned to avoid. We've kind of built our own microcosm. But I have two young associates who still spend time at the hospital because they must.

"Here is a perfect example of what I mean. One of my associates came back after doing a small operation in town, and he admitted that the paperwork probably took five times longer than the actual surgery. The *paperwork* took longer than the operation five by *five* times…not two or three times. So, physicians are spending less and less time looking at patients and talking to patients, and more and more time in front of a computer screen. That is part of the tragedy here. We forgot the basics of medicine: talking to patient and holding the patient's hand to figure out what is going on. Instead, we spend our time on paperwork and ordering tests."

OH CANADA

As we continue to discuss a more socialized solution for our healthcare woes, we again must consult with the clinicians. As we have already noted, outside interference with the delivery of patient care comes with many drawbacks. Many Americans and others who are not consumers of the Canadian healthcare system tout it as a model for the United States to follow. But when it comes to healthcare, cost should not always be the priority. Due to access and convenience factors inherent in their socialized healthcare system, I see many patients from Canada who would rather fly to Miami than visit their local Canadian orthopedic doctor. Let me use an example from my colleagues and our neighbors in "The Great White North" to illustrate my point

Several years ago, I had dinner with the only private practice (or so he claimed) hand surgeon in Canada, following a presentation I had made at a meeting in Montreal on sports-related injuries to the hand and wrist. My colleague and his partner, a shoulder surgeon, planned to travel to Miami to learn a procedure from me that they did not yet have access to in their own country. Neither one of them worked within the Canadian healthcare system anymore. Why did they make this decision? Not because of economics, as many people might assume. For these two medical professionals, quality of care was their main motivation.

You see, in Canada's socialized healthcare system, patients with shoulder rotator cuff tears are seen by orthopedic doctors when the condition is in an advanced stage, thanks to the paucity of M.R.I. magnets in their country. In fact, as I mentioned before, there are more M.R.I.s – a necessary imaging study for the diagnosis of a torn rotator cuff – in Miami-Dade County, than there are in the entire country of Canada. This points to the problematic nature of both healthcare systems. In my city, the plethora of magnets speaks to a converse problem, while in Canada the lack of M.R.I.'s means patients must wait between eight to ten months to undergo an M.R.I. study after they are placed on waiting lists.

In fully socialized healthcare systems this is a common problem, although either overlooked or unknown by a misinformed public that touts them. For example, a sports medicine colleague in Dublin Ireland, informed me it takes a patient in that country's healthcare system three years to see a urologist for a scheduled appointment, in their version of "the waiting list." I doubt the fact we were on our second pint of Guinness® influenced his comments. When the government has full control, healthcare practitioners' hands are tied, and the public suffers further.

While many Americans recognize the major issues inherent in U.S. healthcare – some of them due to government interference – if they had to use the Canadian or Irish system, most would conclude that the government-run solution is worse. In the last chapter, my colleagues and I will share our insights as to how we can improve healthcare in the U.S. However, to move in the direction of Canada or Ireland because we feel we must, rather than fixing our problems, is not the right solution, as you will discover when you take the time to speak with clinicians and patients working within these systems.

As our South Florida pediatrician notes, "The U.S. healthcare system is not properly run. We do not have one system, we have three: a socialized system, a fee-for-service system, and an insurance system. When physicians complain, they get no empathy from the public, which does not regard them as sympathetic figures, compared to their peers in professions like accounting and law. Yet, physicians face more obstacles, especially in primary care when it comes to compensation and reimbursement for work. Much of our work is NOT reimbursed. The healthcare business takes advantage of doctors' altruism. Whereas an attorney can bill for everything, a doctor cannot. The day is not over when the last patient leaves. Once we shut our doors, it is onto emails, calls, and patient education. None of us get paid for this."

We will delve into the insurance aspect later but suffice it to say both the U.S. system and fully socialized systems are bad. Ours is way too expensive and cumbersome; however, if you fight within the system and jump through all the hoops, you will get that M.R.I. very quickly. Yes, you may have to pay – and perhaps placing some of the burden on the person in need is warranted as an excellent price-control method. With a high insurance deductible, an American patient could get one tomorrow. Many clinicians are happy to take these high-deductible patients because they pay for the test and we come up with an answer to solve their problem (imagine that!), much like the plumber or lawyer.

Back to my frustrated Canadian colleagues. They complained that by the time they see these shoulder patients, the rotator cuff is often not repairable. That is sad, and it happens to me, too, when I see a patient. Many times, it is not the insurance company's fault because it has not been that long. Rather, the delay occurs because the patient did not know they had a cuff tear; they were not painful until an aggravating event such as a minor work incident or a fateful football toss with the grandkids. Then when you do the M.R.I., you see the cuff, usually in the supraspinatus portion, is torn at its attachment. When it tears, it sits detached and when the muscle is activated, it moves, and it just hurts. And you reattach it arthroscopically with great success. *Hopefully.*

You see, in certain instances, when the patient comes to surgery the cuff is fully retracted, scarred, and immobile. When I put my instrument in the lateral (side) portal, I have the camera in the back, I pull on the cuff, and it doesn't go to where it must attach. I call it "peek and shriek." You look at it and the O.R. team collectively sighs, "Ugh!" because you cannot repair it. You clean it out, which sometimes offers the patient a little relief. But if that

198 · ALEJANDRO BADIA, M.D., F.A.C.S.

does not work, you must talk about other much more complex operations. It creates a HUGE cost when a rotator cuff tear (like many other medical problems) is neglected or the can is kicked down the road.

The irreparable rotator cuff caused my Montreal friends to depart from the Canadian socialized insurance system after many years. Their decision was not based on money, but the inability to practice medicine the way they were trained. While this is an extreme example, it also happens in non-socialized systems where there is too much interference within the patient journey. The consequential cost of that intrusion is apparent in many areas. With our shoulder patients, the cuff issue can become a rotator cuff arthropathy – arthritis due to lack of humeral head containment, and this requires a reverse shoulder replacement. I perform reverse shoulder replacements outpatient in our A.S.C., but most surgeons do this in a hospital. *Now* you are talking expensive care. Our over-regulated systems have become penny-wise and pound foolish. Stay out of our way, and most patients can have an outpatient cuff repair with three little portal holes versus a major open procedure with expensive implants in a hospital setting.

The shoulder is just one of many examples of how solving a problem earlier is much less costly. Take my dad, for example. He has a prostate problem; one he could have fixed but chose not to because he did not want to take the one in one-thousand chance of becoming impotent. You gotta know my dad; he is a character. It is sad because now he must cath himself. His urethra - the prostate – is so big. Yet it is a self-inflicted issue. Our health system must also accept that fact that many costly problems are partly due to patient inaction, or worse, poor behaviors that lead to hugely expensive medical issues downstream. Poor diet, smoking, inactivity, and high sugar intake are just some of the behaviors that impact our health economy. This is a separate issue from limiting or delaying access.

Whether it is a healthcare system that does not let you see the urologist for three years or our American system, things can always get worse. Think about cancer: if you discover a little lump on your body and it takes you a long time to get a biopsy, then all the sudden, maybe it is metastasized. That comes with huge economic implications because cancer care is expensive. These days, healthcare is much more technological. We cure more diseases. It is not a cheap process, but a patient with an arthritic knee who undergoes a procedure is going to use that knee for maybe another 30 to 40 years. And that has immeasurable value.

MEDICARE, MEDICAID, AND THE 90-DAY GLOBAL

Even though most physicians do their utmost to provide the best care possible at whatever the system decides to pay us (because we have little or no control over it), our exposure is unbelievable. What a crazy concept. In terms of Medicare, let us use the example of a total shoulder replacement, since the most patients who need this operation are over the age of 65. In a total shoulder replacement, the surgeon opens the patient's shoulder, removes the diseased joint, and puts in a new joint. It is a task of vital importance that demands skill, knowledge, and expertise. Yet because most of these patients are on Medicare, the highly trained and talented orthopedic surgeon is at the whim of bean-counters at the C.M.S. in Washington, D.C.

As you might imagine, the C.M.S. is a behemoth organization with complex formulas to determine payments. A hip replacement, Code 27130, pays around $1,320.96. An aortic valve replacement, Code 33405, pays around $2,329.08. A total shoulder replacement, Code 23470, pays about $1,164.56. Notice the specific amounts, down to the penny. Doesn't it make you wonder how they arrive at these figures? Regardless, after the right code is submitted for the patient's procedure, Medicare sends a check in the corresponding amount to the surgeon.

Did you know that anytime a surgeon is paid for a procedure, there is a 90-Day Global attached to it? That means when Medicare or an insurance company pays the doctor a certain amount for that surgery, during the three-month period that follows, every visit and every decision the doctor makes is included in the fee. Guess what happens? Every time that patient comes in, he or she is getting an X-ray because that is the only income the doctor can collect. Every time he sees a patient for follow-up, he tells them, "Well, we'd better check the X-ray." Granted, there are times when an X-ray is necessary, but there are many occasions when that physician says, "We need to get an X-ray on each visit because at least Medicare pays $58 for that." Yes, the X-ray machine and tech come with a cost, but at least you are capturing some income. I know it happens because I am guilty of this myself. With a 90-Day Global, the consultation and the decision-making time is included in the surgical payment. If a case is uncomplicated and a patient does well, it is not so terrible.

But what if a case gets complicated through no fault of the doctor? What if the patient is overweight, diabetic, or a smoker who cannot live with their shoulder pain? If I take that on, all the sudden I have bought a problem since these patients are bound to have post-op issues. I may even have to call their internist. Yet, unlike a lawyer who gets paid for their time (much more on that later) I do not get paid one red cent to handle all the additional complications.

With Medicare patients we must charge five times the amount…not that we expect to get it. As it stands, we must charge more because Medicare and the insurance companies pay us a percentage of our billed charges; they never just pay you what it is, whether it is Medicare or a private insurance company. What other profession works this way? None that I can think of.

Government controlled healthcare, in the form of Medicare, has brought many benefits to our elderly population. It has set the standard in certain areas. However, it is important to recognize the pitfalls and inefficiencies that often come along with big government.

During this week, I had an incident where my billing and collections team told me that Medicare denied payment for one of the digits for a patient on whom I had performed joint fusions on two adjacent painful fingers. When my team phoned C.M.S., they were told they only pay for one finger at a time. Incredulous, I asked my collections supervisor, "Do they understand that if I did the second finger at a different time, they would have to pay for the surgical facilities and anesthesia fees all over again?"

She simply replied, "That is their policy, and of course, it makes no sense." No good deed goes unpunished. I could be unscrupulous and schedule the patients' surgeries several months apart, but I do not think that is good for my patients, nor is it good for our overall healthcare costs. This anecdote illustrates the gross inefficiencies our system not only allows but perpetuates.

Stark Law and Safe Harbor Laws

In 1988, Democratic Congressman Pete Stark introduced an "Ethics in Patient Referrals Act," bill concerning physician self-referrals. Although crafted by a committee of mostly Democrats, it was named after Stark. Those involved in writing the bill took the approach that there would be an over utilization of healthcare if doctors can profit from ownership in something they can potentially refer to. It is a valid point, but as with many things in healthcare, the pendulum swings to satisfy lobbyists in big pharma and big hospitals. And physicians are terrible lobbyists. A pity since it became apparent that many of these legislators thought us doctors where the ones responsible for expensive healthcare. They need to perhaps read this book, and many others. As you will later see, it is nearly impossible to have any discussion with these folks who create policy, even in something as complex as healthcare delivery.

The 1989 law "prohibits a physician from making referrals for certain designated health services payable by Medicare to any entity with which he or she (an immediate family member) has a financial relationship (ownership, investment, or compensation), unless an exception applies," as stated on the Centers for Medicare and Medicaid website. Designated health services include clinical labs, physical therapy, occupational therapy, radiology, durable medical equipment, home health services, outpatient prescription drugs, and inpatient and outpatient hospital services.

When Stark and his fellow members of Congress first created this law, I did not even notice because my nose was in organic chemistry, followed by internship and residency. As I shared with you, for the decade of the 1980s, I spent my whole life in education and then in the early 90s on surgical training. Like any physician, I devoted a decade-and-a-half preparing for an occupation without realizing I would be up against all these ridiculous regulations that are often more harmful than helpful. Let me reiterate that yes, there are bad apples in the medical profession (as in every walk of life) and for that reason, we need some degree of checks and balances. However, it should be a system of checks and balances, not overbearing laws.

In July 2018, C.M.S. administrator Seema Verma announced that her agency hoped to issue a proposed regulation by the end of the year to loosen the Stark rule, citing that burdensome regulations create barriers to value-based care. A few months later, witnesses at a House hearing testified that the law was getting in the way of forming accountable care organizations and other alternative payment models (A.P.M.'s). This past October 2019, the Trump Administration proposed an overhaul of the law against self-referral with the goal of boosting the adoption of value-based care; promoting coordinated patient care; and fostering improved quality, outcomes, and efficiency. To that end, the HHS Office of the Inspector General identified 10 safe harbors in the Stark Law.

At present, the even more complex safe harbor laws allow a physician to bring surgical cases to a surgery center, but it must be one third of their volume. The idea behind it, of course, is "I don't want you to own in 10 different surgery centers, which would enable you to collect some distributions every month. Frankly, if you are busy enough to bring cases to 10 different surgery centers, then, why not? The government stifles entrepreneurship, and instead of taking the approach of, "Hey, let's look at this from the bird's eye view. People who are doing things they shouldn't be doing will be apparent to us," they spend too much time and money going after stuff that doesn't matter. Meanwhile, there are doctors out there making a mint by injecting stem cells for cash and these agencies are only now beginning to look at them because they are policing people who do not need much policing.

I understand the intent. But when you interfere with the free market you create bigger problems. Granted, we could be Venezuela or Russia or China for that matter, but we are not. With all our challenges, we still have the best healthcare system in the world due to innovation. When the government stifles and restricts it, it makes me worry about the future. Which reminds me of a rampant problem among physicians: we have not taken the time to protect our turf, compared with chiropractors, for example, who are brilliant at it. Yet chiropractors do not take emergency calls at 3 am.

How the Government-Mandated HCAHPS: Hospital Consumer Assessment of Health Care Providers, Contributed to the Opioid Crisis – A Uniquely American Phenomenon

Unless you have been living under a rock for the past several years, you know that the United States is dealing with a severe and devastating opioid crisis. While there are many contributing factors at play, one of the root causes is yet another well-intentioned mandate from the C.M.S., a policy known as the "H-caps Scores" (Hospital Consumer Assessment of Health Care Providers). According to the H-cap website:

"The HCAHPS (Hospital Consumer Assessment of Healthcare Providers and Systems) Survey is the first national, standardized, publicly reported survey of patients' perspectives of hospital care. HCAHPS (pronounced "H-caps"), also known as the CAHPS® Hospital Survey*, is a 32-item survey instrument and data collection methodology for measuring patients' perceptions of their hospital experience. While many hospitals have collected information on patient satisfaction for their own internal use, until HCAHPS there were no common metrics and no national standards for collecting and publicly reporting information about patient experience of care. Since 2008,

HCAHPS has allowed valid comparisons to be made across hospitals locally, regionally, and nationally.

"Three broad goals have shaped HCAHPS. First, the standardized survey and implementation protocol produces data that allow objective and meaningful comparisons of hospitals on topics that are important to patients and consumers. Second, public reporting of HCAHPS results creates new incentives for hospitals to improve quality of care. Third, public reporting enhances accountability in health care by increasing transparency of the quality of hospital care provided in return for the public investment."

How does it work in the real world? Dr. Scott A. Sigman, self-described "original opioid-sparing orthopedic surgeon, healer of knees and shoulders, left and right, and social media influencer," explains.

"In this program, the C.M.S. sends out questionnaires to the patient. Three or four of these questions pertain specifically to pain, for example, 'Was your pain monitored carefully?' 'Were you receiving appropriate pain management while you were in the hospital?'

"And if you were getting poor scores as the treating physician, the insurance companies would say, 'Well, you're not doing a good job of pain management, so we're going reduce the amount of money we're going to pay you for the procedures you're doing.'

"I want to be clear: there are some bad apples out there. You read about these doctors who are rolling out these crazy prescriptions in the pill farms and there is no doubt they should suffer the consequences of their actions. However, most doctors were just caught up in this societal pressure of pain relief. We needed to make sure our patients were out of pain and opioids were the most available pain relievers. We were told they were inexpensive and relatively non-addictive. We did not understand the severity of the addiction potential associated with the medications.

"The opioid crisis is a uniquely American phenomenon. No other country in the world has an opioid crisis like we do. The best way to describe what happened to our society is that we were fooled into believing that pain had to be kept to a minimum and opioids were safe, inexpensive, and effective in pain control. The entire medical community got caught up in the wave of opioid pain management and the opioid crisis became an iatrogenic reality. Nurses and doctors were trained to stay ahead of a patient's pain and have them take the medication.

"What happened is that we were created this swath of patients that became addicted. They now have substance use disorder for the rest of their lives. We are treating overdoses routinely in our emergency rooms and intensive care units, and we must arm our first responders with Narcan to save lives. Men and women are dying everyday across our country due to opioid-related events. In both dollars and loss of life, the cost to our society due to opioids is overwhelming.

"Opioid alternatives are much more expensive than opioids. Opioids pills are relatively inexpensive; 30 pills cost about $10. On the other hand, opioid alternatives such as EXPAREL® (liposomal bupivacaine) costs $300 per patient for lower extremity surgery, and $170 for upper extremity surgery. While this increased cost per patient may not seem overwhelming, if totaled over the year for all surgical patients, it can drastically affect the pharmacy budget which is where we have seen push back from hospital systems.

"Yet as we consider cost, we must consider value to the entire medical and social system – not just hospital budgets. If we are operating on patients and saving money on pharmacy budgets and 13 percent of patients are becoming addicted, we are setting up society with an overwhelming financial burden to care for the substance use disorder patients we have created. We are currently spending billions of dollars on the sequalae of the epidemic much less the tremendous loss of life. Money is being spent on substance use disorder clinics and emergency responders for overdoses, not to mention the loss or productivity at work, and the substantial bill to hospitals that must care for the patients that require expensive medical treatment for overdoses.

"The CDC released a study last year that focused on three numbers: six, 13, and 30. If you prescribe a patient a single-day prescription of opioids (24-hours-worth), six out of 100 will still be on opioids after one year. If you write a prescription for 10 days of opioids for 100 patients, 13 out of 100 will still be on opioids after one year. If you are really kind and give them a 30-day supply, one-third of the patients will still be on opioids a year later. Opioids are incredibly addictive, and at this time, we do not have the ability to test for whom will become addicted. The best solution for providers is to operate on our patients and do our best to minimize their exposure to opioids.

"The good news is now there are doctors like Dr. Badia and me, along with key opinion leaders across the country that champion an opioid-sparing approach. And we are making a difference because we are noticing a paradigm shift in post-operative pain management. With the use of opioid alternatives, we're providing significant pain relief for our patients and minimizing their exposure to these highly addictive medications."

How did the mitigation of pain become such a prominent feature of medicine?

According to the National Institutes of Health, the pain as the "fifth vital sign" originated in 1995, "when Dr. James Campbell addressed the American Pain Society urging that health care providers treat pain as the "fifth vital sign" (P5VS) (American Pain Society, 1999), highlighting the essential need for improved pain care (American Pain Society Quality of Care Committee, 1995). Shortly thereafter, the Veterans Health Administration (VHA) introduced a national strategy to improve pain treatment (Veterans Health Administration, 2009) that included mandatory pain screening using the unidimensional Numeric Rating Scale (NRS). As part of an effort to improve pain care, pain-related questions were also added to patient satisfaction surveys. These initiatives were directed at improving pain care broadly, to include patients with both acute and chronic pain."

But as Dr. Sigman notes, "Vital signs are supposed to be objective measurements of vital bodily function. Pain is incredibly subjective; there can be no objective measurement of pain. If you have ever visited someone in the hospital, you have probably seen the whiteboard with the faces on the scale that were used to replace the numbers. The expressions range from a big smiley face with a 0 and the words 'No Hurt' underneath to a teary-eyed face with a 10 and the words 'Hurts Worst' underneath. Here is a sad fact: the only face of a patient that is pain-free while on opioids is a sleeping face. In my opinion, the system needs to be completely revamped. I like to walk into the recovery room and see my patient smiling at me, talking to me, and using their cell phone. I do not need a scale to know when my patient's pain is well controlled.

"A good friend of mine, Dr. Michael Redler, another orthopedic surgeon in Connecticut, is another big fan of opioid-sparing surgery. He believes we should change it from a 'Pain Scale' to a 'Comfort Scale.' In other words, ask the patient, 'How comfortable are you on a scale of zero to 10?' or 'How comfortable are you right now?' Let us eliminate the word 'pain' from medicine and make people comfortable. What a simple but innovative idea."

Unfortunately, most government-mandated programs have transformed the simple art of medicine into a complex juggernaut. The EXPAREL® debate, as mentioned by Dr. Sigman, like so many other positive developments in healthcare, quickly become mired in upfront cost issues, like arguing against the price of a joint replacement, and not looking at the cost of alternative treatments, length of infirmity, and impact to a person's life and productivity. It becomes clear that our decision makers are pennywise, but very pound foolish.

PACs, POLITICIANS, and PHYSICIANS

In 2018, I hosted a political fundraiser for Ana Maria Rodriguez, a former member of the Doral City Council, who was running for state representative in the Florida House. Because she is pro-physician and ran on a platform of preserving our rights, I supported her with a fundraiser at my home, which was organized by the Dade County Medical Association, now run by the same person who runs the Florida Orthopedic Society. We had poor turnout, and in perhaps the ultimate irony, not one orthopedic surgeon attended. Thankfully, Rodriguez won the election and remains one of the few pro-medicine members of the health committee, most of whom have connections to trial lawyers.

As physicians, we can blame government for our problems, but we must also accept fault for not doing enough to push back. While I am complaining, I donate to political action committees at the national and state level. There is a PAC for orthopedic surgeons based in Washington, D.C., but I do not give them as much money as I should. I also donate to the Academy of Orthopaedic Surgeons whose meetings I attend. However, I have reached a point where I think, "Geez, I'm giving and yet others aren't."

Here is an example. I remember standing up at a meeting in Florida and talking about clinical collarbone fracture. After I made my comments, the chairman of the roundtable said,

"Let me understand this. Are you saying you do the surgery outpatient?" And I replied, "Yes, I've been doing it that way for years now." The people in the room were astounded, yet now I hear that this is not so uncommon, and I am proud of that. However, what people in the healthcare community fail to grasp is the significant cost savings.

Another example of the amount of money I saved the system involves a middle-aged male patient who initially presented to a hospital with a humerus (upper arm) fracture. It is an unbelievable story. He sat in a hospital bed for two days, with no clear plan articulated to him by the consulting orthopedic surgeon, after being admitted via the emergency room. He would have sat around in an expensive hospital bed, for another day or two before the busy surgeon could put it on his schedule. Afterwards, he might have stayed in the hospital for an additional two days since they likely will not use EXPAREL® for pain control, increasing his chances of complications like a nosocomial (hospital acquired) infection. The patient spoke to a friend who alerted him to fact that I would likely handle this fully on an outpatient basis, which I did. He recovered beautifully, like the ten humerus fractures preceding him over past few years. If you have a system and teamwork, you can save an immense amount of money while providing better care.

Simply factor in the hospital cost to put in that kind of hardware and the entire operation would be three times the amount of money than it was at our center. Then there are other costs the hospitals add on. For example, they often send things to the pathologist to review and they docpa more imaging studies than necessary. In this case, I did not need a C.A.T. scan; I saw on the X-ray that is was broken. Once I get in, I will fix it. I challenge anybody to look at what we did with Miami hand center in the 1990s and early 2000s, in terms of providing care to thousands and thousands of patients. We saved the healthcare system and our community an immeasurable amount of money and aggravation.

Once, a guy came in at one or two in the morning, whose forearm had been crushed by a forklift at a factory. He was of course brought to the hospital first, but because the E.R. was overwhelmed and the Miami Hand Center had such a good reputation, they put a splint on him and sent him to us. We finished the surgery at five or six in the morning. Granted, I didn't sleep that night but I would have suffered a lot more if I had to make a trip to the hospital and wait for them to give me a room…only to get bumped by a "hot" gallbladder that couldn't wait. That is part of life for a surgeon. And if surgery can be done in outpatient center, it is beneficial for the surgeon and the patient. It is good for the insurer and the overall healthcare system. Nobody, not even the government, can argue against that…although they tried. More on that later.

(LOCAL) POLITICS AS USUAL

About four or five years ago, the commissioner of Miami, who is now current mayor, asked me to put together a financial analysis on the cost of workers' comp in our county, a topic we'll discuss further in the next chapter. As a cross-fit enthusiast, he had more of a personal interest but in Miami-Dade County, everyone complains about crowded emergency rooms. I engaged our OrthoNOW® cofounder, a Wharton MBA whiz-kid who loves data, and we built a cost model surrounding a commonly presenting malady. DeQuervain's tendonitis, sometimes known as "Mommy wrist." It occurs in postpartum in women, due to the fluid shifts. Pregnant women suffer from back pain, swollen ankles, and carpal tunnel syndrome because of the fluid, but they also get tendinitis. While tendinitis occurs in the general population, more women than men suffer from this painful condition. Blue collar workers can occasionally suffer from DeQuervain's tendonitis if they hit their wrist or engage in heavy work. It is not usually caused by work, but it can be primarily related to and aggravated by work.

We decided to analyze the cost of an average case (not an expensive one) if a patient with DeQuervain's tendonitis came directly to OrthoNOW, where we have a focused orthopedic emergency room, versus a typical hospital E.R. where you must compete with somebody who came in with chest pain. Assuming the patient is among the 80 percent for whom the condition resolves in one visit, the cost is $700. Yet this is the kind of case that comes to the hired primary care physicians making an hourly salary. They are much like triage people because they cannot treat most of the things they see. Now, if the primary care doctor has some good hand knowledge, they will pick up on the problem and give the patient an injection. Medical literature shows 80 percent of them are resolved with an injection.

But that is not what happens most of the time. Instead, when the patient arrives to an occupational health center with a painful wrist, they order an expensive M.R.I. test, then therapy. Part of the rationale for ordering therapy is that these chains are incentivized to order physiotherapy from the get-go. Even for patients who come in with a rotator cuff tear, they order therapy before they make the diagnosis. And if you have a rotator cuff problem, the last thing you want is somebody cranking on your arm because it hurts.

Getting back to our DeQuervain's tendonitis patient. Now this person, a blue-collar worker, is doing excruciating therapy. They dread going to the physical therapist, but they think, "No pain, no gain. I'm supposed to be doing this because the doctor told me I need to do this." After a month of therapy, the primary care doctor often tells them it is not better or that they need more therapy. It is a long, painful, and expensive journey, one we figured out costs about $12,000 by the time they are referred to a hand specialist. Now, $12,000 is not much compared to what workers' comp spends on a shoulder. Because that is such a big joint, shoulder patients do months of therapy before they finally send them to me.

Our financial analysis, the one the then-commissioner of Miami-Dade requested from us, proved we could save Miami-Dade County – just our county alone - $9.7 million per year. And we could save the city of Miami $1.3 million per year. Impressive, right? Here is the kicker: I could not get traction for that, even though the local government asked me to conduct the analysis. They asked us to produce a report that they have yet to look at. This was five years ago. This was local government. Are you sure you want the federal government in charge of lowering healthcare costs after understanding this simple example?

The Joint Commission for Hospital Accreditation

Although technically not a government program, The Joint Commission for Hospital Accreditation, founded in 1951, is an independent, not-for-profit organization, founded that wields significant influence over public healthcare policy. From their website, JointCommission.org:

"An independent, not-for-profit organization, The Joint Commission is the nation's oldest and largest standards-setting and accrediting body in health care. To earn and maintain The Gold Seal of Approval® from The Joint Commission, an organization undergoes an on-site survey by a Joint Commission survey team at least every three years (Laboratories are surveyed every two years).

The Joint Commission is governed by a 21-member Board of Commissioners that includes physicians, administrators, nurses, employers, quality experts, a consumer advocate, and educators. The Joint Commission employs approximately 1,000 people in its surveyor force, at its central office in Oakbrook Terrace, Illinois, and at an office in Washington, D.C."

Dr. Mark S. Rekant, M.D. of the Philadelphia Hand to Shoulder Center, advocates for oversight of the Joint Commission:

"It is helpful to have government oversight and administrators that make sure that the centers we work in outside the hospitals are safe. We all want safety. But the way our system is currently set up, there is no one overseeing the Joint Commission for Hospital Accreditation (JCAHO), meaning that the Joint Commission can demand that a hospital change the tile on the floor because of small cracks. This is costly to the patient because these costs get passed down to them.

"The Joint Commission can come to your hospital and say you need to have all these things, even if they are small, frivolous, and not medically related; or non-physicians; or non-practicing physicians. No one can push back. There is no appeal process to say "Listen, listen, the things the Joint Commission are recommending are only going to add to costs while not improving patient safety. We all have benefited from the government setup of checks and balances, yet the Joint Commission does not allow for appeals. All that does is drive up costs.

"For instance, my surgery center is required to have two recovery room areas, although we only use one, because having two is plain stupid. When you do a five-minute surgery, you do not need to have the patient recover twice. They put disposable heating blankets on a patient who is having a 10-minute operation. You cannot lose that much heat in 10 minutes. You have probably sat on the couch longer than that without a blanket. But we must do it because the Joint Commission requires it, not because it is based on scientific evidence.

"While it is helpful to some extent when JCAHO evaluates a hospital for safety and ensures that documentation is accurate, they become excessive with their criteria that is not justified with research and paper, versus if Dr. Badia and I want to do a surgery on a patient. With papers and evidence, we could say, "We looked at 1,000 patients and this surgery works 90 percent of the time or 85 percent of the time."

"With the Joint Commission, there is no evidence half the time. What is worse is that each state also has its own regulatory body. So, there is a state commission that looks at 30 centers, and then there is a national Joint Commission. The surgery centers get regulated twice, adds to the cost and the confusion.

"Like any other self-fulfilling organization, if the organization does not find any flaws in hospitals, then there is no reason for that organization to continue to exist. And the only way JCAHO can justify their existence is to find flaws. It is a catch-22. If there was some oversight of this oversight committee, there would be some checks and balances."

Regulatory Requirements and Medical Devices

I would be remiss if I failed to include the medical device industry among a vital aspect of healthcare that suffers from excessive government regulation. Kimberly Light, Director of Regulatory Affairs at BioPro, an implant manufacturing company founded by orthopedic surgeon Charles O. Townley, M.D. explains:

"I have been in the medical device industry for over 20 years in different capacities. I started as a design engineer and am now working with regulatory. In my role, I deal with the F.D.A. and I.S.O. and quality management systems within the business. I do not have much direct interaction with insurance and coverage and expenses, although I can tell you about the factors that contribute to cost from the inside of a manufacturing company.

"Several regulatory requirements go into putting and keeping a medical device on the market. We must work with the F.D.A. and our I.S.O. auditors. Internationally, there are all kinds of different governing bodies with slightly different requirements for what it takes to get a device approved and kept on the market. Many of these requirements help make to make things safer for patients, so by and large, requirements are a good thing.

"On the other hand, a few rules are in place that have no common sense behind them. They just add cost from a manufacturing standpoint, which is passed on to customers. Where we struggle the most is dealing with the hospitals. From my side of the fence, the hospital seems to be the biggest inefficiency and cost center within the whole process. It is difficult to get devices approved in the hospital because of contracting. They hospitals working hard to minimize the number of vendors they work with. That means, they push out a lot of the small manufacturers, in favor of obtaining contracts with the big guys like Stryker and Zimmer. They do not give the smaller companies a chance to sell into their hospital.

"Yet, you tend to see the most innovation with small vendors. They are usually the ones at the forefront of innovating new medical devices or products to help patients in niche markets. Due to the hospitals' reluctance to allow smaller vendors to sell, it makes it difficult to get off the ground running. As a small business, that is what my company struggles with – getting permission from the hospitals to sell within.

"Recently, we received a contract from a local and relatively big hospital in our area. Built into their contract agreement was a clause that said we would give them the best price anywhere. And then on top of that, we had to give them rebates every quarter, that totaled 13 percent of their total sales. This was NOT a discount; it was a rebate. We had to write them a check back at the end of the quarter for 13 percent of their total sales. And the reason they are doing that as a rebate instead of as a discount off the price of the product is *because then they do not have to claim it to Medicare.* It is a straight up profit, whereas, if it is a discount off a line item on an invoice, they must disclose that discount to Medicare. Basically, the hospitals see this kind of stuff as an additional profit center. It is cash right in their pocket that they do not have to disclose. That makes it nearly impossible as a small business to contract with some of these different hospitals when they build in those types of demands.

"From my standpoint, hospitals seem to be the most archaic, inefficient, and poorly run. It is a generalization and does not include all of them, but most people can see that. If you go to the hospital to get something done, how many different invoices do you receive for different bills that you cannot follow? They intentionally make it difficult. As a small medical device manufacturing company that is probably our biggest roadblock to growing at a rapid pace: getting into the hospitals. To top it off, hospitals have taken away the surgeons' ability to choose the products that are best for their customers – their patients. The hospitals' purchasing departments, comprised of accountants, make these decisions based on straight-up dollars and sales quotas to meet a purchasing agreement. They do not allow the surgeons to choose what is best for their individual patients. To me, that is probably the biggest issue, and the most upsetting. You have well educated professionals who have been through multiple years of medical school. They know what the patient needs and what would be best for them. Yet most of the time, they cannot even use that product, which is very bothersome.

"The total cost of medical devices as a percentage of overall healthcare costs is miniscule. I sat through one presentation at a conference that revealed the total cost of a medical device for a typical orthopedic surgery was three percent, and everything else is overhead: physical therapy, follow-up care, surgical suite time, doctors. But the manufacturers are the ones being squeezed.

"I believe the way forward to improve health care in the in the United States is to get more oversight on the hospitals from a cost standpoint *and* a regulatory standpoint. At BioPro, we get audited by the F.D.A. and the I.S.O.

multiple times a year to various regulatory requirements and quality management requirements to make sure we are doing the right things and have the right controls in place. From what I have witnessed in products coming back from hospitals, the hospitals do not have that same level of oversight.

"We get surgical trays back that have been used in a surgery that are filthy and have never been cleaned. We get products back that have been opened and they are not supposed to send them to us like that. All it does is introduce risk into the system. If hospitals had a little more oversight in that area, it would improve things. You hear about infection rates. And the F.D.A. and I.S.O. are on top of manufacturers to make sure we are complying with all their requirements. Of course, we should have their controls in place. We constantly monitor our cleaning process and our sterilization process. We put all kinds of checks and balances in place to make sure things are as they should be when they leave here. And if the infection rate was caused by the manufacturers in the product that they are shipping out, then the infection rate across the country would be the same regardless of the hospital you are in. But if you research the infection rate statistics, they are all over the place based on where you are. And that is due to hospital practices and their systems. From my standpoint, just that fact alone should drive more oversight into the hospitals.

"And how effective is it? I visited a friend in the hospital this past fall who had a procedure. The daily surgery list and any modifications – everything, was handwritten. There were volunteers checking people in and out that did not know what they were doing. There was all kinds of miscommunication and misinformation that caused multiple issues throughout the whole process. How difficult is it to automate that stuff? Everything is very, very archaic. On the other hand, hospitals are great at other things – the controls they have on medication and the scanning of those types of things are excellent. But any patient or doctor that has done anything at a hospital knows that the electronic health records are a joke because nobody's system talks to anybody else's system. There was no standard put in place to mandate that they talk to each other. One hospital system utilizes System A another hospital system utilizes System B…and they do not necessarily talk nice to each other.

"Nobody seems to know what is going on from one place to the next. So really, how effective was that whole process? In theory it is a wonderful idea, but it was poorly executed. And all those things add costs. All the barcoding we must do to meet the new requirements, add a ton of cost and complexity to the whole process. And I am not convinced at this point that any of that data is being utilized in an effective way.

"Part of that is because the regulators that mandated it did not do a good job of creating that system. That is what happens when politicians create legislation involving healthcare. I do not think they have any place in the discussion, which must be cross-functional. Industry, providers, and patients must be involved if we are to come up with a system and a process that works for everybody.

"Another factor that drives up healthcare costs are the multiple requirements of multiple countries. For example, the European Union is one market with its own requirements, systems, and processes. And it is super expensive to comply with all those different requirements and bring a product to market. Well, that cost gets spread across the entire world. If you must pay all kinds of money to be in the European market, that cost must be distributed across your piece price that you sell in every market. And with the changing tide in the European regulations, many companies are pulling out of Europe altogether. It is becoming such a mess that Europe is prepping for medical device shortages. As they deal with Brexit on top of the European changes, the U.K. is preparing for inevitable shortages. Many manufacturers are either pulling or becoming selective about the product lines they offer. We are going to see the impact of that in the United States, where costs will increase.

"It has not been a fun process to navigate internationally. Whereas the U.S. used to be one of the most difficult markets to get into, prompting companies to go to Canada or Europe first, that pendulum has swung back the other direction. The F.D.A. is much more willing to work with manufacturers to help them. Do not misunderstand. They are still enforcing and auditing and doing everything they need to do. However, they are doing it with more educated auditors, and they are spending much more time educating their staff. And they are doing it with a little bit more of commonsense approach, focusing on what is important, rather than some of the things that were just nonvalue added. I do think innovation might start to increase in the U.S. if we can get the hospitals out of the way.

"Hospitals now are all part of major health systems, and that means purchasing power. Some big conglomerates own hospitals all over the country, with their headquarters in some obscure city in some state that is unrelated to any of the hospitals that make the purchasing decisions. It is sad because it is not in the best interest of the patients at all. Now for some products – if it is a standard off-the-shelf syringe – there is minimal difference from one syringe to the next. In that scenario, I get it. But when it comes to implants, or injections, or different types of procedures and you've got the insurance companies and the hospital purchasing departments making the decisions about what is available to the end-user, and how much they are going to pay for all the options, that is not in the best interest of the people.

"No matter the issue, it never seems to be in the best interest of the patient or the doctor who is trying to give them the best care. And you need to rely on the doctors' expertise and allow them input into the treatment. That is what they went to school for. That is why they should get the big bucks. It should not be somebody in the purchasing department. And now with the Sunshine Act, we have all these controls in place to make sure surgeons are not getting kickbacks from manufacturers. Great. There should be oversight on that, 100 percent. But where is the oversight on the purchasing departments in the hospitals? They have no oversight. And that benefits large manufacturers over the small ones. nothing preventing them.

"In terms of patient education, patients should be informed that their surgeon may or may not have access to the treatment option that is the best for them. And knowing that, they can get a second opinion – outside of the same health system from which they got the first opinion. Because different hospitals and doctors have access to different things, it is vital for patients to do their research. At our company, we have seen a huge uptick in the number of actual patients that reach out to us directly. The increase from last year to this year was just incredible. Patients will say, 'We saw this product on your website, can you give us some information? Can you recommend a surgeon in my area because I really feel this is the best option for me and my surgeon didn't talk to me about this?' The best thing people can do is educate themselves.

"Before I worked at BioPro in implants, I worked in a medical device manufacturer that produced external prosthetics. We made prosthetic feet, a low-risk device. So, there was not a lot of interaction with the F.D.A., but Medicare was going insane: 'You're not allowed to give this patient a better foot, because they're only going to be able to be active to this level, or they're only active to this level right now.' Well, they are only active to this level right now because they are diabetic, and they just had their leg amputated. However, if you would let us give them this better foot, they will have more potential for increased activity, and therefore, increased quality of life. But

Medicare insisted, "No you can only give them up to this foot," which was horrible. Eight years ago, Medicare was doing that kind of stuff.

"People do not realize that this whole side of the industry exists. They do not think about the fact that people do what I do, or that there are companies like BioPro. They think of a hospital when they think of healthcare, but they do not realize that hospitals are businesses that get product from a multitude of other vendors. It is no different than building a car. Ford does not build every single component that they assemble into that car. They assemble it, but their vendors give them everything. It is the same with hospitals. They assemble this healthcare package based on what their suppliers provide to them. When I first went into bioengineering, I wanted to work on prosthetic feet. Everybody I knew asked, 'People do that? That is a thing?' It just does not occur to anyone that this is a career path because it is outside the scope of everyday interaction. Yet it is such an important part of healthcare. I do not know why schools do not educate students about this kind of career path. If you do not deal with it directly, it never enters your thought process that this whole little healthcare microcosm exists."

I will expand much more on the bureaucratic hospital system in the next chapter.

Making Healthcare Great Again?

Government interference, a bipartisan problem, drives healthcare costs up. I can provide an excellent example in a patient who is close to our current president. As you read, consider that if this saga can happen to him, how much worse can it get for the average person with no high-profile connections? In his case, our businessman leveraged his connections to the most powerful person in the United States to salvage his situation to an acceptable – but by no means ideal – degree.

This individual, President Trump's right-hand man in the region of the Florida Keys, was the President's go-to guy in the aftermath of Hurricane Harvey, which inundated the city of Houston with water. He is a logistics guy who knows how to get stuff done…well, achieving efficient healthcare is another story, but I digress. He cut the two flexor tendons in his little finger, causing it to stick straight out. In an understandable reflex action, he went to a local E.R. in the lower Keys.

If you speak to a hand surgeon, they will tell you it is a technically difficult procedure to get a good result. It is painstaking, particularly in the small finger. Mind you, there are no hand surgeons in the Keys. In the span of 180 miles from my old practice in Kendall all the way to Key West, there is not one single hand surgeon. Of course, my general orthopedic and plastic surgery colleagues may cover hand calls at these locations, but each one possesses varying skills, and unless you fix flexor tendons all the time, it is hard to obtain an ideal result. For this reason, I abandoned brachial plexus work over 15 years ago; some issues are too complex to dabble in occasionally.

In this businessman's case, the hospital E.R. contacted the plastic surgeon on call, the same one who often fixes lacerations. He took the patient to the O.R. and tried to repair the tendon but could not find it because it had retracted. He ended up making a big incision in the palmar side of the wrist and forearm, subsequently causing much scarring. Bottom line: the patient never got a decent repair – an understandable yet avoidable outcome.

By the time the guy came to see me, the Mayor of Doral and three other people had called me multiple times to ask, "Hey Badia, can you get this guy in?" Isn't it ironic, it was one of the only times I have every heard from the city administration, despite the many times I had attempted to help our city avoid this exact situation? Yet neither the current mayor, not the past two mayors ever reached out to me, until this well-connected patient had a serious problem that required my services and expertise. That being that I have an excellent relationship with the city leaders, all smart people. Somehow, healthcare just isn't given the attention it deserves. The functions and initiatives are just turned over to the health insurance company du jour. You know how interested they are in the actual nuances of care.

Of course, we extended our customary personal touch and expedited his evaluation. When the patient came in, his condition was so bad it was affecting his other fingers. He had never even been sent to therapy. This is not some average Joe, but a guy who regularly golfs with the president. Yes, in the United States of America, land of tremendous, available subspecialists. Because his entire hand was stiff and not just the small finger, I had to free up a tremendous amount of scar tissue before I could order therapy. And guess what? He went back and he golfs with Trump now in New Jersey on a regular basis.

Taking advantage of the opportunity, I implored him, "Look, the one lesson you gotta get to President Trump about our healthcare, if he really wants to fix it, is there are too many people with their hand in the cookie jar that add to the cost and make it less efficient. Look what happened to you. In the E.R., they had to know that you really needed a hand surgeon. What they should have done is given you a couple stitches in, put a dressing on it, and it would have been fine. They could have simply called me or any one of multiple hand surgeons in the Miami area that could have done it a week later." In a case like this, you must close the wound. You cannot leave it open. And that's the ER's job: to make the diagnosis and stabilize it, meaning, put the dressing on, administer some antibiotics, tie a few stitches in his skin to close it, and instruct the patient, "You need to see a hand surgeon to fix the flexor tendons, then do the rehab." It is a long process and the system failed us, with huge (or, to use President Trump's word, "yuge") consequences. This patient still does not have good control of the finger. I advised him that I could transfer a tendon from here to here to give him more control, but at this point he' is doing everything he wants to do and has declined the offer.

However, suppose he decided to take me up on that. He would have had two surgeries – termed a "two-stage flexor tendon reconstruction," in addition to the first one I did to salvage his overall hand function. Now we are up to four surgeries in total, with hand rehab in between and afterwards. It is the same type of surgery I performed on the famous wide receiver T.O., Terrell Owens, who had been dropping passes for the Dallas Cowboys after he ruptured the ring finger flexor tendon. Because the Cowboys had been in playoff contention, T.O. and the Cowboys organization made a calculated decision to defer repair. During the off-season, he obtained various opinions before Cowboys owner Jerry Jones called me on my cellphone. Not sure how that happened, but T.O. soon flew to Miami, where I performed the surgery. The following season, he led the NFL in touchdown receptions. Sure, T.O. is a professional athlete and they tend to garner attention to these issues, as I heard it discussed on ESPN. However, the care and necessity were not much different for T.O. or my politically connected golfer. The latter did not undergo the necessary therapy after his first surgery, so perhaps this scenario could have been avoided altogether. How much do you think that costs our overall healthcare system?

Once Trump's guy recovered, we spoke on several occasions outside of the medical environment. One occasion stands out in my mind, not only because of the lovely setting but also because of the monumental advice he gave me. "Look, Alejandro," he began. "You have young kids. Enjoy them.

Since you like to practice medicine, don't knock yourself out. Healthcare is controlled by insurance companies and big pharma. That's it."

Perhaps he is right. However, the curse of the entrepreneur is to identify opportunities to remedy a problem. Our government's approach to healthcare revolves around a discussion of who is going to pay for it, not the ways in which we can improve its delivery. This patient's "little pinky" injury presented an ideal chance to get the ear of the president and yet, I got zero traction. On a local level, his injury brought me no closer to obtaining a working dialogue with my local city leaders who implored me to get him in for consultation ASAP. Did they not think this scenario is what I witness every Monday when I see patients? I could tell similar stories from the City of Doral workers, including several policemen who did not know our center even existed, let alone our orthopedic walk-in center. Understand this is happening in a well-run city of barely 50,000 people. And I pay plenty of commercial property tax to boot. I could share similar accounts of work-related injuries that were sustained by city workers, local mom-and- pop carpentry shops, and hotel workers at the now famous, Trump Doral Hotel. If this debacle repeats itself, week in and week out, in our own small microcosm of a city government, imagine the challenge at our county, state, or federal level where my patient has a close connection to the most powerful person in the United States. There just does not seem to be a genuine will to listen to those who live the problem and consider their ideas about how to fix it. Nobody is listening to those of us in the trenches…

Healthcare and Politics
Georgia State Senator Kay Kirkpatrick, M.D.

"As an orthopedic hand surgeon for over 30 years, I spent many days jumping through hoops to get my patients what they needed. These struggles included "peer-to-peer" phone calls that were usually not with a peer and were always inconvenient, pre-authorization for any and all procedures, requirements to do procedures in a less efficient and more expensive setting, and many others familiar to all physicians.

"While serving as Co-President of my large orthopedic group for many years, I did a lot of advocacy at the state and federal levels. Our group hired a lobbyist to help us build relationships with legislators and to represent us at the state Capitol. Many issues that affect our practices are handled at the state level, such as Workers Compensation, Certificate-of-

Need laws, scope of practice, and insurance regulation. These can make a huge difference for doctors in their practice environment and finances. Federal issues are also important to physicians and many times we must rely on our specialty groups (AAOS for example) to represent us at that level.

"When I retired in 2017, I ran for an open state Senate seat and won, becoming the fourth physician in our legislature. I did this to represent physicians and patients and it has been an eye-opening experience. The learning curve is steep, and the frustration level is high, but I have managed to become an effective legislator and to make a difference for my colleagues and our patients. The problems we face are extensive and the solutions not always readily apparent, but at least I can serve as an educated voice on healthcare. Not everyone is interested in running for office, but doctors can still engage in the process by educating your legislators about medical issues and by supporting candidates who are interested in helping physicians."

Although outside forces are making our lives as doctors difficult, there are opportunities to make things better by engaging in the process.

MORE (D.C.) POLITICS AS USUAL

Another local (for me) and national example is Florida Senator, Marco Rubio, an intelligent, fellow Cuban American immigrant (although not born abroad like me), who quickly rose in the political ranks. I first met him at a political fundraiser held at the home of a prominent Cuban American cardiothoracic surgeon. At the time, Mr. Rubio was seeking support in his bid to become Florida Speaker of the House in our state legislature. He succeeded in his goal, which eventually propelled him to the United States Senate.

I supported him and his campaign with a modest check and took the opportunity to explain some of the challenges we were facing. Ever charismatic, he listened intently but once he rose to State Senator, it became impossible to reach him, even though the "Miami boy" and I know many people in common. To be fair, I am not a Miami native, but why should that be an issue? This is not a dictatorial regime, like the one he continually battles in Venezuela. Access to our legislators should not require yet more money, but rather the introduction of good ideas to help our nation solve its problems. I again supported him by attending the ribbon cutting of his senatorial office, located directly across the street from my orthopedic ecosystem center.

That day is etched in my memory. I was in surgery when earlier that morning one of the local business leaders informed me about his ceremony and brief speech he planned to make. Partly due to its proximity, I thought it important enough to attend, and asked our nursing and anesthesia team to delay my next case for another 30 minutes. I hurried out of the A.S.C. O.R., throwing a white coat on over my scrubs, clogs, and all, and made it just in time as he stepped to the lectern. An excellent orator, he uttered some inspiring words and told us he was proud that his office was in Doral, adjacent to Trump's Hotel, and in the heart of a true American melting pot. Doral's demographics consist of over two-thirds foreign-born residents, well over 80 percent of them of Hispanic origin.

Once again, I tried to connect with him via his staff. While polite and receptive, that does not lead to change. True dialogue consists of the average healthcare practitioner explaining what they live through every day in the trenches and discussing possible solutions to prevent out healthcare bill from eclipsing the 20 percent GDP level. Based on my experience, I am not encouraged it will happen.

Still I made many more attempts at the national level. Through Senator Rubio's staff, we managed to procure an appointment at his office on Capitol Hill – amazing when you consider I could easily walk across the street to his Doral office and even delay a surgery to deliver a clear and urgent message. Regardless, I have proven that I can jump through the necessary hoops; the real question lies in the futility of these efforts.

We secured an appointment "with the senator" during a national healthcare meeting we decided to attend. I was not hopeful that much would transpire during the conference, so took the opportunity to make the appointment on the Hill. As I turned out, we were to go to Capitol Hill soon after my second knee surgery. Pretty ironic, huh? In speaking with those who have done prior lobbying activities and attested to the significant amount of walking I would have to do just to approach the Capitol, I decided to stay home and let our team – including my cofounder, Justin Irizarry – meet the Rubio team and a few congressional offices that represented Miami districts.

In every case, my team met with aides, not the congressional rep or the senator themselves – you know, the people we elect to office. I was not surprised. And as expected, nothing came out of it. My intuition, which turned out to be accurate, had told me to stay in Miami because I was still in pain and having difficulty ambulating. If I had felt it in my gut that the trip would have resulted in substantive sessions with our lawmakers, I would have made the arduous sacrifice.

Our modest attempts at the federal level to present a model on healthcare efficiency was understandably met with scant engagement. After all, if I could not get my own city and county to act upon an initiative that would save them $1.3 million and $9.7 million respectively – after they asked my team to prepare a cost-savings analysis on an alternative method of delivering care to their injured workforce – how could I expect more from Washington D.C.?

Undeterred by the advice my patient (Trump's guy) had given me, I decided to keep fighting for reform at the local level. I was soon to discover the exact nature of the problem, which involves much more than money as compared to the private sector level. Due to frustrations in obtaining a follow-up meeting with Miami city and county leaders for the purpose of presenting the results of the study THEY requested from us, I reached out to a well-connected attorney. Like many locals, he was a former patient of mine. Some months after arriving in Miami, I had a dinner meeting with my first partner and the CEO of a local hospital. Hospital CEOs like to meet the new surgeons in town, particularly if they could be a source of surgical cases, if they are on staff at that hospital. I would say the meeting was successful in that I brought a minimum of a thousand cases to this hospital, partly because of its focus and excellence in orthopedics, but also because more often than not they gave me two O.R.s to work out of, maximizing my efficiency.

Near the end of dinner, my beeper alerted me to call the answering service. By then, I had my new clunky cellphone and returned the call. It was a fingertip injury in the E.R. at the old Cedars Hospital, now the University of Miami Hospital. I thanked my dinner host and off I went to the hospital, around 10 p.m. like so many other countless nights. Upon arrival, I happened to see an X-ray of a bad elbow fracture on a lightboard. I attended to the fingertip injury, performed a simple local flap coverage in the E.R. procedure area, a gurney in the corner, and sent the newly fixed-up patient on his way. Next, I spoke to the highly competent emergency room physician who was concerned about the patient, whom I would discover was an attorney and the right-hand man to one of the county commissioners.

The E.R. doctor informed me that the orthopedist had not yet called back. Furthermore, he was not an elbow or upper limb specialist. Being the "new kid" in town, I promptly offered to handle the case and take the patient to the O.R. When the orthopedist did call in, I think he was grateful for my assistance because it was now past midnight. I described the fracture pattern, an intra-articular lateral column fracture of the distal humerus with extension to the trochlea. He said, "Hmm. Likely better that you handle it anyway as I understand you are a hand and upper extremity guy." We both agreed, and he went back to sleep. I, of course, waited around to have the O.R. team come in, open the suites, and get started. This is a multiple-hour process in even the most efficient of hospitals and yet another example of something the public does not understand: sitting around in the middle of the night, waiting to start an operation is not compensated in any way. No whining here, simply stating little-known facts.

I was happy to address the fracture as it was "right up my alley," and being a newcomer, I was pleased to take care of a prominent member of the community. My patient recovered very well and regained full function within months. As the years went on, he helped me with numerous legal issues when I needed counsel.

Fast-forward nearly a quarter century. I decided to speak to him about the obstacles we had encountered in following up with both city and county governments in Miami. What he divulged to me came as a bit of a shock. "To get their attention, you will have to hire someone like me, a lobbyist, to even get a seat at the table," he declared. I argued that we already had the discussion, they understood the value proposition, and had kindly asked me to gather some supporting data. I told him we had the data, for nearly five years now, and simply wanted to report back. Well, this is where I learned the hard truth. My patient and friend informed me that it would cost me $10,000 *per month* to engage his services.

"Whoa," I protested. "Please understand that what our walk-in clinic gets paid can't even cover that on many months in net revenue. This is part of the problem and reason we seek discussion. We cannot throw good money after bad. I am speaking about something that helps our citizens, not trying to sell something. Sure, the big real estate developers and insurance companies do that because they can justify the cost. I am just the guy delivering the care from the trenches. All I want is a discussion so they can understand how we can help these public entities, same ones I pay taxes into." My argument fell on deaf ears and I finally realized that this is what it takes to improve healthcare: more hard-earned money from the folks who do not collect the big bucks for delivering that care. It was an eye-opening experience and something the public is likely not aware of. I just want to point out what happens every day, and the reason I seek a real solution, one that must originate "from the trenches."

Chapter 8 – The Hospital System Behemoths and Bureaucracy

"I will remember that I do not treat a fever chart, a
cancerous growth, but a sick human being, whose illness
may affect the person's family and economic stability.
My responsibility includes these related problems
if I am to care adequately for the sick."

Hospitals are for sick people.

Understand that a clinician uses the word "sick" very differently than the layperson. The COVID-19 pandemic has brought that concept into stark clarity, demonstrating that the delivery of healthcare will be transformed in many countries going forward. When doctors refer to the "sick," we generally mean patients who are unstable and often have chronic comorbidities that obligate them to seek urgent hospital care time and time again.

Contrast this with a patient who breaks their wrist or develops a severe sore throat with fever. The former patient may need a cast or a surgical procedure, while the latter needs an astute diagnosis, followed by a course of appropriate antibiotics. These are not sick patients in the eyes of clinicians because they will receive a course of episodic care, then get on with their lives; at least in most cases.

However, the patient with the wrist fracture could develop an axillary vein thrombosis and then a pulmonary embolus, rendering them sick. The strep throat patient may have neglected their symptoms, or only took two days of antibiotics, and then became septic from uncontrolled infection, leading to an I.C.U. stay. These two complications provide clear examples of "sick patients" who will need further care – and THAT is the role of a hospital.

COVID-19 and other pandemics clarify the distinction between the sick – those who require a hospital visit and admission – and those who can undergo conservative treatment on an outpatient basis. This delineation has a huge logistics and economic consequence and is the reason pandemics are feared by public health officials and politicians, alike. One group does not NEED hospital care and if they seek it, they can overwhelm the system for those who do. Now, think of healthcare with that perspective all the time.

Fortunately, we do not deal with national or global pandemics frequently, but the current escalating costs of healthcare, in the U.S. and abroad, illustrate that we should deal with ongoing medical issues through the same lens. Neither the wrist fracture, nor the strep throat patient *need* the hospital. The former can have an evaluation in a specialty-specific walk-in center or engage an orthopedist willing to see them soon after the injury, as the patient ices and elevates the hand. If surgery is needed, it can take place in a free-standing surgical center. A study in the Journal of Hand Surgery showed that there was a five-fold increase in these types of surgeries performed in a free-standing surgical center versus a hospital-based facility from 1996 to 2006. Both options are "ambulatory." What is the difference? Cost.

I can mention efficiency, complication rates, avoidance of general anesthesia, waiting times, patient satisfaction, etc., but I will not. In a healthcare system like ours that is choking from expenditures, cost alone is reason enough to justify shifting certain surgeries away from hospitals to dedicated outpatient centers not affiliated with a larger, cost-burdened partner. Data from 2016 revealed that Medicare paid an independent ASC (ambulatory surgery center) only 53 percent of what they pay a hospital-affiliated center ASC (whether inside or in a separate location), for the exact same procedure. We are comparing apples to apples here.

I as well as many of my colleagues saw this difference in cost and efficiency decades ago. As an orthopedic upper limb surgeon, if I do that wrist fracture plating or carpal tunnel release – or currently even my shoulder replacement surgeries in an ASC – all my patients go home. I already confirmed that ASCs are much cheaper. I presented data that hospitals are paid about 40 percent more for the equivalent surgery than an outpatient surgery center. *Why?* Outpatient surgery centers should be paid the equivalent as a hospital or conceivably a little less.

Yes, we have fewer expenses, but that is the whole point. Are we not in a healthcare cost crisis? Yet, we continue feeding into a system that is more expensive, which means we end up paying them much more. Frankly, there should not be as many hospitals as there are these days. About one mile from our surgical center, the local public healthcare system is building yet another hospital. No matter that the flagship – a renowned teaching city hospital that includes one of the best trauma centers in the world – is only about six miles away. If patients truly need a full-fledged hospital, including E.R., why not drive a bit farther and save the taxpayers and our entire healthcare system, $300 million to build, not to mention the ongoing expenses?

The U.S. military uses the Ryder Trauma Center at Jackson Memorial (J.M.H.) for its training. A valued employee of mine had her husband flown into J.M.H. by a rescue chopper due to an acute cervical injury where it first appeared that he would be quadriplegic. The neurosurgery team did a stellar job performing the surgical stabilization on a Sunday evening, to avoid paralysis. He initiated his rehabilitation as an inpatient due to the risk of post-op complications and the frequent monitoring he required. This, indeed, is what a hospital does and ought to do: acute, life-saving functions. But you do not need one every five blocks. This is not what I have seen in other countries.

So, this new Jackson West hospital is now a bit closer to his home. Why can't a helicopter fly for five or six minutes more to arrive at the optimal facility? I remain baffled as to why the community accepted this, considering there are several fine hospitals a few miles on either side of the new one being built. Perhaps *that* is the reason. Competition. I feel it has no place in our national healthcare decisions unless it really is going to drive down prices, or significantly increase quality. Neither is the case here, other than convenience due to area traffic. Consequently, there was a major legal fight in allowing Jackson Health System to build the facility. The current administration has done a tremendous job in bringing the system to profitability but you would think they would be more open to discussions on how to improve community access, including Doral, via cost-effective and strategically placed outpatient centers.

To illustrate the real disconnection between "healthcare providers" in the average community, our team has had zero discussion with city officials or hospital leaders about this project. They chose to ignore us, or they were not even aware of what we are currently doing for the community, which is worse. As we outlined in the previous chapter, there really is little interest in collaboration. From what I gather from my colleagues, it is the same in other cities …unless of course they are hospital employees or make a direct impact upon the success of that healthcare system. Yes, the people who deliver the care.

The grim reality is that except for major, necessary inpatient services like an I.C.U., healthcare is moving away from the traditional hospital setting. Two Midwestern brothers and orthopedic surgeons have been performing knee replacements in their two outpatient centers with great success for the past ten-plus years. More recently, they have been performing hip replacements as well, which is astounding. Naturally, they have well defined parameters and indications for inclusion in addition to anesthesia, peri-operative, and post-op protocols to make it a seamless process and deal with any hiccups. As I mentioned, I have been doing outpatient shoulder and elbow replacements in my center, where one of our affiliated spine surgeons did perhaps the first ambulatory A.L.I.F. (anterior lumbar interbody fusion) in the state of Florida, which entails the additional services of a skilled general surgeon who performs much of the exposure via laparotomy. This too, represents a paradigm shift away from the culture of admitting a patient for a routine carpal tunnel release, something I did as a matter of routine in New York City and will detail later.

You know how this cost-saving transition could be accomplished in one fell swoop? By allowing outpatient surgery centers to get reimbursed for implants on Medicare patients the same way hospitals are. This is one simple point I tried to transmit to our current president (yes, "The Donald") via his trusted confidante and golf buddy. This goes above and beyond paying both facilities a similar rate for the exact same service. For example, if a vascular surgeon can perform certain lower-risk procedures on a Medicare patient and that ambulatory facility can receive reimbursement for certain implants and devices, we could push many of those safer surgeries out of the expensive hospital system. Of course, the hospital system does not want that: what do you think the hospital lobby is fighting *against*?

I live this every day, having been performing outpatient shoulder replacements for nearly a decade, in addition to lesser procedures such as a titanium thumb base replacement for painful osteoarthritis. Sadly, not on Medicare patients because the prosthesis in both cases often costs more than the Medicare CPT facility codes reimburse for that surgery, which are frankly, pathetic. That is why I often refer my Medicare patients with these pathologies to a colleague who operates regularly in a hospital. I could make a special trip, but that is not my practice pattern; driving to the hospital and finding a parking spot takes much longer than the 25 to 30 minutes it takes me to relieve that patient's thumb pain. See, the issue becomes a bit more real when we look past statistics and figures.

Now, granted, we all need hospitals. For example, my dad's cardiac episode and my concern about him suffering an occult infarct (MI) warranted him being in a hospital, as did the circumstances of my assistant's husband's neck injury. We, as a society, must help the hospitals stay solvent. It makes me sad when I see a hospital close, however, one can understand why; they are hugely expensive to run. The truth is, the way surgery is done these days, much fewer surgeries need to be performed in a hospital.

Thirty years ago, the first ambulatory surgery center was established by a couple of surgeons in Arizona. So, outpatient surgery centers have only been around for about three decades, which is not that long – it is my same generation. However, every week I run into the issue where I often cannot take definitive care of certain Medicare patients because - forget about breaking even and paying our bills – we would lose money on some of those surgeries, due to the cost of the implants and other factors that are now beginning to change. *Why*? At last, the government figured out, "You know what? We will do this bundle payment for common things like joint replacements." Medicare woke up and declared, Okay, so long as you follow certain guidelines (which are important, of course), we will start reimbursing for knee replacements, (for example), in an outpatient center.

So, one of the biggest surgeries we now perform in our A.S.C. is a total knee arthroplasty (replacement). To some degree, I understood why they were reluctant to reimburse for it, but guess what? Now, they do! It is indeed a major procedure. Furthermore, CMS is approving even hip replacements for outpatient reimbursement, which is simply amazing. Is it going to trickle down at last to the minor ones that should have been approved 20 years ago? Alas, I am still waiting on the thumbs and even the shoulder arthroplasties, body areas not required to simply walk. With exception of my Cirque-de-Soleil patients who do need these to engage in their type of ambulation. If we apply logic to the situation, I – the orthopedic surgeon in the trenches – should be allowed to decide which surgeries are safe or prudent to perform in a surgery center, and be reimbursed for my training, skill, and expertise that facilitates patient care. Why am I waiting on C.M.S., or some insurance company, to dictate when I can do the shoulder replacement surgery in an A.S.C. when knees are now "approved"? Are the clinicians not the best judge of that? The example between shoulders and knees is quite revealing...

Earlier, we discussed the metal plate/screw construct we use when a little old lady breaks her wrist. Well, they come with a certain cost. And Medicare does not reimburse very well for that operation, which means that once you have paid for the implant, the surgery center may even lose money to provide the care. Can you imagine a more ludicrous outcome? We provide a valuable service and lose money? That begs the question, where are all these fractures going? To the hospital, of course. What happens next? Grandma may get a cardiology consultation, or some other test, along with a C.T. scan of her wrist because that is what happens in hospitals – even though most hand surgeons will not require it. The well-intentioned E.R., however, may order it.

Well before COVID-19, we had already been coping with pesky bacteria called M.R.S.A. (Methicillin Resistant Staph Aureus) that often complicates hospital care and surgeries in what we refer to as nosocomial (hospital-acquired) infections. Such cases require a tremendous amount of care, which is expensive. Why shouldn't the clinicians who perform the surgery get a say in the matter? By now, I think you are learning why. In the next chapter, we will get into health insurance…that will be fun.

Regarding safety issues within A.S.C.'s, many have suggested they are not as safe as hospitals, even though multiple studies have proven they are safer. *Why?* Because it is the same anesthesiologists doing the same type of procedures alongside the same surgeons and nursing staff. That comes with immeasurable benefits. What happens in a hospital's cardiac surgery suite, for example? They take the same approach. A cardiac surgeon would never let his patient in the operating room with new staff, novel equipment, or a fresh (albeit excellent) anesthesiologist, for the simple reason that those collective actions could result in an irreversible downside…called death.

While other disciplines including hand surgery may not be life-threatening (although hand surgery could be limb threatening), what I have described above is exactly what happens in many hospitals. The phenomenon usually occurs at night, or after the O.R. morning shift, which is better trained for specific procedures "in their room." Techs and O.R. nurses have literally approached me and said, "No, sorry. I have never seen this kind of surgery before. Can you help me?" I cannot leave, so of course, I explain that they need this instrument here and there during this step, etc. On the flip side, that rarely happens in a dedicated ambulatory surgery center. Now that you know which facility gets paid much more for the same procedures, do you understand why our healthcare system is so expensive and inefficient?

Speaking of inefficiency, let me pose a scenario. Physicians A and B are both excellent technical surgeons who work fast. In other words, they are efficient. Both manage thriving private practices where they see multiple patients and schedule procedures as needed to resolve clinical issues. I will pick on Mercy Hospital of Miami, since I brought them hundreds of cases over the years and made them a ton of money, yet they never grasped the concept I am about to present. Let us be real: they never cared to. I am speaking to the system, not the individual administrators who are mostly wonderful people with whom I have enjoyed a Cuban cafesito in the middle of the day in the well-known Cuban restaurant in the lobby. This is Miami, folks.

Surgeon A and Surgeon B both have eight elective surgical procedures to perform on X day in Mercy Hospital. The typical busy day for them. On that day, Surgeon A gets operating room (O.R.) 1 and Surgeon B gets O.R. 2. They cut skin at 8 a.m., a typical O.R. start time in hospitals, but mind you, due to O.R. inefficiencies, in many cases it is closer to 9 a.m. Whatever. The day goes on. After the first case, which they both complete around 10 a.m., Surgeon A and Surgeon B bump into each other at the coffee machine in the O.R. lounge. They talk politics and baseball, complain about trial lawyers, or even discuss a challenging case if they work in similar specialties. This conversation takes place after they dictate their surgical procedure into the hospital's transcription service, since they will have plenty of time on their hands. They are waiting on what surgeon's affectionately call "turn-over".

After reassuring the patient's family that all went well, they each rush to the O.R. holding area and proceed to urge nursing and anesthesia to head back to O.R. 1 or 2. Once everyone is in place, each begins their second of an eight-day case. You can picture what happens next. After they finish around the same time, the next lounge discussion might center on their kids or their in-laws. It may be quite a while before they see each other again because Surgeon A is about to perform their "big case" of the day, which will not coincide with Surgeon B. One thing is certain: they will both wait quite some time after case #2, hoping soon to start case #3. Their routine is just part of the large, complex machinery we call the hospital O.R. To a degree, it is understandable: the staff is not incentivized, and the paperwork and bureaucracy are stifling. It only continues to worsen as society and medicine becomes more needlessly complicated. By the end of their OR days, Surgeons A and B are tired. They have missed their kids' soccer game or swim meet, perhaps disappointed their spouse or date, and drank a LOT of coffee while discussing more politics than they cared to.

Now, let us consider a different scenario that results from thinking outside the box, coupled with the intrinsic efficiencies that a dedicated ambulatory surgery center possesses. Surgeon A and Surgeon B could arrive to the Happy Days ASC at 7:45 a.m. sharp to cut skin at 8 a.m. However, the pragmatic O.R. nursing director who plans the schedule with the anesthesia director, schedules Surgeon A to come in first. When he gets to the A.S.C. he runs two rooms adjacent to each other. While he finishes in Room A at 9 a.m. (because he started on time), the staff prepares the patient for Room B, which has already been cleaned and set up by the second O.R. team. After speaking with the family of the first patient (and if time permits, dictating the case), he starts the surgery on his second patient in Room B. Notice, no talk of baseball or the A.C.A. debacle with a colleague…oh, and he has already had plenty of coffee, so he is good to go.

Surgeon A repeats this pattern until he completes all eight cases on his schedule for that day. Now at last he has the time to dictate his surgeries, having focused on his main priority, his patients. That is a good thing. He can sit down in his office to complete the never-ending paperwork before heading to his kids' soccer game that afternoon.

As Surgeon A is finishing up, Surgeon B arrives on the scene to see his first patient in pre-op, around 1 p.m. He feels refreshed because he managed to play an early game of tennis before enjoying breakfast with his wife. He also had time to stop by the office to see a few critical patients and of course, fill out the ever-present, ubiquitous paperwork. He begins his caseload in Room 1 while Surgeon A starts his last case in Room 2. If they happen to coincide, due to the duration of the procedures, they might bump into each other in the recovery room as they check in on their respective patients and speak to the PACU nurse. This leaves scant time to discuss politics or whine about healthcare issues, but they do inquire about each other's kids.

Surgeon B finishes his cases at around bankers hours, perhaps 5 or 6 p.m. He still has the entire evening ahead of him and he is not exhausted. Neither is Surgeon A. Both managed to do their jobs well and get other "life stuff" done, yet both O.R.'s remained occupied all day…just like the hospital.

Does this sound like a model for healthcare efficiency and cost-control? Well, if we had true collaboration, it could work to a similar degree within the hospital environment. However, the hospital culture is much different. I could never get a second room at Mercy Hospital despite averaging 10 cases on my O.R. day for years. A pity. In our free-market economy, all I asked for was a sensible solution, even if somewhat constrained in healthcare. Solutions like the ASC will fill that void as this vignette is just one example of multiple efficiencies that are routine in a more streamlined system.

So, you might ask, "Why is the transition to free-standing ambulatory surgery not more rapid and fluid?" There are just too many people with their hand in the cookie jar, and until we acknowledge that the escalating costs of our healthcare system could bankrupt the country, it will not change fast enough. However, COVID-19 is forcing our hands. Many books will be written (not by me) about how the virus will accelerate a new era in healthcare, sometimes termed, "Healthcare 3.0." For now, my account simply represents an effort to point out everyday issues that interfere with my delivery of care – restricted to hand and upper limb surgery – from the trenches.

What is my perspective regarding hospital care and the upper limb? What do I know? Well, my quarter-century of working in two dedicated upper limb practices, developing several surgery centers, and being on staff at over 10 Miami-area hospitals has given me a comparative viewpoint.

Let me reiterate that I can only discuss the upper limb, although this is not a small area considering that some estimates put hand injuries alone at near 10 percent of all emergency department visits. Being more inclusive, the range of upper extremity injuries (hand to shoulder) accounts for 18 million emergency room visits every year in the U.S.A., with 10 percent of those involving hand, wrist, or forearm fractures. These injuries have profound socioeconomic consequences, accounting for an average of eight weeks of time off work per injury. Most are easily managed with closed reduction and immobilization although some require operative treatment, including distal radius fractures previously discussed, allowing improved outcome and earlier mobilization. In another study looking at trends, the majority of upper limb patients were below 44 years old and male. *Ninety-three percent* of them did NOT require hospital admission. It is this last point that we should not overlook.

Considering that 93 percent of upper limb injuries did not require admission, we must ask, "Why are they going to the hospital in the first place?" As you ponder that number, consider that also 93 percent of work-related injuries are orthopedic (more on that later). Most healthcare "consumers," otherwise known as "John Q. Patient", would agree that the hospital E.R. is not a pleasant place. The waits are long, the environment is scary (worse during COVID-19), parking can be a bitch (even for the doctors), and it is not inexpensive. So why do they go? Lack of options, until recently.

The growth of urgent care centers has been near exponential until a recent slowing, which suggests the market is saturated in many areas. Last year, a UCA (Urgent Care Assn) study was published which showed the total number of centers grew eight percent in only one year, from 8,125 to 8,774 in late 2018. There are multiple factors at play, but the paramount reason is that it is a faster and cheaper alternative than the hospital E.R. What many articles do not talk about is the level of expertise when it comes to certain areas of medicine. This is a crucial topic considering that over 25 percent of ALL urgent care visits are from Medicare/Medicaid patients. Keep in mind that the population continues to age and is increasingly active. That has a major impact on musculoskeletal care, whether a painful knee or a wrist fracture.

Specialty walk-in centers are still an emerging trend, rarely discussed in the urgent care industry, yet I had published an op-ed article in our county, and later state, medical journal nearly a decade ago which went unheralded. Interestingly, a financial news website published my thoughts on this in early 2020, using OrthoNOW® as an example, illustrating that the impetus for change may come from the macroeconomics world. Notice it is not coming from the healthcare landscape, nor from physicians themselves. I continue to predict it will come from consumers… and COVID-19 may drive it.

The reality is that orthopedics has a huge economic consequence. HUGE. Most people are not at all aware of the overall cost of injury to our society and economy. Yes, injury includes anything from abdominal and head trauma, penetrating gunshot wounds, or a blow to the eye. While those examples are dramatic, they are not typical. By and large, most injuries are orthopedic.

When you think about injury, the eye is not the first thing that comes to mind. Instead, it is a musculoskeletal injury like a fracture, a laceration, a sprain, or a herniated disc, right? That has a cost…to society…now, hold onto your seat here…of *$671 billion*! Three-quarters of a trillion dollars! What is our U.S. G.D.P., $20 trillion? U.S. annual healthcare spending recently reached $3.5 trillion. Although it is not intuitive, the cost of injury is not simply the medical cost; it is the downstream cost of that productive worker being laid-up after they break their ankle and they can't climb a ladder, stand on your roof, and fix your shingles. Now that roofing company must find a replacement and train them, or they will be short-handed. So, there is an economic consequence to injury. We will not even get into the liability and legal costs associated with injury and its care. That is for the chapter on ambulance chasing – a whole other spectrum of healthcare characterized by unnecessary spending.

The move of orthopedic care away from the hospital to urgent care centers, and perhaps to specialized orthopedic urgent care has been demonstrated, although in somewhat lethargic fashion due to the behemoth size of the industry. We discussed it in the area of outpatient surgery centers and point-of-access issues via the still growing urgent care phenomenon. It was exactly 30 years ago when I was an intern at a private hospital and would admit a patient for a routine surgery like a carpal tunnel release. Dr. Melone, the hand surgeon from N.Y.U., would schedule the carpal tunnel release (still open procedure), I would admit the patient the night before, doing a full H&P (history and physical), the patient had surgery the next morning, and then spent another night in the hospital. Two nights in the hospital for a 20-minute procedure (if that). I did not understand it then, or now.

To some degree, hospitals are struggling because of the availability of many other options. They must focus on their strong suit – caring for truly sick patients and performing higher risk procedures. While the public continues to depend too much on them, hospitals remain a big reason for the high cost of healthcare. Some of it is due to habit, but also the lack of patient education about alternatives. This becomes evident when I meet people in social situations and they ask, "Oh, you are a doctor. What hospital are you at?" I reply, "Why do you assume I'm at a hospital? I am not a heart surgeon. I'm not a vascular surgeon." Of course, a doctor is not going to perform AAA (abdominal aortic aneurysm) resection or cardiothoracic surgery and send the patient home right after. THAT is the purpose of a hospital. Yeah, I'm a real hit at the punchbowl....

John N. Kastanis, M.B.A., F.A.C.H.E., a hospital executive with over 40 years' experience in executive leadership roles for urban-based teaching hospitals and consultative services, offers his insights:

"In the category of hospitals and health systems, labor and supply chain costs are the most significant amounts in their operating expense budgets, representing 60 percent and 17 percent of spending, respectively. The majority of hospitals have minimal or nonexistent cost accounting measures in place, and therefore, their cost-reduction initiatives tend to focus on Lean and Six Sigma, but few look at clinical variation or overall cost accounting, where the most significant savings are found. With a cost accounting system in place, hospitals can track their direct and indirect costs. Examples of direct costs include nurses, physicians, unit clerks, and lab technologists. Indirect costs include administrators, controllers, and overhead. Another best practice within cost accounting is separating all direct and indirect costs into fixed or variable costs. This type of financial data could help establish informative ratios for both labor and supply chain utilization, and yet many hospitals are still years away of identifying more cost savings. This will prove to be a big challenge as health organizations will need to cut their cost structures by at least 25 to 35 percent to compete for a place in a narrow or tiered insurance network and become a provider of choice.

"Other major drivers of costs stem from regional variation in utilization of health resources. For example, the cost of a surgical hernia repair in New York City far exceeds the cost of having it done in Topeka, Kansas. Again, labor costs vary, based on different regions in the nation, with many health care workers unionized, particularly in urban areas, while manufacturing, deliveries, and storage costs tend to be much higher than rural and suburban areas. *Also, U.S. healthcare administrative costs are six times the cost of other rich countries.*

"To date, there are still unexplained reasons for regional variation in utilization of health resources, but over the years, CMS has identified geographic variation in Medicare spending per capita with many health providers in the Northeastern, Southeastern, Southwestern states, and California providing comparable patient care with significantly higher costs to the consumer. Many scholars have concluded that this type of variation is a result of a lack of standardization of clinical procedures and treatments; over utilization; lack of evidence for treatment; and ineffective clinical performance when treatments are known. The landmark IOM (Institute of Medicine) report "To Err is Human" (1999) estimated that 44,0000 to 98,000 deaths occur each year due to medical errors, which sparked serious discussions about patient error. More recent reports suggest that while there has been progress in some areas, significant improvements in preventable harm are still needed. Following the IOM report, the Institute for Healthcare Improvement (IHI) developed an approach to optimizing health system performance. The IHI's belief is that new designs must be developed to simultaneously pursue three dimensions, which they call the "Triple Aim":

1. Improving the patient experience of care (including quality and satisfaction);
2. Improving the health of populations served by each health care organization; and
3. Reducing the per capita cost of health care.

"Most providers have embraced the Triple Aim, but in varying degrees of success, ergo the continuing variation of care throughout the nation.

"Within each hospital, one of the most effective ways to improve overall patient care while maintaining quality is to have management work collaboratively with all the clinical leaders in each organization. Common approaches include the agreement on best practices for each specialty, redesign of order sets, creating new clinical pathways, and then monitoring variable costs; reduction of complications and adverse events; and length of stay. This requires access to volumes of clinical data and perseverance from all involved parties. It is a long and arduous process, but once it is established, along with periodic reviews of quality improvements, overall cost savings result from reduced readmission rates, adverse events and length-of-stay.

"In summary, the hospitals and health systems that consistently provide high-value care share the following attributes: 1. thinking beyond the hospital stay; 2. cutting waste, not safety; and 3. engaging the frontline team in improving the cost-effectiveness of needed care.

"In reference to thinking beyond the hospital stay, many health organizations have embarked on *Population Health* strategies, drawing from one of the Triple Aim dimensions: improving the health of the patient populations being served. This new focus also helps in developing value-based care, inasmuch as it has major health providers looking at social determinants that are the root of many chronic illnesses, such as malnutrition, diabetes, asthma, hypertension and obesity, compounded by mental illness and substance abuse. This process has resulted in health providers aligning with managing agencies in their respective communities that oversee basic services such as Transportation, Housing, Education and Nutrition. These types of collaborative efforts will ultimately result in more denizens within each community improving their health status through improved living conditions, and thereby reducing acute episodes, and urgent/emergent visits to the local hospital's emergency room.

"While hospital-based population health strategies are continuing to be implemented, health care executives are noticing more and more out-of-industry players entering the field with investments in infra-structure, technology, scientific research, and payment and delivery models. As a result, patients are beginning to find more affordable and more accessible options that are transforming the nation's healthcare system. These new players are being referred to as disruptive innovators, as they are a threat to established healthcare providers and will remain so, if their strategies do not change.

"The reasons technology giants such as Amazon, Google, and Apple and mega retailers CVS, Walgreens, Walmart, and Best Buy are entering the healthcare space as disruptive innovators are numerous and compelling. They include: the size and scope of the medical field; the opportunity to engage an already loyal customer base; and the need to fill the floor space that their respective stores already have. With these reasons in mind, these tech giants are well positioned to help customers find medical care more efficiently, and becoming "digital front doors" that leverage artificial intelligence (AI) and voice assisted technology to facilitate health care interactions, including: connecting with care via online scheduling; checking on home delivery of prescriptions; and managing health improvement goals.

"The retailers' interest in filling their floor space stems from the decline in product sales due to online shopping. The increasing empty space is now being converted to in-store primary care retail operations which will bring profitable services in-house, create foot traffic, and feed the pharmacy operation to compensate for the lost retail business moving to online services. Meanwhile, these storefront type services will be helping customers manage chronic conditions such as diabetes, hypertension, and asthma. Some of these new health hubs will have expanded health clinics with a lab for blood testing and health screenings.

"With all these new and disruptive innovations being established, healthcare providers need to be aware, and more so, need to look outside their hospitals and clinics for new ways to connect with patients more efficiently and effectively.

"Commercially insured patients increasingly prefer digital care because of factors related to value, convenience and customer service. Therefore, health care providers who don't have strong primary care presence, need to find ways to do so or partner with retailers that can fill the gap. This way patients with serious illnesses, conditions or diseases, hospitals should strive to be the destination of choice. Also, with everyone's interest in digital services, hospitals should continue to adopt promising new technologies, especially those focused on population health. These technologies include: Disease management using predictive analytics and wearables; home-base health care technology and virtual visits with clinicians; supply chain initiatives to improve delivery of pharmaceuticals and medical equipment. Again, all these types of innovations reduce cost in the short and long run, while increasing patient satisfaction and quality of care."

Interesting that he mentions innovations in terms of today's technology giants, again proving that my partners and I at Miami Hand Center were ahead of the curve way back in the 90s, which paved the way for Justin Irizzary and I to disrupt the healthcare delivery system to achieve the Triple Aim with OrthoNOW®.

Despite clear evidence of the major cost of hospital care to our system, in an ironic twist, hospitals spend more and more money on marketing activities, something that was never seen decades ago. On two stretches of Miami highway, one can see a series of billboards for "competing" hospitals, often one hospital's ad directly in front of their competitor. That would not be needed if they were primarily serving "sick" people as I mentioned at the outset. E.M.S. (Emergency Medical Services) knows precisely where the nearest, and most appropriate, hospital is located for the emergency they are tending to, and internists know exactly where their affiliated hospital is when admitting their unstable patients. Some of these billboards began battling each other in their "real-time" digital declaration of E.R. wait times. Eight minutes versus fourteen minutes and so on. It became ridiculous enough that our local daily paper, always looking to disparage healthcare and doctors, published an expose' on the topic, revealing what we all knew, that it was a lot of smoke and mirrors. Another battle involved the promotion of their possession of the DaVinci surgical robot, a tactic designed to mislead patients about the role and necessity of this high-tech contraption in their ongoing effort to compete with other hospitals in a game of "Keeping up with the Joneses." Most proficient general surgeons will tell you there are highly specific indications for the use of this million-dollar device, while the majority of orthopedic surgeons will tell you the addition of a robot simply adds cost and much more time to the performance of a total knee or hip replacement.

The irony of billboards is that they appeal to the "consumerization" of healthcare with the wrong players. Nobody wants to be in a hospital, and most everyone agrees that they are an expensive, albeit necessary, entity. I rarely see smaller, cost-efficient clinics (other than cosmetic surgeons) informing the public of their services via this high visibility advertising. They simply cannot afford it. I should know. We once paid for several OrthoNOW® billboards along the highway, which turned out to be completely unaffordable relative to our reimbursements, something I will discuss in the next chapter. We will better understand the availability of expansive marketing budgets when unraveling the concept of "non-profit".

What I now understand is that even obvious improvement to our healthcare system happens incrementally, often painfully, and we must accelerate that change, driven by the two voices rarely heard in the debate: "providers" (aargh) and patients.

It turns out that readmission is the single biggest cost problem for hospitals. And yet, why don't they let physicians make that decision as to who even needs to go to a hospital in the first place? I just explained why it is a challenge for me to replace a joint or fix a fracture in a Medicare patient. As I continue to emphasize, most physicians want to do the right thing. If you paid them fairly, there is no issue. The system tries to use the minority who are unscrupulous to justify poor reimbursements. Believe me, we have plenty of unethical physicians in South Florida, with Miami-Dade leading our nation in Medicare fraud. I will touch on this in the chapter regarding opportunists.

HOSPITAL NEGLIGENCE

As I have stated, it is my firm belief that patients will ultimately drive the improvements in healthcare delivery and efficiencies, based on their own frustrations with the current system. With respect to hospitals versus ASCs, South Florida patient Uva de Aragon recounts her own real-life experiences:

"Two years ago, I fell and fractured my femur. After the surgery, I lost a lot of blood and needed a transfusion. And they sent in two students to do the transfusion. I was aware of what was going on. I am 75 years old, I speak English, and I am well educated. These two students fussed around with it and had no idea what they were doing. I remained patient until they dropped the needle on the floor. Instead of throwing it away, they picked it up and started cleaning and wiping it off. That is when I said, "No, this is it. I am tired of you guys playing doctors. Go find somebody who knows what they are doing. I am not going to let you put that needle into my arm."

"But what about an older patient, or a patient who does not speak English, or a patient with less education? They might not know that a dirty needle could cause an infection.

"I had another experience many years prior at another hospital. I had a pulmonary problem, for which I was receiving an aerosol treatment. On a Sunday evening, the aerosol guy came in and told me he was going to give me a different treatment. And I said, "Well, sometimes I have allergic reactions. What you have been giving me so far has been fine." He insisted the new treatment would be okay, but sure enough, after he left, I started to feel like I could not breathe. I called the nurse's station, and nobody came. I had palpitations. My throat felt like it was closing. Finally, since I knew the hospital's number by heart because I had given it to friends, I called the hospital and asked for the nursing station. I told them to get to my room because I was going to have a heart attack and die on their watch because no one was bothering to respond.

"Well, they came and helped me. But it is unbelievable that a patient who had an adverse reaction to medication had to call for 20 minutes... and still nobody rushed to my room. If I had not been smart and figured out another way to reach them, something terrible could have happened to me. I took care of my elderly parents until they passed. And when they went to the hospital, we always had somebody with them because part of the problem is that the nurses are overworked. They are good at what they do, but they are overworked. They are assigned too many patients and it is impossible for them to take care of them all.

"I have also had outpatient surgery for carpal tunnel, for my rotator cuff, and for cataracts and a cornea transplant. To me, this is sometimes a much better alternative to a traditional hospital because you are released to the comfort of your home. You need someone there to take care of you, but you avoid infections. Depending on the type of surgery, of course, a patient might need to stay in the hospital. There is no way I could have gone home after a five-hour surgery for my femur.

"Not all patients are informed, even though we have access to a tremendous amount of information on the internet. But it can be confusing if you do not know where to look. You can get all kinds of information that may not be accurate or from reputable sources. That is why each individual needs to weed out the nonsense to get the right information.

"For many people, it is sometimes hard to get in touch with their insurance provider because one department does this, and another department does that. I have not had that problem. But the doctor or the doctor's office must make phone calls, especially when there are exceptions.

"Everything is fine until there are exceptions. If you need a medication that is not approved, for example, your doctor must call to request an exception. Then things get complicated. We need major changes in healthcare. Insurance companies do not pay doctors as much as they should be paid, which means the patients suffer while the insurance companies and pharmaceutical companies make huge profits.

"Some people do not trust any government-run programs. But I stayed on my private insurance until I turned 65 and qualified for Medicare, which is much easier than private insurance. Most doctors must accept it because the population is getting older; if not, their pool of patients would decrease and become small. I fully believe there must be an option from the government, and if people want to keep paying for their private insurance, fine.

242 · ALEJANDRO BADIA, M.D., F.A.C.S.

"A relative of mine who has a lot of medical problems now has Obamacare. While it is not ideal, before it was passed, she did not have any coverage. Now at least she does receive some medical attention. She is bipolar and cannot hold a job long enough to get insurance through an employer. For people who cannot get insurance through their work and need medical attention, there must be options. Because when people do not have insurance, they go to the E.R. Then the hospital never gets paid because these patients cannot afford the bill. That means more work for the hospital, and more money that never gets reimbursed. You must have an option for people who cannot afford private insurance or do not have a job. Whether it is Obamacare or something else, that option must be available. If not, it is more expensive for society because people do get sick. And then what happens? They wait, they do not get preventive medicine. And then they go to the emergency room, which is not good for the patient or for society."

CUT THE FAT AND SERVE THE LESS FORTUNATE

The logical conclusion is that the army of people who are tasked with policing us costs the system much more than the occasional bad apples. We would have so much money left over in the healthcare universe to care for the less fortunate if we cut the fat. "Medicare for All" would be a laudable matter. We could even expand Medicaid and enable it to offer more reasonable payments, to incentivize more doctors to care for Medicaid patients. We could pay for it easily, if we could only get rid of all the waste in the system.

Here is an example of an email that typifies the unnecessary bureaucratic protocols that contribute to hospital inefficiency:

Dear Members of the Medical Staff,

Good morning. In compliance with Kendall Regional Medical Center Medical Staff Bylaws Section 9.B. Other Medical Staff Documents (2), notice is hereby provided that the Credentials Policy is Amended 2.C.3. Authorization to Obtain/Release Information (3) on page 20, Section 3.A.5. Board Action (3) page 24, Added Appendix A and Appendix B. A note of general information, Section 2.C.3. Authorization to Obtain/Release Information (3) is being adopted throughout the HCA Healthcare System to facilitate credentialing information.

It often surprises people that hospital systems tend to be not-for-profit. However, that is deceptive because many hospitals do make a substantial profit; they just cannot show it on the books. Therefore, they may pay their administrators well, give the staff bonuses and engage in significant marketing efforts. It is not a level playing field for clinics and clinicians who pay a lot of taxes into the system when the non-profit hospitals can afford to place full-page ads in the newspaper or populate billboards. One of my preferred hospitals renovated our surgeons' lounge on two occasions within a few years. I remember thinking, *I preferred the previous look and feel with its cozy rugs and couches, now updated with gorgeous hardwood floors and more fashionable seating.* As I have stated, because surgery is not as efficient in hospitals it results in a lot of idle time hanging out in those lounges. Then I realized, "Oh, they have to spend the money. If they show a profit, they lose their not-for-profit status."

Where did that exemption come from, particularly when you see the bills for care rendered? Why is it important to understand? Nearly two-thirds of the almost 4,000 acute care, non-federal hospitals enjoy that tax exempt status. In 1956, the I.R.S. (Internal Revenue Service) first enabled hospitals to be exempt from tax liabilities by requiring them, if able, to provide free or substantially discounted care to indigent patients, known as the "charity standard." This was amended in 1969 after Medicare and Medicaid came on the scene to be interpreted as the "community benefit" standard, open to much more *interpretation*, and subsequent enforcement challenges.

Our friend, the government, as I discussed in the previous chapter, has attempted to require non-profit hospitals to provide ever increasing amounts of free care, often in response to the growing nebulous number of the uninsured. Even that concept of "uninsured" should be further explored and understood. Forcing uncompensated care to be delivered remains a major challenge and a whole host of laws, including EMTALA (Emergency Medical Treatment and Active Labor Act), were designed to ensure that any hospital participating in Medicare must provide emergency care to their patients and the broader community.

As a sign of major shifts, the IRS revoked a hospital's nonprofit status for the first time in 2017, in line with new A.C.A. Act 501(r) requirements. This demonstrates that there is increased scrutiny of our hospitals, mostly due to the burdensome cost on society, which must be controlled in some manner.

Despite the often-noble mission that hospitals serve, there is a hostile practice that was broadly exposed recently by Dr. Marty Makary, a general surgeon, and Professor of Health Policy at Johns Hopkins Medical School. He had been travelling around the country to better understand why healthcare costs have skyrocketed to write his book, "The Price We Pay". He noted that many hospitals practiced predatory billing and even employee wage garnishing in their efforts to collect debt for care, often with the hyperinflated bill that hospitals have become infamous for. The sole hospital in the small town of Carlsbad, New Mexico became a scapegoat for this practice, and prompted a broader study to determine the prevalence of this surprising tactic.

His subsequent study revealed that nearly 40 percent of Virginia hospitals employed this practice to collect on medical care rendered. More importantly, Dr. Makary stated that 1 in 5 Americans, perhaps an inflated number, has medical debt in collections status, which is wreaking havoc on many American small businesses.

His book makes some very concrete recommendations on how to control healthcare costs, even portraying some of the many disruptors who are innovating how to deliver care. Perhaps consistent with my comments on collaboration challenges in our profession, and broader healthcare spectrum, I was not able to engage Dr. Makary so that he might provide further insight for this book. His views lend credence to my suggestion that our over-reliance on hospitals for much of healthcare can help explain why it has become so costly. His excellent team at Johns Hopkins brought real data and credibility to this debacle. More importantly, his book and subsequent major newspaper articles brought the issue to the public – the one player in the system that will likely achieve real reform. Dr. Makary speaks nationally on many topics, including the opioid crisis (which we will discuss) and disruptive innovation in healthcare. For these reasons, I reached out to him. It indeed takes a village.

Chapter 9 – The Big Business of Health Insurance

"I will remember that I remain a member of society,
with special obligations to all my fellow human beings,
those sound of mind and body as well as the infirm."

Insurance, much like death and taxes, has become an unavoidable component of life in the developed world. The concept is simple. You pay an affordable, recurring fee on a regular basis in exchange for the security of a payout (hopefully) when something unforeseen happens. Seems easy. The insurance company takes the risk, and for that simple fact, they make money, as they should. Somewhere along the way, this transaction has become distorted and even perverted.

In modern society, almost everything involves insurance. Your auto, home, life, job position, belongings, and even your purchases, like airline tickets, can be insured. In many cases, when the need arises, it can be challenging to collect the money you are due. The decision to insure is a personal one in some cases, but in many others like automobile liability insurance, it is the law. Plain and simple. Some of us prefer the "rainy day" concept. I figure if I saved ALL the money I pay into all the insurances I must have and the ones I choose to purchase and placed them in an interest bearing account, I should be fine for that "what if" day. It is not that I am a big risk taker (watch me squirm in Vegas), but I do not consider myself that unlucky. That is why I believe in self-insurance. Alas, as a fellow member of our evermore complex society, I do almost the same as all of you. I play the game…but not always.

After Hurricane Katrina, my waterfront home sustained some damage. I replaced my roof, which probably needed an upgrade anyway, and sustained major tree, dock, and landscaping damage – all of which was "not covered." My insurance covered the roof, but after I paid my double-digit deductible, I had some insurance help to fix it and that was about it. Mind you, I had been paying annual high premiums for windstorm insurance for years until one day we finally got hit. New Orleans fared much worse than Miami, as you know. I did not recover the investment from only the five previous years, which did not make sense. Now, because the banks and insurance companies are cut from the same rug, what do they do? Require you to purchase that same windstorm insurance if you have an active mortgage on your home. What did *I* do? I paid off my home since it freed me from annual premiums that I will probably never recover. It also helped me in another area where yet more insurance is required: the dreaded malpractice. In saintly Florida, I made the investment in my own home since that is one area that the state law protects from creditors or an opportunistic patient and their attorney. And only because I own less than a half-acre. Thank goodness.

So, I have saved outrageous annual home insurance premiums for the past 15 years. Unless my house flies away a la *The Wizard of Oz*, I am happy to take that money and pay for repairs. You see, somebody does not have to make that money off my back. Ditto for flood insurance, another scam I paid into for over 20 years, partly because I had taken out a home equity loan to support my entrepreneurial habits. Sure enough, when Irma hit, I sustained major flooding and damage. It was bad enough that GEICO simply wrote a check to my automobile leasing company, no questions asked. I was disappointed that they could not simply fix the electrical issues of a car that sat in a foot of water for days, yet in one stroke of the pen, problem resolved. All I had to do was find a new car to lease, albeit more expensive. Why did my home flood insurance with Assurant fail to pay for some of the goods that were similarly destroyed? I do not know, but I can show you a seven-page letter from the underwriter that requires a PhD in comparative literature, coupled with a C.P.A., to understand. My response? I paid off the home equity loan JUST so I would not have to pay one single premium more, knowing that it would take a deluge requiring a wooden ark to justify the insurance. Even then, they would probably declare bankruptcy and CC Noah with their explanations.

By now, I trust I have made my feelings clear about insurance in general. Fine. In some cases, as outlined, I was able to divorce myself from that obligation. In others, like auto, none of us can. While I am glad GEICO totaled my car and wrote a check (NOT), I am not so pleased that my ex-wife, with my young toddlers strapped inside, was struck by a commercial bakery van driving the wrong way on a short one-way street in Miami. No brainer, right? The commercial vehicle was at fault AND committed a major traffic infraction. Think again. Despite fighting to get reimbursed for a loaner minivan we needed for the week of Christmas, handled by a grateful attorney patient of mine, we got nearly nothing. Instead, they spend the money on yet more inane commercials involving geckos, cavemen, and silly situations that have nothing to do with reimbursing you for a loss. Such is the nature of insurance.

To stay on topic, what about health insurance? Well, if other types of insurance are frustrating and often recalcitrant to pay, imagine a transaction where the beneficiary is the patient, and the insurance company – whose premiums are typically paid for by a third party known as the employer – is then tasked with paying the healthcare provider. Sometimes. Remember our discussion on T.P.A.s (third party administrators) in an earlier chapter? Can the process get any more complicated?

Why is that? Somewhere along the way, health insurance companies decided to practice medicine and control the clinical decision-making process to mitigate their risk somehow. Furthermore, if they even pay the physician in the first place, the payment arrives long after the physician has rendered the service to the patient. Did they resolve the patient's pneumonia or put a titanium plate in their wrist fracture? No matter: the insurance company can and will second-guess you. They think their concern of "appropriate utilization" and "proper indications" justifies this behavior and practice. However, the part that escapes them and many others in the healthcare universe, is that the actual clinicians are best suited to make the decisions; our years of education and training will generally weed out the unscrupulous from entering our profession. Not always, therefore, oversight is important because there are physicians with poor judgement or even ethics, which results in runaway costs of care. Understood. But why throw the baby out with the bathwater?

One simple example that warrants mentioning yet again is the inane insurance company ad portraying a motorcyclist. It infuriated me every time I saw the United Healthcare (UHC) TV commercial where they depict comments from an aged biker regarding his healthcare. An old *Hell's Angels* looking guy with a scraggly beard and wiry hair expresses gratitude to his insurance company, UHC, for picking up on some possible drug interaction that could have been a major problem. "Thanks to United Healthcare for detecting that..." I thought, *"Hogwash."* A real biker might have said worse. It is not UHC that detected his problem but a physician, nurse, or pharmacist. Sure, they might be employed by that company but how dare they attribute this medical inference to an insurance worker, or more nebulously, the entire organization?

The irony is that the actual people who provide care – the physicians and their offices and outpatient clinics – only represent 20% of the total national health expenditure in the US. The largest component is hospital care, at one-third the total expenditure, which has remained stable. However, the major increase has been in net cost of health insurance and administration, rising from 2.8 percent in 1970 to 7.9 percent in 2018. This five-percent increase is substantial and represents a great intrusion. It is the cause of many of the barriers and obstacles to providing care where there are simply too many middlemen in the equation. If we can simplify the process, it will pay huge dividends we can apply to care itself and not its "administration".

Let us understand the numbers a bit more to better appreciate the gargantuan nature of U.S. healthcare, although many of us remain convinced that the real change must come from the trenches. According to CMS.gov, in 2018 U.S. healthcare spending grew by 4.6 percent, reaching $3.6 trillion, or $11,172 per person. As a share of the nation's Gross Domestic Product (GDP), health spending accounted for 17.7 percent. Those are staggering statistics. And because everybody is aging and people are living longer (which is a good thing), we are consuming much more healthcare. Depending on which economists you read, if healthcare spending reaches 25 percent of GDP, it's going to bankrupt the country. Some healthcare economists, including Pauly, suggest that concern of rising healthcare costs is overblown and that this sector sustains economy due to job creation and the fact that nearly all companies are domestic. Furthermore, the healthcare % of GDP may be a preposterous statistic since it may be due to increased productivity in other major sectors like agriculture and manufacturing, thereby reducing their percent contribution. As the American public ages, it may simply decide it prefers to spend its money on a cardiac screening exam, colonoscopy, or that shiny new knee, as opposed to another plasma TV. These are personal decisions with great consequence.

Think about $3.6 trillion. Of the eighteen industrialized countries on the list in terms of healthcare spending, Norway is number two and spends about 10.4 percent. However, despite the problems with U.S. healthcare, keep in mind that Norway has its issues, too, something the liberal media rarely discusses. I once treated a patient who had traveled all the way from Norway for wrist surgery. Why? He was unable to see one of my colleagues in Oslo who could have resolved his problem because their healthcare system interfered. The Norwegian doctors told him they had to completely fuse (arthrodese) his wrist. When he came to see me, I did a partial fusion to maintain motion while providing pain-relief. Although he is an older guy, he participates in sports like kickboxing and works out regularly at various gyms. After travelling all the way from Norway to receive the medical care he needed, he was golfing within months, and later, he returned to contact sports. If people from highly advanced, first world countries travel TO the USA, we must be doing something right. Perhaps we should focus on that.

When the sheiks from Middle Eastern countries that want to kill us travel all the way to M.D. Anderson or the Mayo Clinic and rent out an entire floor, it proves that the U.S. healthcare system is still awesome. The quality is still there, but the cost is not sustainable because there are too many people with their hands in the cookie jar. Many feel we need a shift to "value based care" but while many talk a good game, roadblocks remain to innovation and fulfilling that mission. The system is too cumbersome, and our insurance system does not *truly* recognize value-based care.

H.M.O.s, whose origins where discussed in the government chapter, exacerbated this downward spiral in efficiency. Let us reconsider the inherently ludicrous concept of an H.M.O: an administrative gatekeeper is required to protect patients from us, the doctors, because we might overspend on their care. It becomes even more absurd when many of these gatekeepers know nothing about medicine, or at least the specialty involved, yet possess the power to police doctors via the process of authorization. As I will share in a forthcoming section, authorization is indeed a "four-letter" word.

The crux of the H.M.O. concept hinges on making healthcare cheaper by assigning a primary care doctor – who sort of knows less and less about more and more – as another gatekeeper. Please do not misunderstand, I am not diminishing the skill and intelligence of primary care doctors; I am pointing out that there is no way they can possibly keep up with the advances in medicine within all specialties. For example, an internist cannot really stay up to date on anything I do as an orthopedic hand and upper limb surgeon. I am now way behind in advances in spine surgery, and I am an orthopedist. So, why would an internist screen a patient with a shoulder injury? Lack of orthopedic knowledge aside, these doctors must be paid, which adds to the cost of healthcare, while making it more cumbersome. The patient journey becomes arduous, delayed, and complicated.

This does not happen in other countries. True, my colleagues in Spain will admit that people wait a long time in their E.R.'s too. In general, though, if they have an orthopedic injury, either an orthopedist will come in to see them, or in the case of a big hospital, there will be an orthopedic doctor there.

It works. Yes, they deal with other challenges, but they do not have as many of these barriers that we face in the United States…barriers that we have self-imposed. Unfortunately, just like the exportation of McDonalds, they too are picking up on bad American ideas. Widespread medical malpractice litigation is another terrible practice they have begun to adopt. We must warn them.

One remedy can be found in the elimination of certain costly protocols like the convoluted process of so-called "guidelines." Medicine is not a cookbook field. By its nature, it is filled with nuances because patients are individuals with their own unique needs, physiologies, and response mechanisms. Even for a trained clinician, these factors can make it difficult to solve someone's medical issues. We examine the patient and review the diagnostic studies in the context of sitting there with them. A third party sitting behind a desk at an insurance company cannot do that. Keep in mind that the gatekeeper employee is earning a salary and benefits. Are we really saving money?

To be candid, much of the time the physician-gatekeepers for the insurance companies are either good doctors who are semi-retired (I am a bit envious) or could not make it on their own in private practice. You do not generally attend medical school to review records of other doctors, right? But the reality is that we have allowed this in our society because the insurance companies have the clout and the money. The people who control healthcare and profit most from it know the least about how to deliver care. Insurance company CEOs will claim that they want to save money, but they have lost perspective. They insist on adding another layer – an unnecessary step – while the public accepts and assumes their motives are all about cost-savings. Let me share a few regulatory issues you may not be aware of. These laws make a huge impact on healthcare.

First, people can make medical decisions from afar, probably due to the influence of health insurance companies that have the financial resources to spend on powerful lobbyists in D.C. and capture the time and attention of elected representatives. And yet, the physicians in the trenches have little voice in Washington. I recounted the story in the government chapter, but it is worth a reframe. I discovered the challenges facing physicians last year in terms of representation when I sent my then-CFO and the CEO of our marketing and PR agency (to transform healthcare, you must inform the public and therefore, hire a PR agency) to D.C. to confer with Senator Marco Rubio in a meeting we had scheduled in advance. Due to my convalescence from knee surgery, I decided to stay home, partly because I realized the intense effort would probably be for naught. Despite having small children, my C.F.O. and the co-founder of OrthoNOW® graciously agreed to take my place. However, when he and the marketing CEO arrived on Capitol Hill, they were greeted by Senator Rubio's aide who informed them that he would not be able to meet with them. Not to worry, though. The aide would pass the information along. How reassuring. Mind you, this is one of my senators from my adopted state of Florida. I wonder if he understands the real-life consequence of the ridiculous rule I am about to present. How could he? He missed our meeting.

A rarely discussed and underreported fact about health insurance company protocol is the M.L.R. (Medical Loss Ratio) rule, another result of the A.C.A. attempt to rein in costs. This is a mandate to spend 80-to-85 percent of their gross revenue on direct patient care, depending on employer size. Sounds noble, right? In a strange paradox, this 80/20 law has the opposite effect. It turns out that often insurance companies are not interested in the most cost-effective solution. *Why?* There is no incentive for them to spend less. If they do, they make too much money and fall out of compliance with the government guidelines. Consequently, even though they impose their own mandates on physicians, their own guidelines are counterproductive to the law's original intent. This is very concerning and would be a great addition to Herzlinger's Harvard Business Review on "Why Innovation in Health Care is So Hard" which I previously quoted. I wonder what the Trump Administration would say about this. It is a pity we cannot ask.

No doubt, executives and other insurance company employees want to make a good living. However, if they are not incentivized to lower costs, it presents a major problem. In my experience, whenever I have approached them with an idea like OrthoNOW® or other cost-effective practice concepts, I have encountered resistance. They do not embrace the ideas systematically, although individually, they love it. I imagine that the bureaucracy and hierarchies in these huge insurance companies preclude any change. Again, what is the reason for networking events and business chamber meetings then?

A recent example comes from a colleague, a semi-retired hand surgeon, who had been following our OrthoNOW® progress on the web via several platforms. Out of the blue he called me and said that our system may help one of the insurance companies that he is consulting for. It turns out they feel they are wasting way too much money in lesser orthopedic injuries that present to an emergency room. "Duh!" I replied, sounding much like my fifth grader. They wanted solutions to an obvious problem that I and several other clinicians had not only recognized but developed a real-life solution for…not that it mattered. While the Blue Cross Blue Shield of South Florida building is almost a stone's throw away from our OrthoNOW® headquarters, there has NEVER been any real dialogue to present this solution to a problem that affects them, the clinicians, *and* the patients: obtaining timely orthopedic expert care in an efficient, cost-effective manner. This is not rocket science as Seinfeld might quip. Communication and collaboration are completely lacking in our system.

What type of communication do *I* have with the health insurance industry? Well, other than constant wrestling to obtain "authorization" or God forbid, payment, allow me to share one very telling anecdote. When I first transitioned to my hand surgery practice, Badia Hand to Shoulder Center, from Miami Hand Center in late 2007, an administrative snafu occurred. At one point, I was seeing some patients in the new office in Doral, and soon operating on them at Surgery Center at Doral. Nothing unusual because many physicians maintain several office locations, and many surgeons, including me at that time, operate in several hospitals and surgery centers for a variety of reasons. Well, due to the strangling bureaucracy, it seems our billing teams had not properly registered me with Blue Cross Blue Shield for that change. Understood. *Mea culpa.* You would think that all I had to do to obtain reimbursement for the surgeries I had performed was to simply submit the paperwork with my new tax I.D. (or whatever method they need to identify me). Wrong. They kindly suggested that they pay me based upon my social security number instead of a tax I.D. for those cases, which exceeded 80 surgeries. Yes, *80.* As I described in Section I, this represents real work for a busy surgeon. It is not "billable hours" or more nebulous services rendered – it is cold, hard steel applied to a patient's skin and innards to solve their clinical issue. I was not even going to fight the consultations or follow-up visits because they were too numerous to recount and bill. I simply wanted to be paid for the 80 surgeries that I performed on *their* insured patients. Keep in mind, I was transitioning to a new center that I built. Ongoing work income was critical.

This wrangling went on for nearly six months, occupying my new staff's time and placing additional mental burden on me when I was developing a new practice location. Due to the close location of Blue Cross Blue Shield's regional headquarters, I jumped into my car, sped over there, and stormed into the lobby. I had to make a scene because they were not responding to the usual litany of letters, emails, and calls. Imagine a plumber not being paid for

80 jobs they performed to resolve customers' problems? Naturally, they called the police. When they arrived, I explained the situation much more calmly. One of the insurance company's mid-level executives then promised to set up a meeting with my staff and me.

When the day of the Blue Cross Blue Shield "summit" arrived, let's call it "Charitygate," my staff had prepared a stack of our unpaid claims for surgical case reimbursements. Furthermore, I prepared a short Power Point to illustrate those cases with before-and-after X-rays, along with some occasional graphic intra-operative photos that demonstrated what I actually did. It was amazing to see the somewhat shocked looks on the faces of people who really control our healthcare – as if what I did was a foreign concept. One person even uttered their distress at the sight of blood. Imagine if I felt the same way. I would not be able to fix that shattered elbow you could sustain if you tripped on the way out of my office into the parking lot. When the presentation ended, they promised they would "do their best" to resolve the situation. Again, I received that *Stepford Wives* glassy-eyed look from the lady who continues to receive awards for her contribution to healthcare in our community. I wish the various chamber of commerce leaders had been in my conference room that day.

To their credit, I was finally paid on most of the claims. Not all, but our team was satisfied. The real question is **why** did I have to go through that ordeal? There is little controversy about a service rendered when I put up an X-ray that shows an 8-hole stainless steel plate on a humerus, or a titanium replacement of a shattered radial head at the elbow. However, this is quite symbolic of the disconnect I discussed in an earlier chapter between the health insurance industry and the actual professionals rendering that service.

If we the physicians are haggling just to get paid fairly, imagine the hurdles we face when attempting to introduce cost savings innovations that benefit all of us in society. The same challenge holds true for many of my colleagues in the trenches who present a myriad of cost-saving efficiencies that provide better care to patients. One example known to me, due to my specialty and early involvement is the informal group known as OrthoFounders, a group of entrepreneurial orthopedic surgeons who each started a healthcare-related company. This was the criteria for inclusion. While most of it involves orthopedic devices, surprisingly it also includes many processes to improve orthopedic care delivery and cost-effectiveness. Why are there so many barriers to progress? One reason is the existence of these third-party companies that erect obstacles between the health insurance company and the clinician-provider. Yes, I embarked upon 14 years of education to be called a "provider" – a term that should only apply to me as a father, not a medical professional.

The fact is these third-party administrator companies (TPAs) make more money if the care is more expensive since they get a percentage of the care costs. They are not incentivized for less costly care, which is another problem lumped on top of the 80/20 rule. It only makes sense (or "cents") that they would want to keep everything in the hospital because the hospital IS expensive. It must be expensive. How can a place that features an expensive I.C.U., 15 to 20 operating rooms, and a huge infrastructure NOT be expensive? It is not a criticism; it is reality. For example, if you are going to have your hernia done, where would it be cheaper? In a big hospital as either a day or overnight surgery, or in a specialized outpatient center, where all they do is hernias? A colleague of mine, Dr. Gilbert, who is now retired, figured this out 30 years ago, in developing the Hernia Institute of Florida, along with colleague Jerrold Young. He was well ahead of his time in creating an ambulatory specialty center that improves efficiency, cost, and quality, simply because they do the same thing, day in and day out. When you do that much volume, in an efficient environment, clinical innovation and protocols will likely result, which is good for patients and our overall healthcare system. Ironic that some of the mesh hernia repair techniques they helped develop have been subjected to predatory lawsuits around the country, and even advertised on network television. The same for the countless ads on Fox News and others regarding failed hip replacement or asbestos exposure. It is simply disgusting. Amazing how THEY have the resources to afford expensive prime-time ads on TV. More on that in the malpractice chapter.

Why is a specialized hernia center a superior option for care? The anesthesiologist, who knows what is safe or unsafe for a patient, is focused on that procedure and assesses the patient for possible outpatient care. The nursing and surgical tech staff have all done the same procedures day after day. Since all the surgeon does is hernia repairs in this scenario, it is the ultimate in specialty care. And of course, their outcomes are better, and their costs are much lower, yet health insurance companies do not often embrace these concepts.

Let us give an example relevant to this hernia center. My shoulder patient, (whose story you'll read in the workers' comp section of this chapter) Kerry has a boyfriend, David, who experienced major challenges simply to find a surgeon for his routine hernia. He told me about his dilemma that required him to drive up to Broward County from Miami-Dade because he could not find any doctors in his own county on his insurance plan. Yet when David reached out to the Hernia Institute of Florida, located in South Miami-Dade, he found out they did not take his insurance either. *Why?* Because the insurance companies do not seem to be savvy enough to realize, "Hey, this is a good thing for my insured patients. This is cost-effective. It is high-quality care because it is repetitive. It is outpatient. Let us negotiate a fair contract."

Instead, what tends to happen is that the patient comes away thinking, "The doctor does not take my insurance. What a disappointment." Most people do not stop to think why. After all, this might come as a surprise, but surgeons like to get paid fairly, like anybody else who works hard. The translation of "not taking insurance" means that the doctor cannot even discuss a fair contract, let alone have one offered to them by the insurance company. The receptionist, office manager, or billing coordinator should tell the hapless patient, "Your insurance company does not give the contract; it is not that we don't accept." It is a matter of perspective and patients do not understand because few, if any, explain it to them. Yet it must be explained by somebody in the trenches.

Why are these discussions not happening in the healthcare marketplace? Would you like to know how much real dialogue I have had with a decision-maker at a health insurance company? ZERO. I do not count the Blue Cross Blue Shield debacle on not getting paid as "dialogue."

How can we decrease healthcare costs overall, if every time I go to a medical conference, there is never an insurance company there? Conversely, when the insurance companies host conferences (the only reason I hear about them is because of blanket emails I get now), there are never any providers in attendance, other than the hired physicians. I mentioned this in my chapter on collaboration, which should be entitled, "Lack of Collaboration." No one who is providing care in the community goes to these conferences and interacts with the people who are paying for the care. Does that make any sense?

Here is the logical conclusion explaining the lack of discussion and collaboration: the insurance industry wants it that way. Do not get me wrong, every time I manage to talk to a decision-maker, they are cordial. They are educated. But nothing ever comes out of it. And they want it that way. Why aren't we talking about this? It is funny, I grew up reading a book called, *The People's Almanac* by David Wallechinsky and his father Irving Wallace, written in 1975. To this day, it remains one of the most fact-filled, interesting books I have ever read (I have always enjoyed nonfiction more than fiction). In *The People's Almanac*, there is a whole section on who runs the government in every country. For example, at the time Paraguay was run by the military and England is run by their House of Parliament, with the Monarchy as a symbol. What did it share about the United States? Our country is run by insurance companies. That is what this book revealed 45 years ago.

Here are the big-picture challenges:

1. The clinicians who work for the insurance companies and make many of the actual decisions are essentially ***immune***. That means, if something egregious happens, there is no consequence for them telling the doctor, "No, you can't do this test, procedure, or operation." The upcoming chapter on medical malpractice (a fun one) makes no mention of an insurance company being sued for influencing a decision that led to a bad result.

2. Insurance companies are mandated to spend 85 percent on healthcare, which sounds like a good thing in the ideal (kind of like communism) but does not work in practice. The way it is written, it accomplishes the opposite of its intended goal.

3. Medicare, one of our biggest payers, is only going to expand as the population ages. That has the potential to bankrupt the country. If our politicians and media are as concerned about it as they claim, why don't we take actual steps to lower the costs?

Keep these three major concerns in mind as we review a few principles and practices of the insurance industry which should be completely overhauled as any physician working in the trenches will tell you.

Authorization is a Four-Letter Word

Authorization is one of the most ludicrous concepts in healthcare.

Who determined that the physician is *not* the best person to decide what is needed? They have done the training and they have certain ethical standards. Insurance companies should appoint somebody who only notices and investigates things that are out of the ordinary. Nevertheless, the current modus operandi is to require an "authorization" on virtually everything we do in delivering care. Need a specialist? Get authorization. That specialist requires a particular imaging study? Get an authorization. That study shows that X is torn and needs repairing? Obtain an authorization. X is now fixed but needs rehabilitation? Pursue an authorization. Get the picture?

Many physicians and I accept the validity of the insurance argument that many people abuse and over-utilize. My proposal has always been to assign insurance company employees to do to spot-checks, like TSA (Transportation Security Administration) should do, instead of frisking 90-year-old grandmas, which makes no sense. It would be more effective for insurance companies to train designated employed clinicians at different levels to detect irregularities because physicians are the best judges of how to spend that money. And most of us are screened to be ethical. We took an oath. Remember Section I of this book? When we say a patient needs to stay another day in the hospital, there is a valid a reason for that. If you do not listen to us, guess what? That patient is discharged but maybe they will be back in two days – hence, the readmission problem that hospitals and Medicare fear.

Every time you hear a denial or even an approval for patient care, you think, "Shit! Why is some person at an insurance company with no education authorizing me to do this?" What I would like to hear is, "We authorize you to see our patient who has our policy." Fine. I get that. If they want to save money, make sure good docs see patients covered by their insurance and let that doctor do what needs to be done. What a novel concept. What a money saver. And time and aggravation. The last part, aggravation, will be discussed in the moral injury chapter, something that should not be underestimated. If you heard something about clinician attitudes on the front lines during COVID-19, you know that we are not going to be society's punching bag any longer. That holds particularly true for insurance companies. I did not see any insurance executives or adjustors intubating patients flush with a virus that can end your life with a bad turn. Enough said.

The authorization issue is so ludicrous and prevalent it is probably best to compare the practice to something we can all relate to: Ordering food in a restaurant. Ten years ago, Dr. Megan Lewis, a vocal and proactive family practitioner from Colorado wrote a blog in a primary care newsletter which imagined if restaurants were run like our healthcare system. The comparison hits home and is so on point that I am sharing it with you in its entirety. Many of us in healthcare reading this will likely belly laugh out loud, some patients will relate, but a few of us may nearly cry out of frustration.

"Imagine going to your favorite restaurant. You are greeted at the door by the hostess, who seats you and takes your drink order. You order through your favorite waiter, Andrew, who recommends the special of the day: prime rib with a dinner salad and a chocolate torte for dessert. Soon after, the food is brought out and it is delicious! You have time to enjoy your food. You then receive the bill and pay for your meal, returning to your home satisfied, all your dining needs met. Let's say, for simplicity's sake, you paid $75 for this meal: $50 for the steak, $10 for the salad and $15 for the dessert.

"A change then occurs in the restaurant industry. A new form of eating out has been adopted. Your favorite restaurant has now contracted with over 30 different "restaurant insurance companies."

"Anticipating another pleasant dining experience, your return to the restaurant with your new "subscriber's card." You pay your $5 "copay." You sit in the foyer of the restaurant. You wait an hour, even though you made reservations. A harried Andrew greets you and quickly takes your order after you briefly glance at the menu. The food arrives at your table. As you take your second bite, Andrew informs you that "your time is up" and the table is reserved for another party. You are escorted outside with your hastily boxed leftovers.

"What has happened to the restaurant? Behind the scenes, the restaurant owner has learned some tough realities of the "new system." During the first month of taking insurance, the owner sends a form to the insurance company requesting payment for the $75 steak dinner: $50 for the steak, $10 for the salad and $15 for the torte. The contract with the insurance company already states that they will only pay $45 for the $50 steak, but the owner decides that the extra customers brought to the restaurant by contracting with this insurance company will more than off-set this small loss.

"The first attempt at collecting the $75 dollars for the full meal is returned unpaid with the note that it was rejected due to a "coding error." The forms for payment from the insurance company require the owner to list the parts of the meal, not by name, but by the numerical codes. The owner had listed the salad by the wrong numerical code. No suggestions for the correct code are offered, so the restaurant owner purchases a series of books, at a cost of $500, to learn how to assign the correct code to the different parts of the meals. These books will need to be bought annually due to the constant changing of the code numbers. After 30 minutes of study, the owner realizes the dinner salad should be coded as a 723.13, not the 723.1 the owner originally put on the form. The salad, it turns out, needed to have two digits after the decimal point, indicating that it was a dinner salad, and not a "main course" salad. The owner mails the corrected form.

"In response to the second request for payment, the insurance company does not send a check, but a detailed questionnaire: Was garlic used in seasoning the steak? Was it necessary to use garlic for this particular recipe? Did the restaurant ask for permission to use garlic from the insurance company before serving the steak? Why was salt, a less expensive alternative, not used instead? The owner submits the answers, emphasizing that the garlic is part of a secret family recipe that made the restaurant famous.

"The owner waits another week (it has now been 3 weeks since the dinner was served). The check arrives three and a half weeks after the meal was served. The check is for $20 and states that it is specifically for the steak. The check also comes with a letter stating that no billing of the patron may occur for the salad, but no other explanation is enclosed. No mention is made of the $15 dessert.

"The now frustrated restaurant owner calls the provider service number listed in the contract. After five separate phone calls to five different numbers (The harried voice behind phone call number four explains that the insurance company has merged with another insurance company and the phone numbers had all changed last week, sorry for the inconvenience...), the owner gets to ask why, when the contract says the steak will be paid at $45, has the check only been written for $20? And what happened to the payment for the $10 salad and the $15 dessert?

"As it turns out, this particular patron's insurance contract only pays $45 when the patron has reached their deductible, which this patron has not at this time. The remaining portion of payment for the steak must now be billed by the restaurant to the patron directly.

"The $10 for the salad would have been paid if the patron had ordered it on a different day, but, per page 35 in the contract, because it was billed on the same day as the steak, it is considered to be part of the payment for the steak and no extra money can be collected from the patron or the insurance company.

"The dessert, the owner learns, should have had a "modifier" number put with its particular billing code when billed with the steak and the salad.

"Realizing that the insurance billing is quite a bit harder than anticipated, the restaurant owner hires a company, who is paid 5% of any money collected to specifically make sure these coding errors do not occur again and follow up on payment rejections. For an additional $99 per month, the billing company will "scrub" the forms submitted for payment to make sure specific clerical errors will not cause future delays in payment.

"The owner now must lay off the hostess and the bus boy to pay the billing company, so these duties are now added to the waiter's other responsibilities.

"In the meantime, the restaurant owner has also had the waiter take on the job of answering the phones due to the now high volume of phone calls from patrons questioning why they are receiving bills for meals they ate over two months ago, and why did their insurance company not pay for this portion of the meal? This extra work is now resulting in longer times patrons must wait to be seated, and grumblings from the waiters who "were not hired or trained to do this kind of work."

"The owner now realizes that, although the dinner originally cost $75 to make, only $25 has been paid. The remaining $30 billed to the patron is now in its third mailing, with the first two requests for payment going unanswered by the patron. The restaurant owner realizes a collection agency must be employed in order to have any hope of receiving any portion of payment from the patron.

"Each meal served now costs at least an additional $20 due to the added overhead of the billing company, coding books, and the collection agency. These added expenses have nothing to do with cooking food or providing any direct service to the restaurant's customers.

"Service to the restaurant's patrons has been compromised with these changes as well. The owner has now overextended the once excellent waiter, who now must take on the roles of host, phone answering, and table bussing.

"To even meet the costs of providing fine dining, the restaurant owner now must seat twice as many patrons in the same amount of time.

"What was once an outstanding business that focused on fine dining and customer service has now been turned into a business in the business of trying to get paid.

"Alas, I wish this were a fictional tale, but it is not. The only fictional portion is that this is not your favorite restaurant, but your favorite doctor's office, which is responsible not for meeting your dining needs, but those of your health."

This humorous portrayal of our system is perhaps not so funny to the clinicians and their staff who must live this experience every day while they try to care for patients. Many patients, particularly those with chronic disease issues, will find this account familiar. A way to perhaps minimize those barriers is to engage patients further and even ask them to share in some of the cost, a growing sentiment in healthcare circles.

As Dr. Roger Khouri notes,

"The insurance companies are in the business to make money. They make money by withholding care, rationing care, or playing games. We as physicians are the only professionals who would agree to work without knowing whether we are going to be paid, or how much we are going to get paid. When I am on-call and I go to the emergency room, I have no idea whether I am going to get paid, and if I do get paid, how much it will be. Would you ever see that in any other profession anywhere else? No, of course not. To add insult to injury, we are the only professionals in this capitalist country whose fee schedule is determined arbitrarily by the government.

"You want to have carpal tunnel surgery? Whether it is the superstar surgeon who does it or Dr. Joe Schmo, it is the same reimbursement, the same price. No other profession works by an arbitrary fee schedule set by the government. Now, we can live with that. I am personally in favor of a single payer system where we erase all the bureaucracy and remove all these middlemen.

"The worst are the Medicare H.M.O's. These guys intercede between the government paid insurance and me to ration care and cut corners on patients. They negotiate my fees to be below what the government would have normally paid me, they ration the care of the patients, and then make millions in between. There is a guy here in town, I know who sold his company for a few billion dollars – a company I helped him to start. When he needed a panel of doctors, I was the first was one.

"How do you make those billions of dollars? By shortchanging one side and shortchanging the other side to make money in the middle. It is incredibly frustrating. I have an army of people in my office that spend their time getting authorizations from insurance companies. We had a guy who injured his finger on a Friday and days later we were still not "authorized" to treat him.

"Another insured patient was already scheduled for surgery but when he came in to have it, the insurance company had still not authorized it. There I was, sitting with my patient whose finger was hanging halfway off. He should have had surgery the previous week, but it had not been authorized. What could I do with the patient right there in front of me about to lose his finger? Refuse to operate on him and risk malpractice, or operate on him, knowing I will not get paid because I did not have authorization? I pay a team of employees in my office with the sole job of obtaining authorization for care.

"Now the problem, of course, is abuse. We cannot control the abuse. And let us face it: we have bad apples in our own field; hence the amplification of stories of Medicare fraud, etc. Negative stories travel much faster and farther than positive stories and add to the false perception that most doctors are crooks. They have no clue and still hold the perception that doctors make tons of money. If they see a doctor driving a Rolls Royce, he or she must be a crook because it is unacceptable for a doctor to drive an expensive luxury car."

According to Dr. Robert Terrill, our orthopedic hand surgeon from Massachusetts,

"I would say that the last five years have become especially challenging to be in practice, just in general. The various insurance plans all have different requirements and regulations. Insurance companies have gone from organizations that collect premiums; group patients; and provide and pay for healthcare, to companies that make as much money as they can while not providing care. Insurance CEOs make ridiculous amounts of money for managing a business. My understanding is that in the first quarter of 2019 United Healthcare made $2 billion in profit. That sets up so that the CEO makes deferred income annualized in the range of $500 million. Those are rough numbers. Insurance companies should reduce their patients' premiums and put some of that money in a pool for people who do not have insurance or are uninsured for whatever reason.

"I love taking care of patients. I love doing surgery. The thing that is killing me is the administrative bullshit. And I guarantee I am not the only one who feels this way. I keep it very lean. I have four staff members in my office: a medical assistant/secretary; a second secretary; a third person who deals with the insurance companies and booking surgeries; and my office manager who does most everything. She used to be a middle manager at a local insurance company, so she gets it. She knows some of the people and understands how these companies operate. By contrast, I am still astounded by some of the stuff that goes on. I have a letter that is currently being reviewed with various cases to go the Attorney General here in Massachusetts regarding patients and stuff with me. It is becoming like a chess match between the MBAs in the insurance company saying, 'Hey, let's change this,' and the providers, who are going along, taking care of folks, doing surgery, or seeing them in the office.

"Then the insurance company declares, 'Oh, well, that's not covered.' And you are like, 'What? What do you mean it's not covered?' Some of the insurance companies just take the money back, and then you must chase it down. I can give you a couple examples. One is a patient who did not get injured, but had carpal tunnel syndrome, which is a common condition we take care of. The insurance company sent out a subrogation sheet with questions like, 'Could you have fallen?' 'Did you do it at work?' to see if they could get out of paying for it. And the patient said, 'Well, I already had surgery and I'm better. I'm back working, and no, it wasn't a work-related injury.' So, the insurance company threw the sheet away and claimed, 'We did not get the sheet back and we are taking all the money we paid you back. You must chase the patient down and get them to fill out the sheet.'

"When we contacted the patient, she was mad and told us she did not care. We had to threaten to take her to small claims court to fill out the sheet so that I could get the money. There was no penalty on the part of the insurance company for this deception; the penalty was for me because I had to ask my staff to chase this crap down.

"In a second case, I had an infant born with extra fingers, a common occurrence in the African-American population. I usually tie them off and remove them in the newborn nursery, so the parents do not have to deal with it at home because they can be unstable, twist and fall off, and things like that. I billed it to one of the local insurance companies. And they said, 'Oh, we only pay one of those codes a day.' I replied, 'Well, they had two fingers. I billed it with the code and bilateral. Did you want me to keep them in the hospital an extra day and do the other finger on a different day?' For 91 days, they played games back and forth. Ninety days is the line that you cannot bill beyond. When we reached 91 days, they informed me, 'Oh, you should have billed this code, but it's too late. Too bad. You don't get paid.' These are two simple examples, but this is happening several times a week.

"My concern, and it would be interesting to do a cross-sectional study of primary care physicians, orthopedic surgeons, hand surgeons, plastic surgeons, etc. is that there is going to be a large brain drain in the next five years. A lot of people are just going to say, 'Screw this.' The governor of Massachusetts announced that he's doing a big push – and I applaud him for it – to pay primary care doctors more because they work their butts off chasing down all these different cases they have to do on people every year, in addition to paying more for behavioral health issues because, here in central Massachusetts, I think we're number two in the United States for overdoses.

"It is extremely high. For us, as hand and upper extremity surgeons, we see a lot of IV drug related hand problems. Last spring, there was a batch of heroin mixed with fentanyl that came into the area. The reason the pushers were using fentanyl is apparently (I cannot speak from experience) if you have one big hit, you are addicted. It is basically building their population, but it does not have a good safety profile. There are people overdosing everywhere. I mean, at the library, all the librarians are trained in giving Narcan, and they probably do it a half-dozen times a day. In the hospital, we have IV drug folks. We see at least one a day with various infections, and sometimes needing surgery from shooting up with dirty needles. It is a huge problem.

"As I said, I applaud the governor for at least trying to look at some of these issues. He has been in the forefront in solving the opiate problem and so on. But I worry and I look at other things I can do. While I enjoy dealing with patients, my income has been adversely affected. Another phenomenon I have noticed in my younger colleagues tends to be an attitude of, 'Let me do as many cases as I can, in as short time as I can.' Maybe that is their way of dealing with being paid less by insurance companies.

"Maybe I am old-school, but I like to see all my patients. I do not have a P.A. I had a P.A. for a while, but then he went back to work at the Shriners Hospital. I see every pre-op and every post-op patient. I am there when they go to sleep, and I am there when they wake up. There is not any kind of 'now you see him, now you don't, because for the total joint, surgeons are being rewarded to do surgery as fast as possible.

"An orthopedic surgeon in upstate New York is being sued. One of his patients broke her femur. And he said, 'Well, that wasn't me; that was a P.A. They were closing.' But he was doing 10 total hips in a day. And there is no need. If there was that much of a shortage of people being able to do total hips, then you get another surgeon. I hate to say it, but that was greed. And it is also greed on the part of the hospital because the hospitals are part of this as well. They get paid about $30,000 to $35,000 for a total hip replacement. They pay that for the hip prosthesis but by allowing this guy or gal to use two different rooms all the time, they make more money.

"Physicians as a group have not been out in front with respect to what is going on with healthcare. My sister-in-law has nothing to do with medicine, so I will use her as an example of "Susie Average." I asked her, "Well, what do you know; I just operated on this guy with a bad infection in his finger from a piece of wood. How much do you think I'll get paid for that?"

"Now, this patient was on one of the lower paying Medicaid plans. She answered, "$10,000." I replied, "No." She countered, "$2,500?" and I said, "No. Do you want to know how much? Two-hundred bucks." She was astounded. I mean, I once operated on somebody who had such a shitty plan, I got $26. I cannot park for that amount of money.

"What patients must understand is there are two entities making the most money in the healthcare arena right now: insurance companies and hospitals. Yes, there are plenty of physicians driving nice cars. I drive a Subaru; I am not a big car dude. One of the anesthesiologists drives a Maserati SUV that cost about $120 Grand. I'm like, 'Well, shit. I could buy four or five cars for that amount of money.' Cars may be important to some people, but not to me. But in general, the average person has no idea. They assume the doctors are just rolling in it, and yes, we make an OK living, but it is much less than they think. My guess is that my income has probably gone down 60 percent in the last six years. That is significant.

"Thank God, my kids are educated and gone because my son went to private boarding school in New Hampshire for ski racing and his boarding school now is $61,000 a year. I could not afford it right now. He is 30 years old now, so that was 15 years ago. I ask myself, 'How are people doing this?' 'How are they going to do that?'

"And I think that's why some of my colleagues do as much surgery as they do. I have never changed my indications for a given procedure. One of my colleagues did a total joint replacement on a patient that was actively using cocaine. Well, I would not do it, period. It would not be a discussion. It is going to be a nightmare, which it was for the P.A. However, physicians have done a poor job of communicating what's going on in healthcare, and that they are not rolling in dough.

"On the flip side, expenses have gone through the friggin' roof. Liability insurance is the single biggest ticket item I have. I do not do spines. Thank God I do not do OB/GYN. But still my malpractice insurance costs me around $40,000 a year – more than a staff member. Then there is the rent. I am sort of negotiating with the hospital, which is part of Tenet, the big for-profit group, where the rents are high. I spend about $7,000 a month for my space. And I am getting paid less. Expenses are higher and we are getting squeezed. That is why doctors take moonlighting jobs, another big problem people do not understand. The health insurance industry has been marked out as part of the evil empire. I do not think that is inaccurate. They do very well for themselves. Whenever I update my health insurance, the plans pay for less while my co-pay is higher. My deductibles are higher. And you wonder, 'What exactly are they paying for? My premium went up by 10 percent.' I can tell you, as a provider who accepts many of these plans, neither I nor my office staff has seen an increase in the rate we have been paid over the past 10 years.

"In 30 to 40 percent of the premium dollars used, it is 'overhead' for the insurance companies. Why is the Vice President of Government Relations (or some such title) making $150,000 a year? What exactly are they doing? And for every insurance company, there are hundreds of these types of positions.

"I have not looked at all the details with Medicare for All, but I'm leaning more towards a single payer, simply because of the gigantic overhead and unending bullshit I deal with from insurance companies. I had patient, a lady with a mass growing in front of her elbow and I wanted to do an M.R.I. The insurance company told me, "Oh, we need a peer to peer." Fine. I wrote all this stuff out and my staff called the X-ray organization, which I think was AIM for Blue Cross. I know from experience Blue Cross wants me to call for 100 percent of them. And again, it is just another means of blocking care. They know the physician may not be able to call, which means they may not have to pay for it, or they may be able to delay it.

"When I called and talked to the nurse, she said, 'Well, I don't cover Unicare.'

"'Why am I talking to you then?' I questioned.

"Then, she put me on the phone with the doctor – somebody or other – and I told them what was going on. "Oh, we didn't have the information," he told me.

"I said, 'My secretary read it to the people.'

"'Well, I don't know.'

"But as soon as I said, 'mass growing in the elbow' – boom! Approved.

"I asked, 'Well, why did I have to do this? I am not doing my regular work. I cannot see patients, I cannot dictate office notes, I cannot do the stuff that really is the practice. I'm just doing this crap.'

"She replied, 'I don't really know.'

"This is an example of the unending hassle factor. I talked to my brother, who is an attorney in Philadelphia. He represents many ophthalmologists who are getting paid less for what they do. I think the insurance companies look at procedures and say, 'Oh, there are too many cataracts being done. Let us reduce what we are paying. We've decided to change it from you know, $1,000 bucks to $500 bucks.'

"Explain to me why you're paying it half as much as you used to. Then we have more doctors not interested in doing them. The insurance companies make more money but then their clients, the actual purchasers of insurance raise hell because they say, 'Geez, we cannot find a doctor that takes United Healthcare.' I worry about that. Perhaps a single payer type of system like Medicare would be better.

"Obviously, Medicare is not perfect, but as a doctor you do not get nearly as much of this crap, the insurance company hassle. Then comes the secondary, 'We have reviewed what you did, and we are going to pay you half.' And I think, 'Wait a minute, that is your fee schedule.' They have already taken the money back and demand that we tell them why we think we should get that money. This kind of hassle is partly why I have a letter out to the Attorney General. I have had a bunch of patients that have been hurt by delayed treatment, delayed therapy, etc. I would love to be a consultant for the Attorney General because I know all the crap that they do. And I do not really mind battling with them that much; I know I am in the right in most of the cases."

Authorization is not limited to medical tests and procedures, as pharmacist Aileen Gonzalez recounts below:

"Healthcare is part of corporate America: the pharmaceutical companies and the insurance companies have taken over. A doctor prescribes a medicine they think would benefit a patient, but their health insurance company does not want to pay for it. Then, the doctor must explain to the insurance company why they need it in what we call a 'prior authorization.' The patient must get their doctor to answer the insurance company's questions before they will approve it. It is not even that the doctor gets to dictate what prescription he wants for their patient. It is more like, "Oh, is this covered with my insurance?" Insurance plans have tiers: tier one, tier two, and so on. It depends on the copay and all insurance plans are different. There are thousands of different insurances and different groups of insurances within those insurances, so it gets complicated for every individual. They all want to know, "Is this covered?" and I must explain to them that until I process and submit the claim, I will not know. It is impossible to know off the top of my head if they cover it or not...and I get tons of prioritizations every day.

"We submit them via fax to a third party called 'Cover My Meds.' But I always tell my patients, 'Look, this can take anywhere from 24 to 72 hours. It depends how hard they are working at your doctor's office. If they have somebody in the office who just handles authorizations, it depends on how busy they are.' Yes, the pharmacist can do it the old-fashioned way and get on the phone. But we lose a lot of time because we deal with, 'Press one for this department,' then wait on hold before someone else gets on and says, 'Oh, let me get you to the right person.' Then the patient gets upset and takes out their frustration on us. I always explain to them, 'Look, I'm the middle person here. This is between your doctor and your insurance company. I am here to fill your prescription and give you your medicine. I want to give it to you. But if they do not pay for it, I can't.' We see a lot of that in the pharmacy. Some patients end up paying out-of-pocket if they can, but it is an everyday battle.

"After working in corporate America for Walgreen's, CVS, and Publix, I took a job near my home at an independent pharmacy. While Publix was a bit more organized on the back end than either Walgreen's or CVS, they still demanded way too much. There are countless tasks to perform. As a pharmacist, I had to complete the task of the technician, which encompasses about 15 tasks. Then there is a checklist of tasks for the pharmacist, in addition to giving flu shots and vaccines, checking orders, taking the prescription and typing in it, consulting, answering the phone...I mean, the list goes on. And it was just me doing all that in an 11-hour shift. I barely had time to eat some days. It was not human; there is no way a person can work in a pharmacy by themselves. It was crazy. Another employee helped me, maybe six hours a week, while I kept up with a volume of almost 100 prescriptions a day. In addition to doing vaccines because Publix demands it. They told me I needed to meet a specific quota for vaccines and if I did not meet their quota, they could fire me. It got ugly but I eventually left on good terms and accepted the job at the local, independent pharmacy, where I only do 11-hour shifts every other Saturday. I work four hours a day, for a total of 30 hours per week. The difference is that it is not as intense, and I have the assistance of techs and clerks.

"Another huge contrast between the independent pharmacy and corporate America pharmacies is that the independent pharmacy must count every dollar and make sure they're not losing money. As a pharmacist, I still deal with the same customer problems. For example, sometimes they want everything quick, as if it is a fast food restaurant. They have no problem waiting at the doctor for an hour, but when they show up with that little piece of paper, they demand, 'I want my medicine now.'

"On the back end, we get tons of prescriptions electronically. In another year or so, they are going to do away with handwritten prescriptions altogether. Everything is going to be electronic. Nobody knows the value we have in our computers when they drop off their prescription at the front of the counter. There is a lot going on in the back.

"When I graduated back in 2001, the insurance and pharmaceutical companies started huge marketing campaigns, like, "Oh, if you are feeling sad, try Lexapro," featuring a happy person in those TV ads. I thought to myself, 'What did I get myself into?' I enjoyed pharmacy school and I was thrilled to get out and work my first job in a mom-and-pop retail setting and interact with people on a one-to-one basis. My whole view of pharmacy was shot since I started. In the commercials, they tell you about the side effects. Guess what? They will manufacture and prescribe another medicine to counteract the side effects of the first medicine.

"Yes, I believe that sometimes you need your antibiotics or certain medicines; for example, if you have cancer, you do need certain prescriptions. However, most prescriptions manage symptoms...unless it is an antibiotic that kills the bacteria. It hurts me to see so many people on antidepressants because I grew up with a mother who was on several of them. I saw what it did to her and thought, 'Wow, I want to help her and other people to know there are other ways to heal.' That is one reason why I am moving into an area of healing that focuses on the energy centers within, because all diseases come from the inside. If you can clear the emotional pain from your energy centers, you can live a much happier life. To me, this kind of work is more rewarding than standing behind a counter like a robot, just counting pills, answering the phone, and trying to smile in between. I am a big, free-spirited, happy person. And when I go to the pharmacy, I become the opposite of who I really am."

Certainly, the holistic part of medicine would demand another book entirely; it is not the aim of this account. Suffice it to say that most physicians and pharmacists embrace significant holistic components in their care of patients, although those patients often do not realize that fact. We are too busy fighting for standard care to even explore other areas that we know can be beneficial. If we can barely get approval for certain cutting-edge surgical procedures, how are we going to embrace more controversial therapies?

AN OCCUPATIONAL THERAPIST IN NEW MEXICO SHARES HER EXPERIENCE WITH INSURANCE AUTHORIZATION

Kristin Forno is an occupational therapist in New Mexico who runs her own private practice clinic with one other therapist. She set it up that way on purpose after working for a busy therapy clinic, where she could not dictate how many patients she could see and how much time she could allocate toward their treatment.

She observes, "I set up my own practice where I can spend a full hour with a patient. I do not see as many people as I used to, which is nice. The people who own the business are trying to make an income. They pay the salaries of the front desk staff, the billing staff, and everyone else who works there. There are a lot of administrative costs to cover, and the therapists are generating that income. At the same time, insurance companies are decreasing their reimbursement rates. What ends up happening is that these therapy clinics schedule more patients. They shove as many patients as they can into the therapist's schedule because the more patients they treat, the more income they generate to pay for the staff and other overhead.

"In my current situation, I do not have any staff. I work with one other therapist, but I do not have a front desk person that schedules patients and does all the prior authorizations. The other therapist and I do that ourselves. It is not hard, but most therapists hire somebody else to do it. We do not get paid quite as much as our colleagues because we take time away from patient care to obtain prior authorizations and handle other administrative tasks. But I do not feel like I can treat the number of people that I am treating now and support like a front desk staff salary.

"The unfortunate part about insurance is that it does not always cover everything. For example, a tendon takes 12 weeks to heal. The insured patient needs therapy for 12 weeks, but their insurance will only cover six visits. That is when I feel as if I am leaving these people because they cannot pay out of pocket. And their insurance will not cover more than about six visits, so they are left to heal on their own. In these situations, I do my best to outline what they need to do.

"However, it is not ideal. Thankfully, it does not happen to too often because most of my patients have Medicare, which provides adequate visits. Many practitioners will not accept it because the reimbursement rates are a bit lower, but Medicare does not require any prior authorization; therefore, I never have to appeal for a denial. For me, the time I save by not having to deal with appeals or prior authorizations is worth the decreased reimbursement rate.

"Many times, patients who have private insurance will walk through the door believing that they will not have to pay anything because they already pay a high deductible every month. They think their therapy should be totally free, and that is not the case most of the time because patients tend to have a co-pay. And when I tell them, 'You have a $50 co-pay,' they think I am the one setting that price. They do not understand their insurance coverage because nobody sits down with them to reviews their insurance plan details.

"That is one thing that I would like patients to know: your therapy is most likely not going to be free. You are going to have a copay or coinsurance or deductible, and it might be months down the road that you get this bill in the mail. Many people get upset with me about their payment responsibility for occupational therapy services, or because they receive the bill three or four months later, after their insurance company processes it. They call me up to express their anger over their high bill. And the bottom line is they do not understand the terms of the insurance plan they have enrolled in.

"If somebody needs a splint or something that is not covered, I will just go ahead and make it, then hope that the insurance company will retro reimburse me. And if they do not, I end up writing it off, which is not ideal as a business owner. However, I want people to get the care that they need. Thankfully, that does not happen too often. I do my prior authorizations a week ahead of time and tell the patient what to expect when they come in, for example, the amount of their copay, to avoid any upset.

"While I try to get the prior authorization ahead of time, sometimes I get into a pinch, like when my husband, orthopedic surgeon Dr. Philip Forno, sends over a patient for a splint to be made. If I do not have time to get the prior authorization, I will make the splint, then attempt a retro authorization with the insurance company. If they deny it, then I must go through the whole appeal process. And I have a billing company that helps me out with all of that because I just do not have time to write appeals. Generally, if I ask for the retro authorization in a timely manner – about a week – they will give it to me.

"My clinic is quiet; it is not a hustle-and-bustle clinic. Rather, it is more of a healing space. I am not contracted with all insurance companies but some people value what I offer and will pay out-of-pocket to see me. About

10- to- 15 percent of my patients are self-pay. I have contracts with all the primary insurance companies, but I am not contracted with the smaller ones. Occasionally, a patient will come in with insurance that I do not take and choose to pay out of pocket, instead of through their insurer."

PHYSICAL THERAPIST LINA PETERSON

Lina Peterson is a native Colombian with a professional American backdrop by which she adopted the prevailing culture to begin navigating the health care "Everest" system. Her professional denomination as a Doctor of physical Therapy (DPT) with more than 20 multicultural years of eclectic clinical and managerial experience, provided her with the privilege to engage daily challenges as she navigates "The Villa Pisani maze" of the physical therapy (PT) practice in the United States.

"Let me begin by unfolding *the transformers* of the healthcare system, the Managed Care Organizations (MCOs) known as the evolved healthcare. The MCO system claims to manage cost, utilization, and quality with an efficient multiple provider reimbursement system under plans like Health Maintenance Organizations (HMO), Point of Service (POS) and Preferred Provider Organizations (PPO) in addition to the capitated plans for large practice groups. Sounds successful and dynamic.

"Now to explain the abysmal zone of the cost component applicable to the capitated plan. This model of care is a hurdle to access to skilled physical therapy services. The daily bread of my practice as a DPT is assessing the needs of each patient for PT skilled services during which I create an *individualized* plan of care with a functional diagnosis, frequency, and duration of treatment for a long term resolution and prevention of any musculoskeletal (MSK) pathologies. At the end of the day, the patient's restored independence of function saves millions of dollars by side-stepping the healthcare system with the physical therapy practice as the Point of Entry (PoE), avoiding additional costs for hospitalizations, ER visits, nursing, surgical care, diagnostic testing, pharmacology expenses, DMEs, among others.

"Conversely, the capitated plan forecasts specific therapeutic procedures/interventions, duration/frequency of treatment on a written referral to save costs, ruling out the physical therapist's expertise and the component of evidence-based practice, using a "cookie cutter" rule to manage the costs. In other words, it knocks down individualization of patients and their needs as determined by the skilled professional, bundles the best practice codes to use for treatments, and frames the rehabilitation time as a forecast prediction, resulting in an increase budget expense.

"On the other hand, with the shifting to a cost-sharing healthcare model, in which patients have to share part of the cost, many patients have to make decisions between what providers to see and what type of service they need, based on out-of-pocket monies and deductible met consequently affecting the compliance to a full course of treatment.

"The other fact is the utilization component. The multiple provider option could deceive beneficiaries into accessing the best personal option of care (certified professionals, traveling distance, rapport with the professional) which are important reasons for treatment compliance. Not to mention that the HMOs, POS, PPOs networks are closed to new providers in certain geographical areas which limits the providers to a partial reimbursement when the beneficiary's choice is an out-of-network provider.

"Lastly, the ongoing cuts on PT service reimbursements negatively impact the quality of care – driving the PT practice into concurrent patient treatments in addition to the overwhelming detailed documentation to justify medical necessity of treatments and the liability restrictions limiting the use of ancillary personnel leaving a burnout fingerprint at the level of the professional practitioners. The certitude of threatening the well-being and balance of the professionals ends with a high employee turnover rate directly affecting the marketing investment of the company due to a short term commitment to the jobs, or for independent PTs to shut down their practice.

"At sunset, I dare you to overcome the Everest system adventure."

HIGHER PREMIUMS, HIGHER DEDUCTABLES

In the past decade, largely since the A.C.A. experiment, insurance companies figured out there is good incentive to get patients more involved in paying for their care. Good idea...but not at a $2,200 monthly premium. Over time, they increased the deductible, which used to be about $500. Now the average in the United States is somewhere around $4,500. I, and many physicians, are on board with having patients pay their fair share for care. There is a growing movement for engaging patients further in their healthcare by hitting them where it hurts: the pocketbook. Now this must be commensurate with their income level and the insurance plan that they or their employer (another problem) choose. However, the industry cannot have it both ways. If patients are to pay for a significant component of their care, then stabilize or decrease (heresy) their premiums. Most importantly, make care more efficient and cost-effective. That way, everybody pays less while improving the quality of care. I have suggested ideas in the one sector I do know, musculoskeletal care. These are the type of debates we should be having but it is not what I hear in the media.

It is a commonly accepted fact that making something free invites abuse. Remember my V.A. patients who would show up to the emergency room in the early morning hours with a chest cold? The out-of- pocket cost should not be so onerous as to discourage utilization because delaying care often leads to even greater cost downstream, not to mention the human factor. Someone should not die of colon cancer because they put off that colonoscopy. The role of the primary care physician is critical here. We must develop better practices and strategies to compensate these colleagues more fairly. These type of preventive health measures should be well covered as it is perhaps an insurance companies best "insurance" to decrease their exposure in future years from their collective patient pool. Besides, it is the right thing to do for patients – and society. The benefits and some misconceptions about the push for preventive health is beyond the scope of this book but is also rather intuitive.

Now they make you pay a deductible up front because people were not paying. I am not against that. Almost every medical office manager in the country would stand up and cheer for that standard. Granted, people do not like to pay for routine or even complex healthcare, unless it is for elective cosmetic procedures like liposuction, breast augmentation, eyelid surgery, and facelifts. According to The Balance.com, since 1997, the number of cosmetic procedures among women increased by over 538 percent, and among men by 325 percent. This is a staggering number, considering most insurance plans do not cover these types of procedures because they are not deemed a medical necessity to maintain quality of life and bodily function. In our youth-obsessed culture, perhaps it is time to get our priorities straight. Instagram is creating a huge societal problem for the near future as these young people age given their expectations of youth and beauty.

The bottom line is that experiencing a health challenge is bad enough and having to pay for it simply adds salt to the wound. Like death and taxes, we must suck it up and realize that many expenses are painful, pun intended, and often unexpected. Paying our share comes with many benefits. We have already seen that depending solely on a third party to pay comes with major downsides. Should we not participate in paying for our own bodies' mainte-nance and repairs when there is a breakdown?

One of my colleagues related an amazing story to me many years ago. A young lady, barely out of adolescence, had cut multiple flexor tendons in her right, dominant hand with a knife injury. This is not an uncommon event as you will recall from Trump's buddy. She presented to the office with all four fingers outstretched, unable to flex (bend) them. She had, of course, been seen in the emergency room where the injury was "stabilized," meaning the wound was cleansed and skin stitches and a dressing were placed. Fine. I wonder how much THAT cost. Now she needed definitive care by a hand surgeon. Let me reiterate how disastrous this injury is. She cannot bend her fingers or con-trol them at all, let alone approximate a fist. As typically associated, she also cut multiple digital nerves since they run near and parallel to the flexor ten-dons. Hence, she had no sensation, let alone protective sensibility to detect a hot stove, or the sensation of holding an object in her hand. As I type this sentence it is easy to imagine the impact this would have on your entire life. No typing, no gripping, limited ability to work and even attend to your daily tasks, however routine or simple. Makes me chuckle a bit as many ask me, "A hand surgeon? What is there to do? Remove wrinkles and make the hand look better?" This is the type of question I hear in South Beach circles in Miami, which is why I share this story. Well, let me simply say that I would rather lose a leg and get a good prosthesis than cut all my flexor tendons.

This young lady, along with her parents, came in with nearly no function in her dominant hand. As often happens, she had no insurance because she was fresh out of high school and not yet working. However, her parents were not destitute. She did not qualify for Medicaid. It was understandable that she did not have insurance as a young, beautiful, healthy woman. Why would she need it? Well, she has saved money on expensive monthly premiums for quite some time, but now it is time to pay the piper. This is a commonplace problem for the patient and the specialty clinicians who must take it from there. It is not the E.R. where the busy physician simply tacked the skin to-gether with some nylon stitches, something my surgical tech could do in under ten minutes. Of course, they got a fat bill from the hospital for hours of wait-ing and some suturing. They were not happy about having to pay again, even though this time it was for the real job of restoring her hand function – one that requires much more than ten minutes of the hand surgeon's time, not to mention, expertise. Such a procedure demands years of training and the surgeon likely has a huge overhead. Thanks to bureaucracy, I, a solo practitioner have ten employees alone.

Back to our patient. We have a young lady with her fingers sticking straight out, as if she is dancing "the robot" from the 1970s. If not repaired perfectly in a timely fashion, she will deal with severe impairment for the next 70 years of her life, assuming life expectancy advances. What to do? Well the surgeon, naturally, gave them some type of fee beforehand, usually a global package, to do the procedure. Why talk money first? To avoid another Blue Cross Blue Shield situation where you are trying to get reimbursed (we should simply say PAID) after the fact. Once those tendons are fixed, nerves repaired, or a steel plate inserted, the work is done. Now try getting paid when countless people believe, "Oh, the doctor is rich anyway, and besides that is expected of them".

A global package, usually offered in an outpatient center, saves a lot of money, and does not allow any surprise bills. The surgical scheduler in the office will give the family one fee, which will of course be substantial (I would say after all we are not plumbers but based upon my last big job at the house, it might not be so far off). That global package will include anesthesia, surgeon's fee, any specialized equipment/implants and the facility. The latter is typically the largest component since keeping the lights on in a surgical facility is not cheap. However, this package is FAR below what a hospital would charge. *Why?* Think what it takes to keep the lights on in that behemoth complex. Regardless of whether the family is happy about paying – which they are not – it is inevitable. But think again. Remember our oath. Remember that physicians tend to be altruistic and while we deserve to make a good, no *great* living after the years of sacrifice I described in the first section of this book, we tend to put the needs of the patient first. However, this should not be taken advantage of, neither by insurance industry or even the public. You see, true altruism comes into play if the family suffered from abject poverty (which we sadly see in sectors of our own wealthy U.S. of A.) in many countries around the globe. However, if that family pulls into the parking lot with a mid-series BMW, with the young lady sporting a designer purse, yet they quibble with the bill, it demonstrates avarice and gaming the system. There is nothing altruistic about that.

What transpired? I believe the family refused to pay anything, but my colleague knew this was disastrous for a young person about to go into the real world and job market. She did not have funds, so he simply performed the surgery. Here is the kicker – as the nursing staff applied the surgical tourniquet on her upper arm, near the axilla, and anesthesia placed cardiac leads on her bare chest, the O.R. team noticed something peculiar. This young lady, still in her teenage years, had two breasts pointing straight up to the O.R. surgical lights, defying gravity and appearing like a Himalayan skyline. I am certainly not averse to the breast augmentation procedure, as a doctor or red-blooded male, but I am quite certain that the family did not negotiate a price with the trained aesthetic surgeon, who did not do it for free. After all, this is not "Operation Smile", where children without resources or access can have their cleft palate deformities reconstructed by a charitable organization. I remember sharing a cold beer with the founder, Dr. William McGee, and even he has a practice where he is fairly compensated for his laudable plastic surgery skills.

I don't believe my colleague, or the center, was ever paid for the intense surgery which required many hours due to its extent and complexity, and I am not clear what happened during the hand rehabilitation process which is prolonged and extensive for this injury and reconstruction. Our hand therapy colleagues also deserved to be well paid for what is one of the more labor intensive rehab processes, leading to the prestigious designation of CHT (certified hand therapist). Any hand therapist, usually an OT (occupational therapist) by training, will tell you that flexor tendon rehabilitation is an arduous process, even in a single digit particularly if a zone 2 injury.

The breast augmentation surgery was reportedly a birthday gift from the family. My colleague did what he felt he had to do, and sometimes that is its own reward. But that (hopefully grateful) family and the insurance industry must realize that we have expenses. When something is "free", given that scenario and perspective, it is not intuitive that the physician actually PAYS to do the surgery. If you divide the total practice overhead by number of work hours, you come up with an hourly figure that is quite impressive. And daunting.

A simple example for a busy, state-of-the art private practice with facility costs, equipment leases, insurance costs (the other types) and staff can be nearly $200,000 a month at the extreme. Let us say that a surgeon works 200 hours a month. That is not a lot for any physician in private practice but understand that many of us participate in extensive academia, so I am often out a week or a month on average, teaching and learning. Therefore, 200,000

/ 200 = $1000 dollars an hour, about what some local healthcare attorneys earn hourly; with much less overhead.

If that surgery took three hours, not even including the assessment, peri-operative discussions with patient and family, and extensive follow-up care (including some hysterical phone calls), this signifies the surgeon PAID the family $3000 for the privilege of operating on that young lady. Think about that for a minute. Think about what I basically paid Blue Cross Blue Shield for the 80 surgeries that I would not have been paid on unless I fought (those contentious hours not included), for the privilege of caring for THEIR pre-mium paying patients. Sounding absurd and grossly unfair at this juncture, right?

As healers of any type, we must often find solace with the sheer satisfaction of helping our fellow man. However, we must be content and fulfilled to be able to give our best, and yes, often donate our services. When I have travelled to Bolivia, Guatemala, or Ghana to donate my time and expertise, it is perhaps as much for me as it is for the patients' whose lives I touch. Many of us see it as our role to give back but understand the expense for us is simply the airfare and possibly the humble lodging and simple meals, often granted to us by the host organization or hospital. I do not think of the opportunity cost of being away from my busy practice, as overhead continues in my absence, much like I do not agonize over this when I attend a conference, mainly to sharpen my skills. We are happy to do it, but it is a much different scenario when a prof-itable insurance company, or a patient with financial means does not recognize our worth or the expense involved in providing that skilled service.

Let me share a relevant example. A prominent surgeon colleague of mine, who works two hours away, was paid ZERO dollars to work on a pa-tient who had an uncommon surgical minor complication. "You didn't give antibiotics preoperatively during the surgery," the insurance company told him. We're not going to pay you for managing that complication." Yes, it happened to be an infection that simply needed to be washed out. This case illustrates the art of medicine. The jury is still not out regarding this issue in many clinical scenarios. For example, about four years ago I stopped using routine pre-op IV antibiotics on certain minor cases because the literature supports that the infection rate is not any different. The appropriate indica-tions and procedures are beyond scope of this book but I, the physician, made a decision according to evidence-based medicine. Yes, the antibiotics add cost and time, but more importantly, it can be deleterious to overuse antibiotics because our population can develop resistance. W.H.O. (World Health Organization) has called for stricter criteria on the use of antibiotics, particularly prophylactic antibiotics in minor surgery and the overtreatment of simple viral URIs (upper respiratory infections), or complex ones like COVID-19. While some in our administration take issue with the W.H.O., they possess data that is used to guide our decisions as a global species.

Consequently, there are physicians who say, "I don't use antibiotics for this or that, either." That should be their prerogative unless the patient is in dire medical condition. But in this case, the insurance company said, "You know what? We're not going to pay you for having taken care of that patient for that infection because you should have used antibiotics at the first surgery." That's a real slippery slope for some armchair medical director at an insurance company, and many times it is just an excuse not to pay. Thank you, but I will follow the literature, and the W.H.O. guidelines, not some insurance company representative on the other side of the country. If the industry is serious about saving money (as they should be), we can talk about the sensical solutions, already present, that can achieve significant cost savings if implemented on a large scale.

The insurance industry phenomenon of "denials" is a much more monumental issue than the public realizes. A qualified clinician (physician, P.A., A.R.N.P., therapist etc.) provides care, and while not everyone is equally trained, he or she has a license and an agreement with the insurance company. It is implicit that not everything goes perfectly all the time, and just because something does not, it is no justification for the insurance company to withhold compensation from the clinician for their time and expertise. I often tell my patients who want "a guarantee" that medicine is often more art than science. I cannot even guarantee I will get home in one piece, although I wish I could. Oncologists, for example, treat patients who die on them all the time – God bless them, but it does not mean they did something "wrong." Should they not be paid? Or worse, should they be sued? My childhood friend died like a dog within months of his osteosarcoma diagnosis, despite an immediate amputation, followed by another, and ample chemotherapy with what medical science knew at that time, 40-plus years ago. He might be alive today, perhaps even with his leg salvaged. Should the doctors back then not be paid? Or worse, sued??

Alternatively, once a doctor has a lot of infections, or a heart surgeon has a high mortality rate, the insurance company, or even the community, might say, "You know what? You don't really want to go to this guy or gal." Of course, we need to understand why. I previously discussed that our mortality rate in cardiac surgery was a bit high at N.Y.U., compared to some community hospitals, because we took some of the sickest cases. That is fine. But not paying people even when they provided the service is wrong.

Physicians also need to do a better job at policing our own profession. We should work with attorneys and the judicial system, not against. Sadly, the current toxic system discourages cooperation, while for-profit insurance companies call the shots, not the so-called "providers".

Denials are not the only problem. Thank goodness that is not the norm as we would eventually lose all of our clinicians. We are naïve, altruistic, and resilient, but not stupid. Usually.

The issue of underpayment is much, much greater and that, sadly enough, IS the norm. Anybody who has taken the time to read, and maybe understand, that confusing statement called an EOB (Explanation of Benefits) will quickly grasp what I am referring to.

In a nutshell, this confusing document lists a series of codes (CPT, ICD, etc.) which correspond to something clinical that was performed; a consultation with physical exam, an X-ray, an injection, or even a surgery. Most surgeries involve several codes since often several different, albeit related, procedures are being done at the same sitting.

The young lady with the robot hand with all flexor tendons cut, had a major surgery where the coding and billing process would list out the debridement (cleaning up the damage), repair of the different tendons (2 in each finger X 4), micro repair of the nerves, and repair of the laceration. She had a global package, which is handled differently, but for insurance companies, this MUST be done. And it must be done perfectly as to not invite multiple denial responses. Mind you, the work was completed. We understand that there is a billing process, but it has become so complex and finicky, that a whole host of cottage industries spawned up to "help us". More on that in the chapter on opportunists.

Let us present an example of an older gentleman with a significant clinical problem or host of issues, who sought relief with me, as an illustration of how even innovation and cost-saving measures are not rewarded by the insurance industry. *Dr. Barnard, we are not going to pay you for that heart transplant simply because it's never been done.* Talk about stifling progress.

Lew Streeter was a jovial, 60-year-old retired Midwestern gentleman who was now living on a boat in the Florida Keys with his lovely, devoted wife of many years. The American dream. He also suffered from diffuse, debilitating rheumatoid arthritis (RA). It caused him increasing difficulty with boarding his boat, handling the ropes, and attending to needed manual tasks. As an avid boater with my own boat, I understood. Boating requires relatively good function of your limbs. Due to his positive personality, I took a liking to him. You might recall that this dreaded disease is one of the main reasons I became a hand surgeon. My beloved paternal grandmother, Consuelo Badia (RIP) suffered from this malady during my entire childhood. I was eager to help Lew.

Lew presented primarily with severe pain in both wrists. While X-rays showed the typical destruction pattern we see in this rheumatologic condition, his pain was out of the ordinary. He had prior injections which gave short lasting relief, and he did not want to consider a fusion which would greatly hamper his function, particularly since both wrists were similarly involved. He had sought me out because he knew I was one of the few area surgeons who did much wrist arthroplasty (replacement) surgery and wanted to know more about it. It is important to know that Lew had an acute fear of hospitals, having suffered a hospital related infection. He was aware that I used our adjacent ASC almost exclusively. My office team and I told Lew that we could certainly do the surgery that way, once I received anesthesia approval, but the insurance carrier, Blue Cross Blue Shield presented a challenge as I had suspected it would (innovation is not an insurance company's strong suit, even when it benefits them and the lives of their insurance customers). To our knowledge, a total wrist arthroplasty (TWA) was never done outside the hospital environment, certainly not in Florida.

As usual, my focus was on the patient and the surgical challenge ahead. We performed the surgery, replacing his right wrist with a shiny new titanium/polyethylene press fit prosthesis. This was done under region block anesthesia; there was no need to intubate the patient, as is often done in many hospitals. This would have been risky since he had prior cervical fusion, typical of many RA patients. He did beautifully and soon afterwards, he sent me his running internet blog, *Capn's Log Living out of the Box and off the Grid*. An independent guy who wanted to stay that way, he kept a running account of his progress for friends and loved ones to see.

On his two-month follow-up visit (a long drive from his home in the Keys in the days before I did telemedicine) he asked, "When can we do the other side, doc?" I was incredulous. "Lew," I explained. "You just had a complete wrist replacement and you are recently post-op." He told me the pain was completely gone and he could board his boat easily, using a protective intermittent splint. He was eager relieve the pain on the other side. I wanted to do more conservative treatment but in looking at the X-rays, there was little point. His mind was made up. Lew and his wife, Deborah were convincing people…in their friendly, Midwestern way.

Three months almost to the day, we replaced his left wrist. Again, within months he came to my office for his follow-up, beaming as he showed me his excellent function. This time, he asked me something curious, "Doc, do you fix shoulders?" I replied, "Gee Lew, I guess you are not sitting in my waiting room (we call greeting room) long enough, because the sign reads *Badia Hand to Shoulder Center* in nice big wooden relief letters."

"Well, mine are killing me."

With that, he showed me how little motion he had, due to a condition that was getting progressively worse. X-rays showed marked narrowing of the joint, indicative of advanced arthritis, although the anatomy was still maintained. He related that his excellent primary care physician, Dr. Collins, had injected his shoulders and the relief was short lasting. Lew convinced me once again.

Within months, I performed a resurfacing hemiarthroplasty replacement of his right shoulder, applying a titanium cap to the denuded humeral head bone. I had done quite a few of them in outpatient manner, but this was a unique situation given the recent wrist replacements. That procedure is akin to what the tennis champion, Andy Murray, had done to his hip, allowing him to even attempt a tour comeback.

Technology is amazing, but the insurance industry certainly does not keep up. During this time, it soon became apparent that Blue Cross Blue Shield was not treating us fairly in this process. Of course, they had an excuse because there was little precedent for reimbursing a total wrist in the outpatient environment, nor the surgery center facility fee. Be aware that there are only about 500 total wrists done a year in the U.S. market. It is not a common surgery and many hand specialists have not been exposed to the technique. While I do not recall well, I believe I was never paid on one of the wrists. Nothing, zilch, nada. But you know us doctors…

I went ahead and did his right shoulder, naturally as an outpatient, and you can guess the next part.

Some months later, Lew and Deborah again came up from their boat in the Keys. Lew announced that the three joints were doing great and demonstrated that for me. Then he showed me how he could barely lift his left shoulder to chest height and his external rotation was markedly limited. "Doc, could you work your magic and resurface this darned left one?" What was I to say?

The following year Sweet Lew came in for his one-year follow-up visit alone. However, that day I was having my left shoulder scoped for painful AC (acromioclavicular) joint osteoarthritis (I too was getting older). My staff had tried to phone Lew and Deborah, but unlike most of us in modern times, they are not glued to their phones (hey, they live on a boat for goodness sake). We never reached Lew to reschedule. When he arrived in the office, my excellent team, including Gigi the X-ray tech, proceeded to take follow up films of all four joints. By that time, I was out of the O.R. and in the recovery room. Having an excellent O.R. team and anesthesia protocols, I was quite awake by the time I hit recovery. My then office manager informed me that Lew was in the office and just had his films. "Should we reschedule?" she asked.

"Heck no," I replied. "He came all the way from Islamorada. Have him come over."

At my bedside, me with the silly bouffant cap on, dressed in the embarrassing patient OR garb that is contrarian to Parisian fashion, I proceeded to examine sweet Lew from afar. "Lew press your palms together and show me your wrist extension. Now flexion. Okay, great. Now bring both arms over your head." Like an eager Jack Russell in the Westminster dog show, Lew last showed me his external rotation and his internal rotation which allowed him to reach his wallet…which did not matter since he had not made any significant monetary contribution to his care.

As usual, I would remain in the dark for quite some time about what our ASC center and I were compensated for his excellent and progressive care. We NEVER received a thank you letter from Blue Cross Blue Shield for saving them money by not taking all FOUR reconstructive surgeries to the hospital where the cost would have been at least five-fold. Furthermore, the difference amounted to much more than that as the facility did not even collect $2,000 dollars to do the joint replacement. Thank goodness most commercial carriers, unlike Medicare, pay for the implant – which is at least three times that amount – as a separate cost. But $2,000 dollars?! To avoid hospital costs, a probable overnight stay, possible consults from other doctors as typically happens once a floor nurse is worried about X vital sign or lab result in a post-op patient. The decreased risk of infection should be obvious as COVID-19 has brought to light among the lay public.

I do not know what I as the surgeon was compensated. It was actually he and his wife who pointed out that I was never paid on one of the wrists, and it bothered them more than I. After all, they were not accustomed to the insurance game as was I. Yes, I am eternally grateful I was given the chance to come into Lew's life and he entrusted me with something so valuable as is upper limb function and lifestyle. However, it did not pay the bills or cover my high overhead at that time…which is all irrelevant now. What matters the most are the emails he sent me thanking me for his care.

Dear Dr. Badia,

I am doing fairly well but due to the RA not as well as I would like. My left works as well as a normal one would, my right only will go as high as my shoulder but that's ok with me.

The wrists are both as flexible as normal.

Send me the prescriptions for the x-rays and I will get them done. I have an appointment with an orthopedic surgeon on July 3 to start the process to get the left hip replaced before we head back south for winter.

Thanks for the concern. Your whole approach to care has made it the best experience I have had.

The last line meant a lot to me, as it does to anybody in the healing professions and our dedicated staff without whom we could not function. I do not get many of these, but when I do, I tape the note onto our conference room fridge, where it is sure to be seen by my team.

Lew died some five years later, after having both hips replaced, but also doing well. His wife, Deborah, wrote me a very poignant email the very next day after his death. I could not believe it. She told me how grateful she was that her Lew could live out his last years without pain, boarding their boat and enjoying sunsets without popping pain pills. As I write this, I called her today. I found his old cell number in my medical record which is certainly easier these days. There are some benefits to EMR (electronic medical records). Mrs. Streeter told me she had gone to the University in Michigan where Lew's body, his skeleton precisely, was preserved after his autopsy after gaining her permission. She could see all four shiny implants I had put in, fully exposed, as well as both hip prosthesis and even the femur plate he had in since he had a periprosthetic fracture complication. He handled that like a champ too.

She then reminded me that they were upset that I had never gotten paid on one of the surgeries. She believed it was the second wrist replacement. They did not take for granted what our team accomplished. Lew had written an unsolicited letter to Blue Cross Blue Shield explaining why an outpatient surgical center is a much a better option. I do not believe he made mention of the underpayment or lack of payment, but the message was far more important.

To the best of my knowledge, he did not receive a response, which did not surprise me. Most of my messages to this group of people go unanswered. It is their M.O., much like the celebrated Humana executive I wrote of earlier.

I did, however, keep part of Lew's letter in a Power Point presentation that I have shown as example of outpatient arthroplasty surgery. It sometimes pays to be a bit sentimental as I can now share Lew's sentiments for posterity through this book:

Blue Cross Blue Shield

Dear Ms. Shaffer,

I am writing this letter because of a very positive experience that I had at Dr. Badia's Hand to Shoulder Surgical Center. He partially replaced both my shoulders and totally replaced both of my wrist joints.

The use of a surgical outpatient center makes logical, physical, financial, and medical sense.

Logically a surgical center is much less intimidating and patient friendly than a huge hospital where you lose your identity. You are not treated as just another case, you are treated as an individual patient with your own peculiar set of needs that are addressed on a personal basis including your family, friends and loved ones.

Use of a surgical center is a lot less expensive than a hospital, with all of its available services that you do not need nor do you have to pay for.

Medically, a surgical center can control all the factors that lead to infection, which can be fatal for a relatively simple procedure. Patients obviously want to make sure they get the best treatment possible but getting some additional benefits certainly can't hurt either. This means they will not only need to choose whom they should have for an Anesthesiologist, but it also means weighing the differences between an Anesthesiologist practicing in a hospital versus one working from a surgery center. The question is which is the better choice.

The end of the letter is cut off in my presentation, but it highlights Lew's sentiments that are most likely shared by many patients. If he wrote a restaurant, hotel, or department store, he would have surely received a cordial and perhaps helpful response. Customer service and perhaps marketing departments would have been apprised, and some changes instituted, however minor. Not so with much of healthcare. Those of us who deliver care feel this must change.

Going forward, many of us will not continue playing "the game". We will practice medicine but not be constrained to the bureaucracy and insulting reimbursements from being "in network," essentially granting permission to give us the shaft. I wish I had seen this sooner, like my interventional pain colleague, Sanjay, who I will mention later. He has been "out of network" (OON) for the past 25 years, as long as I have been in practice. Most practitioners are not that wise or pragmatic.

At the time of Lew's procedures, I was apparently "in network" with that insurance company, performing all four surgeries within 10 months' time with excellent outcome and cost utilization.

Fortunately, I was not too late to see what was coming. I think it is important for me to cover that a bit. I am referring to my own upper limb surgical practice...not OrthoNOW® or any innovation that is geared towards trying to work with the entire convoluted system, challenging as it may be. I made a substantial shift because I simply will not "work with" commercial insurances anymore, certainly not in network. I did not want to play the game. I did not want to be hoodwinked with another demanding case such as Mr. Streeter's.

At this point in my career, a quarter century in practice, I do not want a bureaucrat calling the shots for my patients. I am not perfect, but I am confident I know much more about the hand, wrist, elbow, and shoulder than

ANY of the folks I have ever encountered within the insurance paradigm – medical directors included. I now know a lot about little in medical terms. That is okay because it is the nature of being a specialist – actually a subspecialist. I admire my primary care colleagues who must know material in multiple disciplines. Funny, as a swimmer I swam IM (individual medley). I was good in all the strokes but not great in one. As a doctor, I am quite the opposite. I am a sprinter – 50-meter butterfly only. Nothing wrong with being a specialist.

While it is primarily control I seek, no insist upon when caring for patients, it is also the reimbursement. The reality is that what they pay you in network barely covers your costs…unless you become an assembly line and see a ridiculous number of patients. When I was at the Miami Hand Center, we participated in almost every network, but we did not have to contend with electronic medical records. Furthermore, we had eight patient rooms lined up with an amazing team. We provided excellent care, despite some patient complaints about "the wait." However, I had little time to ask about the family, or how their injury was affecting their hobbies and their life. I did not enjoy it as much. The slim margins now prevalent have caused physicians to align themselves in large "supergroups." Why do we have to do that? I am not yearning for Marcus Welby days, but the pleasure and personalization of medicine is slowly being eradicated by the insurance industry. Some of us do not necessarily want to practice in a 50-person group, where decisions are made painstakingly slow, and one must deal with even more bureaucracy, this time internal. But current challenges explain why 90% of current medical school graduates/residents are taking jobs as fully employed physicians, mainly in a healthcare system. That number was less than 10 percent only a few decades ago. The surprising fact is that current graduates of residency programs want to be employed. They have spoken to their mentors and resigned themselves to the fact that the system is too difficult to take on alone. That is indeed sad. I will be curious to see their response to the message this book imparts.

I must confess I do not have to deal with a lot of the stuff my colleagues are complaining about. Sometimes I feel a bit guilty, but I am compensated by going to another country or providing care through some local charitable clinics (Open Door, Liga contra el Cancer), or volunteering for local organizations such as Special Olympics. But then I stop and think, *why should I feel guilty?* Is it not inherent in human nature to want to be treated fairly? To be recognized for your good work? To be paid according to the value and worth you bring? Not to mention the long preparation. The insurance industry has largely eroded that sentiment.

It is not equitable for somebody to drive into my parking lot with the latest automobile and saunter into my office thinking they have this great health insurance, when their health insurance pays me squat. The patient *thinks* I am being reimbursed well, which is really part of the game. This same patient likely pays his accountant, lawyer, and plumber very well, or at the minimum, fairly. So, the independent-minded physicians are getting out of network. And that is a problem.

Just yesterday, as I wrote this chapter, I spoke to a prominent interventional pain management specialist who practices in the New York City area. He does minimally invasive procedures on folks with intractable back pain. There are a few of those. He told me he was out of network for the past 25 years; the entire time I have been in practice. I felt a bit better. He asked, "How can one be in network with what they pay?" Should he feel bad that he did not play the insurance game for past quarter century? I, for one, admire him.

The simple reality is that insurance companies prey upon physicians' altruism. As I tell my staff, once a patient makes it through the door and sees me, then I feel like I am stuck. Not necessarily in a bad way but I am now compelled to fully establish that venerable doctor-patient relationship. Even if it is a complex and time-consuming pathology to address, I feel like I must take care of them...and I do. Despite the economics. The insurance companies know that. Once they get you on the ropes, they know that you are going to do the best thing for the patient because that is in our DNA.

It is one thing to take an oath. The point is most physicians want to do the right thing for their patients. But one has a business to run; otherwise, you cannot provide care. There are many independent doctors around the country who are closing their doors, or becoming employees at a hospital or large group, after 20 years of running their own practice. Some are just retiring early, which is more common and harder to calculate prevalence. The result? The AMA declared last year that more than half of ALL physicians are employed by someone else. Much of this is contributing to what is being termed "moral injury' as opposed to burnout. This critical issue, and a cornerstone of this book, will be explored in Chapter 13.

SELF-PAY PATIENTS AND COMPARISON SHOPPING

Julio Gonzalez is an orthopedic surgeon in Venice, Florida. Born and raised in Miami, he trained at the University of Miami and served nine years in the United States military, deploying twice as a flight surgeon. He is also a member of the Florida Bar and has served as state representative for his Florida district for four years. As you see, he is eminently qualified to comment on the hurdles of delivering healthcare in our system. Furthermore, he is about to release his 4th book on the subject. Below, he describes a common scenario that takes place in his practice when dealing with a self-pay patient versus an insured patient.

"Healthcare is expensive because there have been a lot of interventions made by outside forces. The bottom-line problem is that the free market has not been allowed to dictate or influences prices. That means, patients use other people's money to pay for their healthcare. Individuals do not have a direct stake on the cost of the procedures and the work ups that are being done. The government made a huge effort to cut prices and make healthcare more accessible to others to protect or insulate providers from the influence of the market and competition. To me, that is the reason why prices have been skyrocketing out of control every year over the past 40 years.

"The conversation between my patient and me take on a totally different tone when they are paying for the care. When it is their pocket we are dipping into, all of a sudden, we have conversations about prices and what facilities offer lower prices, while remaining amenable to negotiation. You can easily tell what healthcare would be like if the patient were involved, just by observing the limited interactions my practice receives between a consumer whose wallet is at stake in negotiating and agreeing to treatments.

"If it is a self-pay patient, I will either know about it from the beginning because it'll be on the sheet where we document their insurance (or lack thereof), or the patient will volunteer the information. They will tell me that they would like to have their wrist fixed or their knee scoped or whatever the case may be, but they are worried about price. Next, I ask my office manager to come into my office because everything is done generally with CPT codes (current procedural terminology) that dictate what gets billed. Unless I have a super photographic memory, there is no possible way that I can know what each code means and what each insurance company is willing to pay me for performing the procedure that correlates to those codes.

"For example, if it involves a surgery, my office manager gets the code for the procedure that I suspect we will perform. Then, the patient will have a discussion with the office manager about financing and price. I must decide if I am willing to do it for X amount as compared to the usual and customary allowance from the insurance companies. In most cases, it amounts to more than what the insurance companies allow but tends to be much less than the usual and customary. The patient and the office manager have that discussion. I also give my patients phone numbers for the multiple facilities where I perform the procedure, so they can call to decide which one gives them the best price that includes anesthesia. If the anesthesia is a separate charge, we give them the phone number for the anesthesia, and so on. Self-pay patients negotiate not only with me, but with the various entities from whom they may receive care, for an appraised price that is acceptable to them. That is something that does not take place with insured patients. When a patient is covered, they agree to the surgery. They may ask about their copay, which is not negotiable and that is it. And off we go."

The difference between Dr. Gonzalez's approach and mine is simply the place of service. He allows – no, encourages – the patient to shop around for the best surgery center and anesthesia package. This is a true free-market approach. In my case, I went through the considerable expense and energy to build an adjacent A.S.C., as discussed in section 1; hence there is only one place that I am going to perform procedures. However, I know the cost and value we bring; thus, I feel supremely confident when my staff discusses their overall cost package for said procedure. Soup to nuts…. It is one-stop shopping and that alone saves on cost, not to mention quality of care, something not to overlook.

Dr. MARK REKANT ON THE COST OF HEALTH INSURANCE

"The cost of people's health insurance is somewhat troublesome. From a grassroots perspective, I do not know if that is right. If you compare health insurance to other types of insurance like homeowners or car insurance, there is a big disparity. With homeowners or car insurance, if you are unhappy with your insurer, you can call them up, cancel your policy, and sign up with a new company tomorrow. By contrast, if you are unhappy with your health insurance, you can only change your plan once a year.

"This arrangement gives the health insurance company tremendous control while it takes power away from the consumer. It is analogous to Walmart: if Walmart were the only game in town and you could not shop at other venues, it would be interesting to see the effect on prices. The other real question with insurance companies is that maybe they should run a zero profit or a 20 percent profit. They are private and heavily incentivized to make as much profit as they can, which is sort of counterproductive. For a situation where there are limited choices, fine. If I could switch insurance companies tomorrow, great. Let them make all the profit they want. The consumer's ability to switch carriers would provide a checks-and-balance for them. Furthermore, if we could buy insurance across state lines, it would give people more choices and help reduce costs, in the sense that it would create more competition."

DO HEALTH INSURERS OR DOCTORS KNOW BEST? SURGEON A.J. DIGIOVANNI RECOUNTS A REAL CASE WITH SERIOUS CONSEQUENCES

"Insurance created problems in terms of entry into the hospital. Patients had to come in the day of surgery, whether you as the doctor thought it was better that they be admitted prior to surgery for preliminary work or not. We eventually got to the point now where all these outpatient preoperative studies are done. In many instances, it is appropriate.

"But there are times when you must apply your expertise as a medical professional as to whether it is applicable or not in a situation. I can refer to one patient, a rather charming lady in her late 50s, with no history of heart disease. When she came into my office as a patient prior to admission, I observed that she was extremely anxious. Considering her anxiety issues, I knew it would cause a problem to bring her into the operating room for surgery. I wanted to admit her the day before surgery to work her up, but her insurance denied it. When she came into the O.R. to be sedated, she was visibly upset. To my dismay, she developed a heart attack, post-op. She had no history of heart disease prior to this incident.

"Yes, it could have been something going on that she had not yet been diagnosed with. On the other hand, because her insurance company denied her the ability to be admitted the day before surgery, she was put under the intense pressure of coming into the hospital the same day of surgery – a patient who was so anxious, we had to heavily sedate her. And I believe some of that was because I did not have the jurisdiction or control for a patient, who in my professional judgement needed some other help aside from applying the surgical knife. There was an issue here of adapting to her emotional state and it was just denied because of this kind of thing where everyone had to come in on the same day for elective surgery. It is one of the many privileges that has been taken away from physicians: the ability to make their own judgment when a patient should be admitted."

The Billing Game from the Trenches

My in-house director of billing, Tina Rodriguez, gives a perspective that is rarely heard, certainly not in the media or any so-called debates on health–care challenges.

She shares, "I've been doing this for a long time and as has my colleague, who previously worked at a large hospital collections department. I have been here with Dr. Badia for 11 years at our hand and upper extremity practice. Part of our job is to call for benefits. We get the benefits over the phone, the patient has a deductible and a co-insurance and once those two requirements are met, we're finding that the insurance companies are still putting most of the responsibility on the patient instead of paying based on out of network benefits. This is because we are now out of network with all commercial plans. Dr. Badia can tell you why he made that decision, but it is obvious.

"We try to explain this to the patient, that we are fighting for the money that is due to the doctor and the practice. What we are finding now, too, is that a lot of the commercials are saying, "Oh, there's this MNRP (Maximum Non-Network Reimbursement Plan) that's in the patient's policy. And when we go to verify benefits online or even on the phone, they are not saying anything about this.

"It is kind of like saying, 'Well, we have you on a contract, but we don't really have a written contract, and we're going to pay you what we think we should pay you and that's it.' So, they are not really going by the patient's out-of-network benefits. They are just paying whatever they want; and they do not pay consistently. They pay some patients correctly and they pay a lot of patients incorrectly. When we try to explain this to the patient, they do not know because they have not spoken with anybody. They just bought a plan. They just want to be seen by a doctor; they do not really understand their policy. They leave this burden up to us even though we are not the insurance company. We provide the actual care. We try to collect from the patient up front, so that we do not have this issue. But then, you know, we do have some insurances where there will be a patient responsibility that is higher than what we collect, so we turn around and bill the patient. Then, the patients get upset because they do not understand the process.

"Another problem that I see is that Dr. Badia does some unlisted codes. He is a specialist. He does some innovative procedures that do not necessarily come from the CPT (Current Procedural Terminology Book) cookbook. He feels that these procedures help the patient. They help the patient, their recovery, and the overall outcome. And the insurance companies do not want to pay for these unlisted codes...even though they are in the CPT book. And they do not want to pay for them because they say it is investigational. They do not have enough information, so on and so forth, yet it is still listed in the CPT book as a covered service. What is amazing is that Dr. Badia has published papers on some of these techniques so it's not 'experimental' as they claim.

"A lot of customer service reps just read off their customer service script. I am sure that is how they are trained to do it. Then, we must turn around and ask for a supervisor; somebody who might know what we are talking about. It is becoming an ever-increasing time-consuming battle. He does surgery on the patient. The patient has an excellent outcome and is doing well. We simply have the insurance companies not paying the way they are supposed to.

Another big problem we get is, "No Claim on File," – when we know darn well, we sent the claim. It really is just one lie after another.

"We often do a reconsideration or an appeal for something that's not processing paid, or not paid properly. First, they tell us, 'We don't think it's worth this amount of money.' Then after we put in the reconsideration or appeal from our end, back to the insurance, instead of accepting it as an appeal or reconsideration, they process it like a duplicate claim when it clearly is NOT a duplicate claim. You spend all your time on it, and you must do it all over again. It is busy work. All these employees taking all this time on one case, when you think about it, is costing the practice and the physician even more overhead and money. It is incredibly frustrating.

"Any time a claim must be sent back to the insurance company it is either a reconsideration or an appeal. This depends on the denial reason. Even when the insurance company denies in error, they still make you take the time to do an appeal instead of simply reprocessing the claim correctly. This allots more time for them before they must pay the claim.

Many times, after taking the time and resending all supporting documentation along with the claim, they will deny the claim as a duplicate submission. When calling the insurance company, sometimes they say, "I do not see the reconsideration in the system," or "Oh yes, I see the reconsideration right here". Our question: why did they deny the claim as a duplicate then? Does the insurance company even look at the reconsideration, or anything else submitted? They have people who are not subspecialists auditing the claim.

"I would say 90 percent of our patients don't even know how their insurance plan works. They do not understand the policy or the coverage. We try to educate them as we go. As we talk to the patients who are trying to understand why this is happening, we encourage them to call the insurance company on their end about their policy. Since the patients are not familiar or aware of what is going on, it makes the providers look like we're the ones chasing down money, or not processing claims correctly, but it's really the insurance company. We must explain that to the patient.

"One of the biggest complaints we get from patients is that they must pay out-of-pocket. The reason is because they really do not understand the benefits of the insurance plan *they have* chosen. Especially now, seeing Dr. Badia, who is out-of-network, like many other good doctors. They are choosing to see a doctor that is not contracted with the insurance company; therefore, the insurance penalizes the patient for choosing the doctor they prefer and feel most comfortable with by imposing a higher deductible or a higher co-insurance. Then, it is our job to explain that to the patient because they are under the impression it is just co-pays for office visits and things like that. The insurance company washes their hands of that.

"Additionally, the reason Dr. Badia became out-of-network for most insurance companies is due to the issues the billing team has with insurance – issues they created. Now, instead of having our team fight for reimbursements and covered services, we see our patients out-of-network. Seeing patients out-of-network, we collect more of the cost upfront than having to bill the insurance and depend on the payment after.

"A frustrating thing also happens when you call for authorization, let's say for a surgery. The insurance company authorizes it, but their little spiel is always, 'Well, you know, an authorization is not a guarantee of payment.' Then, what is the point?

"If they know that code is not going be authorized, they should let us know ahead of time so that we can either collect from the patient, or we can let Dr. Badia know. Instead, they wait till after the fact. Then they just deny it altogether. They deny the whole surgery and we will have to fight for that as well. It is a risk that the doctors take, accepting the authorizations written or verbally, hoping that the insurance company honors and processes the claims correctly based on all the medical necessity that was done.

"A lot of patients feel it is simply better to go to self-pay because they pay a high monthly premium and they still have to come out of pocket for their procedures or visits, and after we bill, sometimes they still have to come out of pocket for the patient balance. They are typically out of network. You're already paying your monthly premium, you will see a doctor, you pay your copay or some percent of your deductible, if you have a procedure or a diagnostic study, then 30 days down the road, you're at home and you receive yet another letter saying you still have a patient balance. It does make you wonder, 'What is the point of paying for insurance?'

"For many self-pay patients, we accept finance plans through Care-Credit. We do offer patients a discount if they are private pay because we have room to work with them via a direct contract between the office and the patient. We usually offer them discounts if they need it. In terms of surgery, we offer them global packages, which is an all-inclusive package. So, we try to keep their costs down, offer a discounted rate, and include everything in an all-in-one package. They do not get billed after the fact. They know exactly what they are paying for, what's included and not included, and there are no hidden fees.

"The issue of denials is particularly puzzling. The insurance company will deny something, and yet they will put at the bottom, "Paid, per contract agreement." We do not have an agreement. We are out of network with everyone. We have no written agreement with the insurance company. Where do they get that from?

"Since Dr. Badia is a hand surgeon, a high percentage of our patients are workers' comp patients. Workers' comp insurance is quite different. It is even more complicated than general insurance and commercial insurance. Agents are depending on the insurance company, or TPA, for approving everything. Sometimes it could take even up to a month or two months for a patient to get authorized for a procedure, a test, anything the doctor is recommending – just because the adjuster is taking their time with it. That is another frustrating thing we go through in the office with the Workers' comp patients. It's out of our control and out of the patient's control, because everything is dependent on that in Workers' comp. There is really nothing you can do with moving forward for the patient, unless you get an approval, and the approvals take long many times. For some reason, we get the brunt of the blame from the patients.

"Workers' comp sends them to a specialist, then somehow they don't want to authorize what the specialist recommends for that patient. We have a patient right now – she called yesterday and was quite upset and wanting an appointment to see Dr. Badia again. When I checked her chart, she was pending an MRI study that Dr. Badia had ordered a month ago! One month later, we finally got the authorization. I let the adjuster know how long we had been waiting and the stress it had caused the patient. And all they said was, "Okay, yeah, it's approved." For those 30 days that we were waiting, this adjuster was just sitting on it. The lack of empathy is astounding.

"In those 30 days, her condition could have potentially gotten worse. The waiting period delayed her therapy. She did not want to go back to therapy unless she knew what was actually going on with her arm. So, the MRI was an important part of determining her next treatment option.

"Many of the carriers make it difficult for their OON patients. One of the biggest offenders is Blue Cross and Blue Shield when we try to call to see what's going on with the claim since we accept the out of network benefits and file on behalf of the patient. We don't just say, "Okay, here, we're going to charge you 100 percent and you've got to file on your own." Theoretically, we can do that because we are out of network, but we don't because we want to get the patient the care, they sought from us. We want to get them well and taken care of. So, when we try to call to get benefits, or we try to call on a claim that we haven't been paid anything on, they do not want to help you over the phone. They don't even want to send you any EOBs (Explanation of Benefits). They will send you a complex letter and you have to even call to get that. That is another thing we have to explain to the patient: 'Okay, this is what we billed. This is what the insurance paid for. This is what they denied and why, and what the patient responsibility is supposed to be on that EOB.'

"One of us spent an hour-and-a-half on the phone the other day for ONE patient who has a BCBS plan. You are speaking with somebody, trying to explain things to them, and they have no clue what you are talking about. They do not even understand. Then they come back with some answer out of left field. And you ask, 'Did you hear what I just explained? I mean, is there an issue with the phone, with the connection? You're not even understanding what I'm telling you.' Then, we must ask for a supervisor and wait on the phone for another 30 minutes for them to find a supervisor. Or, many times, they will tell us nobody is available. How convenient. 'There's nobody available for me to talk to in all of Blue Cross and Blue Shield? There's not one supervisor we can talk to?' It is crazy.

"Dr. Badia is really good with us. We explain things to him and he says, 'Girls, let me know where you're having an issue, I'll try to get on the phone with whoever I know, and do whatever I can do.' He is supportive and helpful in that aspect. And you know, I see it in his face every day. He is getting very frustrated because he is the one in the O.R. for hours, making these patients better.

"Many of the main commercial carriers go through third-party payers. For example, Cigna will go through Multi Plan. It will say, 'Multi Plan' on the back of the patient's card. Now we have a direct contract with Multi Plan. But Multi Plan is going back and forth with the carrier, and Multi Plan sends us a fee agreement. Since we have a contract with them, we sign on the fee agreement. They always want to deny cold. So, I send the fee agreement back and they reply, 'No, this is the payable code. This is what we will accept, based on the terms of the contract that you signed. This is what we will accept.' Finally, when we get them to get anywhere near the amount they're supposed to pay, they sign it, it's great, they send it back to the carrier...and then we never get the amount that they promised on the fee agreement in the first place. In other words, they breach their contract. It really is a game full of deceit."

Workers' Compensation

As Tina mentioned, a major group of patients I (and many other orthopedists) treat is workers' compensation. Talk about a money pit. Take the complexity and inefficient processes of commercial health insurance and triple it. So, you might ask why do I deal with this given that you likely surmised my tolerance for nonsense and abuse is low? Fair reimbursement. It is a plain and simple concept where, again, everybody likes to be paid fairly for their work.

Workers' compensation is run by the states and each one handles it quite differently, including the payment to us "providers". Fortunately, in Florida it is still quite reasonable and hopefully it stays that way. In Massachusetts, despite the near socialized medicine quandary many doctors are facing, they are some of the best compensated for work related injuries. California? Terrible. Their "Terminator" ex-governor overhauled the system in 2004 with the intent to curb abuse, which was indeed substantial. However, the result is that doctors were paid even less for a now overly complex system where the insurance companies fared much better, since premiums from employers were not touched, but the payouts decreased. Yes, ridiculous settlements to workers were reined in but at the expense of increasing the review system where insurance companies reviewed the doctors' decisions and in the end workers' compensation judges made many of the medical decisions. Can you imagine if I, or my buddy the cardiac surgeon, had the final word in a complex legal argument regarding the hedge fund industry? It is so preposterous that I will not even comment on it any further.

The result is that the quality of clinicians willing to deal with the headaches of workers' compensation ultimately depends on fair reimbursement. If you asked one of your employees to start cleaning the office toilets in addition to serving as the receptionist, or perhaps your insurance coordinator (apropos), it would likely come down to price. What are you willing to pay and what will they accept? It is possible. That was one of my jobs at my Cornell fraternity house. We divided house chores and I often selected cleaning toilets in a house of 30 guys as that was less time consuming, albeit less desirable, than some of the other needed tasks. That was a sort of compensation. Less infringement on my time to study and enjoy college life. We all have our price.

Despite the complexities of workers' comp, I choose to do it and it is a substantial part of my practice. However, there is one additional reason not to overlook. As a hand surgeon knows, most complex injuries occur on the worksite. Typically, industrial injuries require expertise to not only reconstruct, but get them back to their challenging job in the first place. Sports injuries are often knee or ankle, for example, but those areas are much less injured in job-related trauma. Frankly, I enjoy that challenge and others may choose not to pursue that. The fact that it certainly compensates me better than Blue Cross Blue Shield is gravy.

Another advantage (and this is where it gets ugly) to treating those patients is that many of them sue their employer, not their doctor. Let us surmise that I truly did something wrong and the outcome was not good. The patient typically brings a suit against their employer, which kind of shields me a bit. The system encourages the employee to bite the hand that feeds them, literally. That principle is so perverse, and complex, that I do not have the time or the gusto to even explain it. I am not referring to actual negligence where an employer lacks the safety protocols or materials in order to minimize injury to his most valued commodity- his workers. I am referring to the simple fact of WHERE an injury occurred is quite enough to permit litigation.

We have a fairly equitable system in our country to pay for ALL the medical expenses of a worker once an injury is deemed "work-related". Sticking to hand issues, if a secretary slips in the bathroom and breaks her wrist, it is work related. Granted, this could have happened at home or at the gym and would be an entirely different paradigm – for the patient, provider, insurance company, and the overall system.

If a factory worker catches his end in a punch press, or circular saw, that is certainly a clear-cut work-related injury. Now, if that worker has basal joint arthritis, and they claim that the job caused, or even aggravated, that commonplace osteoarthritic process, this is where it gets slippery fast.

I will present one example, painful as it is, to illustrate the problem and how there is immense waste in the system. I assume you have heard of "carpal tunnel". Well, the entire workers' comp industry, and most patients, refer to the condition this way due to the inaccurate myths and urban legends surrounding this extremely common nerve compression at the wrist. The name is "carpal tunnel syndrome" since a syndrome is a collection of symptoms that are related to an underlying pathologic process. In this case, it is a compression of the median nerve within the carpal canal (tunnel) of the wrist and leads to numbness, tingling and sometimes pain in the thumb to ring fingers. The compression can be due to many factors, including a clear history of a wrist injury, but usually it is a metabolic or hormonal phenomenon which causes thickening of the lubricating sheath (tenosynovium) that surrounds the nine tendons that run with that little, itty, bitty nerve. Tendons get thick within a closed space; the nerve pays the price. It is like sciatica of the wrist, so common that many women will experience symptoms during the third trimester of pregnancy due to hormonal factors and fluid shifts. A JAMA published study discussed the common incidence among women, less so with men, and how this differed according to age group. Chronic conditions such as diabetes, hypothyroidism or obesity all play a major role, obviously nothing to do with their occupation.

So how was CTS associated with work? If you have underlying median nerve compression, many tasks will aggravate the symptoms and we might construe that as causality. Typing for example, for many hours and holding the wrist in a flexed or hyperextended position, will put pressure on the median nerve. There has NEVER been a good study that confirmed any association of casualty of CTS to computer use, or even job tasks. Myself and many hand specialists have written on this but get lost in the cyberworld since it has become much more of a legal and occupational issue. Let's face it – there are many more lawyers and insurance adjustors than hand surgeons. To prove that, realize that a large Swedish study actually showed an inverse relationship with intense keyboard use and CTS symptoms.

So why is it considered job related? Money.

A very revealing epidemiologic article compared the Australian incidence of CTS to American patients in a Social Science & Medicine journal article in 1990. It basically concluded that the explosion of workers' compensation claims regarding CTS, and similar maladies, was largely due to the societal response in Australia, at one point even being considered an epidemic hysteria. Sounds familiar during Covid19, right? The term RSI (repetition, strain, injury) was coined in 1982 in a small pamphlet by the National Health and Medical Research Council essentially relating a common metabolic condition, tenosynovitis, to work activities although many of us perform repetitive tasks at work or play (or writing this book). Essentially, the existence of a simple term and catch phrase (RSI) gave legitimacy to the issue in the public mind, regardless of the actual science and causality. A letter to the *Australian Medical Journal* declared "currently there is no similar epidemic of upper limb pain anywhere in the world". The media fed into the hysteria with skeptics using the term, "kangaroo paw" and labeling it an Australian disease. I can only imagine what my Australian hand surgeon colleagues thought, many of them being close friends and extolling hard science. The incidence of the condition being reported, and subsequent workers' compensation, skyrocketed in the early 80s until guidelines and science helped rein in the problem by 1985. The damage, however, was done and the near universal myth of CTS and typing association became global affecting healthcare systems and workers' comp systems worldwide. Understand this was before common usage of personal computers and well prior to the internet, or mobile technology. The current Covid19 pandemic continues to fuel ridiculous claims on either side of reality and hard science.

Unfortunately, most workers' comp systems rely more on legal and public opinion than knowledge by subspecialists. Nearly 25 years ago, I began a quest to educate the local workers' comp community on the known pathophysiology of CTS, tendonitis and related common issues that have little to do with work, other than perhaps aggravating symptoms. Granted, that aggravation often suffices to justify a workers' comp claim in many states, but science rarely has a seat at the table. Those of us in the trenches are rarely involved in policy discussions regarding the conditions we treat and have a real cost to our economy and society.

As we will see later, legal interests often rise above medical facts and science. Naturally, we are caring for patients and not making policy or arguing our case. I once had to walk out of a deposition because of the berating by a claimant's attorney who absolutely blasted me for my stance on the etiology of CTS. *How dare I say that her median nerve compression is more related to her diabetes, obesity and perimenopausal state than the fact that she types 8 hours a day?* What was the consequence of his action and my participation in the process relying on evidence-based medicine and my 20 years as a hand specialist? I ceased doing IMEs (independent medical examinations) altogether. It was an adversarial chess game where what I said and how I said it was more important than the scientific literature. I even pulled a book down from the shelf, *Carpal Tunnel Syndrome,* right behind the attorneys right shoulder, where NO chapter suggested that this was primarily an occupational condition. Ironically, my contributing chapter 35 was on "Median Nerve Compression Secondary to Fractures of the Distal Radius". In THIS case, I told the counsel, it can be related to work since many wrist fractures occur in an occupational setting and a related CTS would clearly fall under the workers' compensation realm. No matter. Science and medicine do not matter when money is involved. So, I no longer do IMEs. You can only beat people up so much.

The public has some blame here as well, but naturally, we cannot fault the masses who are not expected to understand wrist anatomy, let alone the pathophysiology that leads to median nerve compression and symptoms. However, the media does have some blame. We will touch on this in a later chapter, but I will relate one story that helps explain why.

A reporter from one of the local Hispanic networks asked me for an interview. I was busy with patients, but I am passionate about patient education so agreed to take a few minutes. We stood in my office where she informed me that she would be asking me questions about "blackberry thumb." I shook my head and commented that there is no such thing but we could certainly discuss causes of thumb pain, one of my major areas of interest in hand pathology, which would be of great interest to her viewers since it's a very common affliction. We did not even get to sit down. She packed her bags and scurried out of the office, cameraman in tow, uttering "Muchas gracias por tu tiempo, doctor"! She was clearly not interested in science or dispelling myths, but rather feeding misconceptions and sensationalism. I was not about to feed into the "kangaroo hand" scenario and propagate the so-called "blackberry thumb".

I have since learned. Now when a reporter or blogger asks me what you can do to avoid CTS from typing so much, I first validate their question by simply repeating it. Then I go into the anatomy, prevalence, or typical causes of the condition, not disparaging their misconception. I finish by saying if you suffer from A or B, it is certainly common that being on a keyboard all day will aggravate or bring on *symptoms,* which is true, but I never affirm that it is caused by computer use. Somehow, I am naïve enough to think that science, evidence, and common sense will prevail.

However, do not underestimate the power of legal circles, money, and the media. Little has changed since I first started to try and dispel myths in my own Miami community and I now focus more on trying to control the related costs due to those misconceptions. Even that mission has been a monumental challenge and earlier chapters discussed the challenges on fruitful collaboration in the healthcare arena. This cause has been particularly challenging with workers' comp insurance companies, TPAs who control the process, and even the employers, who stand the most to benefit. After being in the trenches for so long you start to realize things and it can be discouraging.

If you look at the data, 93 percent of work-related injuries in the US are orthopedic. What are the rest? An eye injury, a chemical burn, a coal miner's lung. The last time I checked, there were no coal mines, chemical plants, or manufacturing hubs in Miami, unlike Pittsburgh or northeastern New Jersey. Therefore, in Miami-Dade County, a workers' comp injury is de facto an orthopedic injury. Furthermore, the upper extremity is THE most common location for work-related trauma, accounting for over 50% of ALL injuries, worldwide. Hence, I do feel a bit qualified to speak about this issue. Yet these patients are not seeing someone who knows about orthopedics until late in the game, let alone the upper limb.

When we started OrthoNOW®, I made it my mission to engage the business community, and relate why healthcare has become so expensive for the employer, particularly in the area of work related injuries, subsequent lawsuits from said injury, and the downstream costs of not having your optimal employee at their position for X amount of time to recover from their injuries. I often explained to business chamber members, even on occasion from the podium, that when an employee has an orthopedic injury or even just an ongoing pain that needs to be assessed, this can cost a company significant amounts of money. When the injury occurred on the job, this initiates a complex cycle of events known as workers' compensation, which you now better understand. Depending on where the patient starts that journey can lead to significant time off, wages paid despite the person not working, and even a payout at the end if a patient engages an attorney.

I explained it many times, yet it is worth reiterating the story I presented earlier. I finally realized that my message had little impact when that employee came to me from a nearby major retail center, a member of the local business council, who had amputated the tip of her finger in a heavy freezer door at work. I had related this story when discussing lack of real community and employer collaboration in healthcare. After all we could have avoided this scenario if the employer had simply considered, or cared, to pursue a better solution for these injuries. Consequently, the patient with the finger injury, employee of the business council president, was transported to the emergency room where they simply bandaged the finger and said she would need surgical care. Because it was a work injury, she was then referred to a typical Occupational Health Center, where of course the person seeing the patient is not even an orthopedist, let alone a hand specialist. And then finally the insurance company sends her to me directly. Why, why, why....

What if it was your finger? Your mother's? Your child's? Speaking of children's finger injuries, I will relate a curious anecdote in a later chapter. Municipalities are also subject to this issue and inefficient process, now costing us taxpayers, not just private corporations, a great deal of money. More importantly, that needed policeman, firefighter, schoolteacher, or sanitation worker is now out of service to us for a MUCH longer period. It is not simply about the cost although that is reason enough.

In the chapter about government, I recounted the story about how two highly respected city leaders, a father and son, asked me to calculate how much money we could save our city of Miami as well as the greater county. We did that promptly, being that we maintain data and our cofounder, a Wharton MBA and Cornell grad, has worked as an analyst and was able to provide eye-opening figures. That was never looked at, nor did the respective workers' comp carrier ever heed our concerns and at least discuss options. The employer, this time our own city, simply shifted the responsibility to the insurance company du jour. I think this chapter points out that this is a very costly mistake.

The calculation was based upon the average cost of assessing and treating a common type of wrist tendonitis called DeQuervain's. The fact that this is even considered work-related is another issue and I already expressed my resignation at not being able to influence what should be compensable in the swamp that is the workers' comp universe. However, I was hoping our team could share strategies where at least we make that process more cost-effective and efficient to get the worker back to productivity faster, and cheaper. No dice there either.

We compiled that data around 2016 and since that time our team has seen innumerable cases of DeQuervain's tendonitis that was sent to us via workers' comp even though clearly due to underlying metabolic or hormonal causes. Sometimes there is a clear etiology, as when a water and sewer department worker is struck on the wrist by a valve handle, or errant wrench. Regardless, the current focus is not determining causality but rather streamlining the system so that the worker is seen by a clinician who clearly understands the pathology. This does not happen. The patient is seen by a well-meaning general or occupational health physician, they often order unnecessary tests such as an MRI, and almost always reflexively send them to therapy. This can go on for months and our rough calculations showed that this process costs nearly $12,000 whereas the majority of patients, at least 80% in the literature, would respond to a single injection, which we estimate at $700 dollars total. Discharged, back to work within a week, pain-free and no money bag at the end of the process.

Why is this important? Well this ONE little but common diagnosis has been estimated to cost the U.S. economy $13 to $20 billion dollars. With a capital B. No matter that the prevalence among the general population is estimated at 1.3% for women and .5% for men. The risk factors are similar to CTS as the same underlying pathology of tenosynovitis (tendonitis), but this is never challenged or even discussed.

I can spew statistics and data, not to mention science, all day long but those in charge will not change course. Like the drug war, there are too many people involved who benefit and there is little impetus to change. However, the public may be better moved by concrete examples of patient care that clearly embodies the problem and why we spend so much on healthcare, not to mention it's frustrating inefficiencies that we have all experienced.

In mentioning just one example of poor management, DeQuervain's tendonitis, I described that I continue to receive referrals, often months after onset where the patient had tests and inadequate treatment leading to delay and high cost. Soon after the onset of the COVID-19 pandemic, a city cop was referred to me via workers' compensation. Due to fears and social distancing concerns, I saw him via telemedicine, something I had espoused years before. Now all the sudden more than half of all physicians are using this convenient option.

The police officer was walking his beat, holding his cell phone by his chest, so I was staring up at this chin. He did not skip a beat. Within minutes, I digested the history, listened to what had been done already for the past month (which was ineffectual), and remotely examined his wrist. I could see the swelling near the base of his thumb and asked him to show me where it was tender. Then I instructed him to perform a Finkelstein maneuver, the sine quo non finding of this painful tendonitis. After yelling "ouch" into my ear, we quickly determined that he was probably in time for a corticosteroid injection, which I determined once distancing restrictions were relaxed via a quick ultrasound exam in my office. I could then inject him at that moment if warranted. It was that simple. He understood the next steps and thanked me. Pretty fast and cost-effective, huh? However, I also informed him that due to the delay in receiving appropriate care, the injection, there is a higher chance of him needing the wrist procedure, simple as it is.

I have been doing telemedicine for some years with few carriers or referral sources engaging with me on this simple concept that many other industries already use. Credit goes to the workers' comp system in Monroe County, where the Florida Keys are located. This is largely due to several case managers, nurses, and other clinicians, such as Raquel, who have been tasked to increase efficiency of the injured worker's treatment journey. She ensured that approval for a same day M.R.I. was obtained, allowing a patient who drove four hours from Key West, to get a nearly immediate diagnosis of their shoulder pain. IF that patient had an injection, usually done same day as well, we could do the follow-up visit as well via telemedicine. Why have the patient drive a total of eight hours to simply tell me, "Thanks Doc. The injection took my pain away two days later, just like you said. When can I go back to full duty?" Conversely, the patient may tell me that the injection gave little relief and that ample work with the local trusted therapist, Rosie, did not resolve the issue. I can then schedule the arthroscopic shoulder surgery during that tele-visit. Granted, I cannot do the surgery remotely, but even that day is coming...

I wish I could say that this is the norm. Some folks in the workers' comp system, like nurse Nancy Williams, see the challenges and care enough to do something different. They, along with some workers' comp insurance carriers, and even TPAs, realize that working with the clinicians, together, can lead to better, faster, and even less costly outcomes.

"My name is Nancy Williams. I am an R.N. and B.A., with a certification in C.R.R.N. (certified rehabilitation registered nurse). I have been in the workers' compensation arena almost 24 years. Before that, I worked in the hospital on the surgical floor as a nurse, and prior to that I worked in the laboratory at MedTech for about 15 years. In the workers' comp arena, there are field nurses and telephonic nurses. As a field nurse, I act as a liaison between the injured employee, employer, and the providers (the doctors). I make sure that the injured worker receives the medical care they need related to the injury to get better and go back to work.

"Along the way, there are many roadblocks, beginning with the injured employee. Sometimes the patients want to recover and get back to work and sometimes they do not. Some patients will hire an attorney, and their attorneys will allow us to remain with the patient to help them to get the care they need. And I am very much a patient advocate. Whatever they need, I am going to fight for them and get it for them. With respect to the patients that do not want to return to work and hire an attorney, it can present a challenge. In catastrophic cases, it makes it even harder to get them what they need to move forward. I understand that everyone is different. Whether a patient has an attorney or not, it does not bother me because I can work behind the scenes. I can escalate it and get the notes, the orders, and everything else that is required.

"If the patient does not want to follow through; for example, if they do not want to go to therapy, to the doctor, or back to work – which means they are noncompliant – it leads to another can of worms. These kinds of patients always have an excuse, like 'I do not have transportation.' So, we give them transportation. That is how I work as a case manager, though I cannot speak for other nurse case managers. More than anything, I love a good outcome. I advocate for their proper care to get better and move on with their life. Sometimes they appreciate that and sometimes they do not. If their attorney tells me to leave them alone, I say, 'Okay.' It does not stop me from doing what I need to do, and cases often proceed much more smoothly with an attorney. No matter what, I do my best to help them recover and move forward. If I must fight with the carrier, too, I do not care.

"Health-minded patients who like their jobs tend to recover and get back to work. At times, there will be a psychosocial overlay where they think there is something wrong with them. Because the doctor told them they have a herniated disc, they believe they are sick. I try to be as proactive as I can and advise them, 'You're not paralyzed, you don't have cancer, you didn't lose a limb, and you're going to get better.'

"Now on the employer side, it is great when they care about their employees, because some of them do not. Most of the time, the employer will offer them light duty, which makes it a little easier. On the provider end, they want everything 1, 2, 3. They want it yesterday. That is a difficult result to achieve because we must fight on the other side of the equation to get the carrier to authorize the care and treatment the patient needs. They physician sometimes gets upset because we cannot obtain the authorization fast enough for them.

"In some patients, other body parts are included, in addition to the injured parts. Let us say you hurt your right knee and the other extremity hurts. After we treat the right knee, the left leg hurts, which means we must bring them level again because your gait has been altered. It complicates things a bit because we must ask the doctor to address whether it is related to the injury or not.

"During the 17 years I worked as a nurse case manager for an insurance carrier in corporate America, we were very proactive in providing whatever needed to be done to help the patient get better, go back to work, and live a normal life. If it is related to the injury, we will authorize it just like that. However, if some red flags come up, the medical director must look at it a little closer to make sure it is, in fact, injury related.

"For example, I had a gentleman who hurt his knee, and the doctor wanted to do an A.C.L. repair. Before we do anything, we must get medical clearance. This patient's medical clearance showed some very abnormal lab results. We had to send him to another specialist that did the $1 million workup on him. We knew he had some crazy stuff going on, but the doctor decided it should be authorized, which left us no choice but to authorize it. He needed the knee surgery.

"Before I discuss doctors who over-utilize testing, let me say that I love Dr. Badia. He does an excellent job and he can do surgery on me any time. He does what he is supposed to do: treat the patient and move on. He is excluded from the pool I am about to talk about. However, there are doctors in Miami-Dade, Broward, and Palm Beach counties that overutilize diagnostic testing and medications. I have dealt with patients that have had as many as ten, eleven, twelve, and thirteen knee surgeries. Other doctors order medications in their group, meaning they prescribe medication and deliver it in their office, versus writing a prescription and sending them to CVS or Walgreen's, which makes it easy for the patient. However, it makes it hard for the carrier to keep track of how many medications they are dispensing in their office.

"It was rough in corporate America. We used a first help list of doctors. Workers' comp pays a fee schedule that the doctors must accept. When the insurance carrier refused to pay the fee, it upset me. These educated providers have gone to school to be orthopedic surgeons, for example, and they were getting paid nothing to perform complicated surgeries. It was not right.

"Now I have a better understanding of it all. I have been in this arena for so many years, it is a breath of fresh air when a patient recovers and goes on with their life. But that is not how it goes most of the time. I have dealt with everything from little finger splinters in the thumb, all the way to quadriplegics and the removal of extremities. Sometimes, the attorneys add to the burden. In my mind, I wonder if they are thinking about the patient or all the money they are going to make.

"I will never forget what one doctor told me. 'See this room? This room is workers' comp. The next two rooms are not workers' comp. Nancy, I did the same surgery on the patients in rooms 1, 2, and 3. Room 3 was workers' comp and the others were regular patients. The patients in rooms 1 and 2 are doing great, but the patients in room #3 are not doing well at all.' And that is just the way it is. Are the people who do not want to get better ruining it for the patients who are in bad shape?

"I once had a patient, a man who slipped and fell and was in excruciating pain. It was hard to get him in to a doctor. I knew Dr. Badia was an upper extremity guy, but we could not get the patient in to see him ASAP. So, we sent him to this orthopedic clinic, which was upstairs. We got him in the next day for the M.R.I. which showed some abnormal findings. In the next couple of days, we got him in to see Dr. Badia, who needed to do surgery. We got everything done fast and for that I am grateful. Because this patient had a reverse shoulder replacement, Dr. Badia wanted him to go to his physical therapy center, so he could monitor his progress. However, we did not get the right direction at the outset of the case. Had I known Dr. Badia wanted this patient to have the therapy there, I would not have had a problem with it at all. When it at first appeared that the carrier was going to send this patient somewhere else for therapy, Dr. Badia was upset. This patient had undergone a complicated surgery and I agreed with Dr. Badia that he should remain under his care. We got Dr. Badia's center authorized, and the patient progressed, recovered, and went on with his life."

As Ms. Williams attests, good care is often ultimately delivered through the arduous workers' comp process. The question simply is, "Why should it be that hard and costly"? I will now present what is, sadly, the norm from a patient's perspective. Kerry Anderson works as a waitress at a sports bar my dad frequents often. He loves their steaks, which are inexpensive and delicious. He even brings home food for his dogs. Kerry and the staff know my father well and take excellent care of him. She suffered a work-related injury when she fell at the sports bar, causing significant damage to her shoulder. It took her a year to see me. Why?

As you now understand, almost everyone with a workers' comp injury gets sent to a general urgent care or occupational health clinic, according to workers' compensation policy. Keep in mind, it is not policy because it is better. It is simply because it has always been done that way: the injured patient sees a physician (most often family practice doctors earning an hourly rate) who is usually not at all trained in orthopedics. As we already pointed out, well over 90 percent of workers' comp issues are musculoskeletal. Kerry's story, recounted below in her own words, provides a classic illustration of the disastrous disconnection in healthcare.

Kerry Anderson's Story

"I work at a sports bar. In October 2017, I fell on a wet floor. I went home about a half-hour to 40 minutes later, just feeling bruised and banged up. I did not feel as if anything was broken so I did not go the emergency room. I did not go to Urgent Care. I went back to work the next day. I bruised my shoulder, arm, hips and felt like I had been in a car accident.

I just worked and did not think anything of it. However, I stopped working out. I stopped riding my bike and all activities we like to do, so I could heal. Then we got into the holidays, Thanksgiving and Christmas, and I did not really think much about it. Then my boyfriend David told me, "You really don't sleep. You toss and turn a lot." I would get in a position and feel uncomfortable.

January came around. I had informed my manager about the fall when it happened and the owner of the place the next day. I had it on video. In

January, I started the process of submitting the paperwork for the workers' compensation claim. My boss submitted something, then a week later, somebody contacted me, and two weeks later somebody else contacted me. It was a slow process.

We started at the end of January and in February they told me I had to go to Urgent Care first. I followed their directions and went to the Urgent Care Center they directed me to go. There, they judged my mobility, my pain, etc. The doctor said that I needed to go to physical therapy.

I went to physical therapy, but in between these visits where the doctor says this, a week and a half later, somebody contacts me, and then in another week, I show up. There are huge time gaps in between. I was scheduled for physical therapy for three weeks, three times per week. I believe I did the two weeks, but I kept telling them it did not feel good. I was sweating and in pain every time I came out of there. I was confused, thinking, "You don't know what's wrong with my shoulder?" It was out of order: I thought a patient would see an orthopedic doctor first, then maybe have an M.R.I., and then physical therapy to see if you can rectify the problem before you must have surgery.

It seemed to be an ass-backwards process because I saw an Urgent Care doctor who told me, "I'm not really schooled in this. I think you have a sprained shoulder." I was sent to physical therapy, where they assessed me. But they had me lift weights and do motions, and I was like, "Man, it hurts more now than it did before I came to you."

I went to physical therapy for two weeks, before I went back to the Urgent Care doctor, and then they scheduled the M.R.I. At this point, I still had not seen an orthopedic doctor. I had the M.R.I. that was prescribed by the Urgent Care doctor. I would later find out in the process that he did not order a full scan. There are two-to-three-week time lapses in between going to the doctor, getting results, going here and there. So, I went back to the Urgent Care doctor with the M.R.I. results and he advised me, "Yeah, I see something there, but I'm not an orthopedic so I can't tell you if there's something wrong. I'm going to suggest that you see an orthopedic."

I said, "Okay." Another couple of weeks went by. Remember, we started this process in late January/early February and my surgery was in July. Because it was workers' comp, I jumped through all their hoops. Unless you are going to argue that you don't like where you're going, they tell you, "Here's where you're going to go next." I followed their instructions and went where they told me to go next: Dr. Badia.

When I saw Dr. Badia, I brought the M.R.I. scan. He looked at it and said, "Oh yes, I see a small tear in the rotator cuff, and it'll probably be a

45-minute surgery. I am going to put in a little mesh. You will be out of work for the month of August, and maybe another week or so after that. But let us see how you heal, and we'll proceed from there."

I followed what they told me to do and went to the doctor they wanted me to see for a pre-op. After I got cleared, I went to Dr. Badia to have the surgery...but my 45-minute surgery turned into over three hours! I totally messed up his surgical schedule for the day. Remember, Dr. Badia had not ordered the scan; the Urgent Care doctor – who admitted he was not schooled in orthopedics – did. He did not order a full scan. So, when Dr. Badia got in there, he saw a tear in the rotator cuff but he also saw that the whole labrum was torn off the back – something he could not detect from the M.R.I. scan I supplied him with.

Dr. Badia wanted to send me to physical therapy the next day, but I said, "No." He replied, "Okay, I'll give you a day. The second day you must start physical therapy. All they're going to do is put electrodes to stimulate the muscles, and then I'll see you on Monday." My surgery was on a Tuesday. I had Wednesday off. On Thursday, I went to a physical therapy center assigned by workers' comp – not Dr. Badia's office – where he has his own physical therapy center.

When I was in recovery after my surgery with Dr. Badia, I was very aware of what he told me. David was also there to hear the doctor's instructions: "Do not allow them to remove your bandages, and do not allow them to move you. All they are going to do is put the electrodes on to stimulate the muscle until I see you on Monday. You're going to go twice."

When I showed up at the physical therapy place, the first thing the therapist did was take off all my bandages. "No, you're not supposed to do that," I told her.

"It's okay. I have his orders," she insisted. "I'm going to put on clean ones."

Mind you, I cannot even describe how much pain I was in, so I just followed orders. She took off my bandages, then proceeded to have me shrug my shoulders. Then, she started moving me. Next, she raised my arm. I began to hyperventilate. "I don't think you're supposed to be doing this," I repeated.

"I have your orders. I've read your case," she repeated.

I followed orders. Before I left, they gave me pain medication, maybe eight or 10 pills. I only took them to sleep because I was in a recliner. I have never been in so much pain in my life...and I have two children. I have had other surgeries. I could not sleep. That happened on a Thursday and as much as I did not want to go back, I knew I had to follow the process and returned on Friday for more physical therapy.

That day, she moved me even more than the day before, to the point where I got so nauseous, I had to cut that therapy session short. That whole side of me was black and blue. Over the weekend, I swelled up like the Hunchback. The whole side of my body – my hip, my stomach – swelled more from the physical therapy than the surgery. I did not sleep the entire weekend. When I walked through Dr. Badia's office door on Monday, he took one look at me and asked, "What the hell happened?!"

"I don't know. The physical therapy girl was brutal."

"What are you talking about? Where are my bandages?"

"I told her not to take them off," I replied. "She said she read your reports and she took the bandages off. She moved me and raised my arm."

"Oh my God, you need an emergency M.R.I. right now. She might have undone my surgery. I may have to go to have to go back in tomorrow."

My caseworker, who had accompanied me there, implored Dr. Badia, "Don't make me call the insurance adjuster. Look at the messages on my paperwork. It says, 'Do not call. Do not ever call.' I can only text them or email them."

"You need to call him," Dr. Badia replied. "She needs an MRI because the physical therapist compromised my surgery."

Both Dr. Badia's staff and my caseworker tried to call the workers' comp insurance adjuster. After about five or six calls back to back, he finally answered the phone for one of Dr. Badia's staff members. "The surgeon would like to speak to you," she informed him.

To which he responded, "No."

"Excuse me?" she said. I was standing right in front of her.

"No, I have nothing to say to him," the adjuster retorted.

"But the surgeon would like to speak to you" –

And he hung up on her. "They won't approve it," she informed us.

That is when my boyfriend David took out his credit card. "Here, do whatever you need to do. They hurt her and you need to find out what's wrong." We paid out of pocket for the M.R.I. I was in the M.R.I. machine for 55 minutes. It was awful. I was in excruciating pain because I was lying on my shoulder.

Once he read the results, Dr. Badia announced, "Yes, she compromised it, but no, she did not undo my surgery. However, I would like you to talk to the workers' comp people about staying under my care with my physical therapy department."

Later at home, I called the guy from workers' comp a couple of times and left messages. He would not answer. Then, he finally called me back. "I don't understand why you denied my M.R.I.," I told him. "I don't like the physical therapy place you sent me to. She disregarded Dr. Badia's instructions altogether, and I want to stay with Dr. Badia's physical therapy department. Why would you have one guy do my surgery, then let somebody else undo his surgery? You should keep me with the same doctor for all the care. You are not going to send me to another doctor. This one is going to say, 'Oh, this happened because he didn't so something,' and the other one's going to say, 'This happened because she didn't do something.' I need to stay with the same person."

"Well, that doesn't make sense. You just need to go where we tell you."

"Of course, it makes sense," I countered. "Even if it comes down to liability, you need the same person liable for my care, instead of sending me to multiple people that are doing or not undoing what Dr. Badia did."

He told me I could have had an M.R.I. the day I talked to him. "I wasn't denying you the M.R.I.," he explained. "I was just denying you the M.R.I. at that location."

"Well, you didn't tell the case manager that I had a chance to go to another place. That was never communicated to me. The communication was that you were denying the M.R.I. altogether."

"No, I was only denying the M.R.I. at that location. "I don't like him (Dr. Badia). He is an asshole. I've been working with him for 15 years."

"Oh! So, it's personal?" I exclaimed. "You are compromising my care because you don't like Dr. Badia, or the office, or whatever you've been involved with him in, in the past? I am out-of-pocket for that. You never communicated that I could go somewhere else for an M.R.I., and the physical therapy people you sent me to, compromised my surgery. They just disregarded his orders and did whatever they wanted. They said they knew what they were doing. I want to stay with Dr. Badia and his physical therapy department. You sent me to that doctor."

"I didn't send you. I don't like him."

"Whatever. Your company sent me to Dr. Badia. I did not choose Badia; your company assigned me to him. Your company needs to do whatever they need to do to continue my care with him until I am finished. You are making this hard because you are making this personal. Somebody is going to have to reimburse me for the out-of-pocket because that should not have happened."

By the way, when I paid for the M.R.I. at Dr. Badia's office, his staff member asked if I was related to him because he charged me so little. He charged me $450 and I am sure he took a loss on it because I'm friends with his father, a regular customer at the restaurant I work at. "I'm going to give you extra care because you take really good care of my father," he told me. "I'll charge you the least I can, but we must do this test." David and I were willing to pay the regular charges for an M.R.I., which are easily three times that amount, but Dr. Badia felt bad about the whole situation. He knew that I had been compromised by other people.

When I got home and called my workers' comp guy I said, "Look, I don't know what you need to do but I cancelled my appointment with your preferred physical therapist on Monday. I am not going back there. You need to find out how to approve my care with Dr. Badia's physical therapists; you started me with this surgeon, and you are going to finish me with this surgeon. I am not going to somebody else who will say, 'Dr. Badia didn't do the surgery right,' or this other person did not do the physical therapy right. Do not put me in the middle of that. But I need to be reimbursed. Where do I send the information?"

He said, "You're not going to be reimbursed. You chose to do the test when I told you 'no.'"

I replied, "I hope I don't have to make it a legal issue," sort of joking. With that he informed me, "If you are being represented, you are being represented. I am done with you." And he hung up the phone. I have never spoken with him again.

Again, he claimed he informed my case manager that I could have an M.R.I. at another location, which was a lie. Afterward, my case manager called me to say he was sorry for everything that was happening and asked what he could do to help. A Hispanic man for whom English is a second language, he asked me to stay on the phone with him to dictate an email to Roger, the claims adjuster who had hung up on me and refused my reimbursement request. I have no doubt that when Roger read the email, he knew it came from me, due to the wording and the command of the language. I stated that I didn't say I had a lawyer; I made an off-the-cuff remark about how I hoped I would not have to make it a legal issue, because under workers' comp, everything in my care should be reimbursed.

The next day, my caseworker called to tell me I had been approved to stay with Dr. Badia for physical therapy. My comments in the email did not say directly that I was going to take legal action, but it put the liability on them to make one person responsible for my care. They sent me to Dr. Badia. Their company chose him, not me. Since they had chosen him, I needed to stay with him for the duration of my treatment.

In the end, I remained with Dr. Badia for the physical therapy. He told me that mishap with the workers' comp physical therapist set me back about four to five weeks. I was on a no-movement order to make sure it attached because she had loosened it. I had a lot of unnecessary bruising and swelling. They gave me anti-inflammatory medicine. I knew they meant well, but I did not take it because I didn't want to upset my stomach. I did not want to take one medicine that would mess me up, then take another medicine to counteract the effect of the first medicine. The process was a little slower without sleep and pain meds because I did it naturally.

Three times a week, I went to Dr. Badia's physical therapists. Every six or eight weeks, I went to his office for follow-up X-rays and M.R.I.'s. I followed all the protocol that workers' comp expected me to follow, and I never heard from that guy again, the one who hung up on me. I just dealt with the guy who came to my doctor visits. He had to hear from Dr. Badia how many more visits needed to be approved and so on.

My surgery was July 24. I was signed off December 10, I think, as being through with physical therapy. I am still in pain, but I think it is just a matter of time. And I had a frozen shoulder. Dr. Badia had said at the time that there was a high possibility that they were going to put me under and do manipulation therapy so they could move it and do scar tissue and whatever they needed to do while they knocked me out, because trying to do some of that in physical therapy made me sweat and cry. But as I said, he signed me off in December. That is when I finished my travel log and sent it off to the workers' comp insurance company so they could reimburse me for the miles and the Sun Pass.

Other than that, I probably lost about $600 to $700 a week in wages. The issue at my workplace that is causing the wet floor still exists, so I am cautious when I walk through that way. I am not one to sue. That would be my only recourse, I guess, to sue my employer for negligence. It is just not my personality. I make tips. I make my wages. Workers' comp paid 66% of my paycheck. I do report my tips according to a government formula or a state formula for my taxes, but it does not incorporate 100 percent of the tips. It varies. I did have excessive lost wages.

I am sure there are multiple stories with patients regarding workers' comp. Just seeing people at physical therapy who were there under workers' comp, there are some people who want to do the exercises and follow the routine because they want to go back to work. Then there are some people who do not want to go back to work.

Dr. Badia is wonderful, as is his entire operation. But the whole workers' comp process was backwards. The way OrthoNOW® is set up, the specialist is there, the M.R.I. is there, and you can get answers right away. By contrast, the workers' comp process was two weeks, then three weeks, then somebody called me and sent me to physical therapy before an orthopedic doctor even determined what was wrong with me. They had me lifting weights when the whole labrum was torn off my back. When the primary care doctor finally ordered my M.R.I, he neglected to order a full scan, then admitted that he "saw something," but could not say for sure because he wasn't an orthopedist. Why didn't workers' comp send me to Dr. Badia right away? Why not start the process with an orthopedic doctor?

With Dr. Badia's concept of having all the specialists in one place, it is less pain for the patient and less money spent for the insurance companies. Within two hours, you can know what is wrong with you. For David, it was a nightmare to watch me being torn apart. What bothered him the most was being blindsided. He could not believe an organization could be run like that. The patient was the last thing they thought about. It was sad for him. He felt helpless. He even got proof that the workers' comp approved physical therapy center received the orders from Dr. Badia but chose to ignore them.

Dr. Badia and his office were the only bright spot in this entire ordeal."

This patient account is quite harrowing. In fact, I was not aware of many of the details until I read it as the patient wanted to recount her story. I found it intriguing that the CCMSI insurance carrier's adjustor, a Mr. Roger De-Mello, had commented that he worked "with me" for the past fifteen years. I have no idea who is he is and I consider people who work "with me" as my staff, fellow clinicians, and those in the insurance industry, usually nurse case managers who help me obtain the care our patients need. This gentleman sits at a remote desk and as you see, was not even willing to speak to me about a much-needed patient issue. I would love to know what his perception of NOT working with me is. Furthermore, I found the personal attack on my character as perplexing since we again, never met. Of course, when the doctor fights for his patients, that can be construed as very negative by some on his side of the desk. I was, however, surprised that he would make this statement to my patient, one who went through a major ordeal just to seek the care she deserved.

My referral and workers' comp coordinator, the one who enjoys the arduous task of requesting authorizations from people like Mr. DeMello, provides this account, copied word for word:

Ms. Anderson is the patient that Dr. B had requested get an MRI done here in office back on July 30th and got denied by the adjuster." Hal" was the case manager accompanying the patient to the office that day and he was the first to speak with the adjuster when this happened, he asked Mr. De-Mello who simply said no and Harry let me know straight away. I told Dr. Badia and he said to call Roger because he wanted to speak on the phone with him personally.

Mr. Socias and Ms. Anderson as well as her husband were all present when Dr. Badia requested this. When I called Mr. Dimello and finally got a hold of him, he told me "If you're calling me to talk to Dr. Badia, I'm not going to do it. The patient is not having her MRI done there". I again pleaded for him to just give Dr. B two minutes and he said he "was very busy and didn't have time for this", then hung up on me.

I let Dr. B know and he started defending the patient because she and her husband wanted to have it done here to Mr. Socias. The patient's husband then said he would pay for the MRI without contrast out of pocket if he needed to if it meant she'd be able to have it done in the office that same day and then try to get reimbursed by worker's comp. Our office manager said to charge them $450.00 for the MRI which the patient paid with visa.

There is an update to Kerry's story. Sadly, she sustained a second injury at work, this time involving her knee. However, the bright side is that based on her previous experience, she knew what to do and went straight away to an OrthoNOW®. At the time of publication, Kerry is recovering well and undergoing therapy following a broken patella (kneecap). Her experience was completely different. I ought to know because I was in the adjacent therapy bed rehabbing my right shoulder after surgery while Jorge, our PT director, worked on her knee, which healed with conservative treatment. Unfortunately, she had to learn the hard way. But we can all learn, perhaps even "the system".

In Network vs. Out of Network from the Patients' Perspective

Breast cancer survivor, three-time author, and medical office manager Cindy Papale-Hammontree shares her insights and experiences on in network vs. out of network, plus higher copays for specialists.

"With respect to healthcare and insurance, co-pays are not consistent. For example, to see a specialist, you might have to pay $100 to $150 versus your own primary care doctor, which can range between $10 to $40. Yes, I understand that a specialist has spent more time in school, but all doctors go to school. I am spending the same amount of time with a specialist, yet I must pay more. I do not think that is right, because a physician is there to help a patient – whether they are a primary care doctor or a specialist.

"Another issue people share with me all the time is that most, if not all HMOs require a referral to see certain doctors. The patient is at the mercy of her primary care doctor because if he or she does not feel they need to see a specialist they can deny the patient's request. Today, people are more proactive than ever; not being able to get a referral from their primary can lead them to seeking another primary care doctor on their plan – or even worse – going to the ER to get special care.

"Insurance costs are also astronomical, especially individual groups and/or plans. A friend of mine pays $980 dollars per month – and if that is not bad enough, sometimes insured patients still cannot get in to see a physician early enough because they are already booked with other patients. Many physicians are overloaded, which is another issue.

"Imagine being diagnosed with cancer and listening to the coordinator tell you there isn't an opening until eight weeks from your call. This has happened to me on a few occasions, leading me back to my primary to inquire about how well he knows the physician to whom he referred me, to see if he can use his influence to get me a faster appointment. How sad that, unless you know someone, you must wait.

"As a breast cancer advocate, friends often come to me for help. Either they need to see a doctor they cannot get in to see, or they do not have the money to pay the high co-payment because their medical bills alone are already unaffordable. I feel their fear and frustrations. As most people know, a cancer diagnosis is serious. Our healthcare system compounds the problem by making it nearly impossible to see a specialist – which is devastating for the cancer patient. While they wait, they live under a cloud of fear and uncertainty as they wonder if their cancer is spreading throughout the waiting period imposed on them to see their doctor.

"Another issue is whether your doctor is in your network. If you are lucky enough to have out-of- network benefits, your insurance company would require you to pay the higher cost to see the specialist. However, most people choose a specific plan because their primary care doctor provides excellent care.

"The most concerning issue arises when you get sick, for example, with cancer, and must see a specialist: is that specialist on your plan? Most physicians take both in- and out-of-network benefits. But if they are not in your network, you could pay up to double the customary fee to see the specialist – and God forbid, you need treatment! That is when you hope and pray that the hospital accepts your in-network benefits.

"I remember getting my mastectomy and asking the hospital administration how many days I would be required to say in the hospital. They told me my mastectomy would be performed as an outpatient; however, if I had any complications, I would be admitted. How comforting was that! A lumpectomy and mastectomy should require at least a 24-hour stay post-op. In fact, many physicians will indicate a 24-hour stay, only to be forced by the insurance company to justify it. For example, because I have high blood pressure, I require 24-hour monitoring after almost any surgery.

"Finally, there is the added burden of facility fees. One year, I went for my routine visit with my oncologist and was greeted warmly at an amazing facility. I paid my co-payment ($40 dollars at the time), saw my oncologist, and thanked God that nothing was wrong. A few weeks later, I received a bill for $350 dollars from her office. Thinking it was a mistake, I called the billing department number to inquire about this new charge. To my surprise, they told me it was a 'facility fee' I had to pay. Shocked that a facility fee could be as high as $350, I responded, "Oh, is this to keep your building looking beautiful?"

"While I felt bad responding to her in that way, a facility fee this high is criminal. I would have agreed to a $50 facility fee, not a $350 one. Either way, I had to pay the bill; otherwise, I am positive they would have sent me to collections. My credit is important to me and I did not want that to happen. As I made the payment, I wondered, 'What do weekly chemotherapy and/or radiation therapy patients do? Do they have to pay an additional $350 every week?'

"I hope we can make many positive changes in healthcare in the future. It is both sad and alarming that many Americans will die without proper medical care because they cannot afford insurance. I pray we reform the United States healthcare system within my lifetime to better serve the needs of patients."

Patient Uva de Aragon agrees,

"After a rotator cuff surgery by Dr. Badía, I needed therapy, but the insurance would only approve four sessions at a time, which caused unnecessary delays, and paperwork. The system is harmful both for patients' health and the doctors' ability to dedicate time to his or her practice and not to have the office staff mangled in a bureaucratic mess. Years later, in May 2017, I had an emergency surgery due to a triple fracture of the femur performed by a different doctor. At the end of that year, when I was just starting to be able to put weight on my leg, and had for the first time been able to go up a step, my therapy was interrupted in December because I had exhausted the amount allowed for PT that year. I had to wait more than a month to resume therapy the next year. I am not completely well and have always wondered if that hiatus in my care was detrimental to my recovery. It should be doctors – and not administrators who decide medical issues. Healthcare in the United States needs a complete overhaul. I believe the current pandemic has shown how ill-prepared the country is and how much underlying health issues in the population affect us all."

Erica Pacey says,

"I took care of my mother for a few years before her passing last August. During this time, I had my fair run-ins with Medicare, and their doctors. I had a tough time finding a primary for her, but when I did, we went to her first appointment together. He kept us in waiting room for over four hours! When we finally got into the room, I checked, and he did own a watch. When I asked him how he thought that was okay, he told me "Old people have nothing better to do than to wait...they are on Medicare and they are used to this." I took her files and left.

Towards my mother's last year, she had progressive pain on her lower back. Her doctor from Baptist Hospital prescribed a few cortisone shots to her lower spine. After finding that the last few injections were not working at all, I called SEVERAL times and never received a call back from him. The call back was always a nurse or assistant wanting to blow me off. Eventually the pain was so intense, she could no longer walk.

I was told the cause of this could be many things - pancreatitis, loss of muscle, osteoporosis, and even her Alzheimer's. I knew my mom and the athlete she had been and was sure there was something worse. At this time, I felt they basically had written her off since she did not qualify for surgery. If they had searched years back when this first began, and listened to her, I feel they might have found it sooner.

I eventually had to move her into a home. About three months later, when I was out of town, she collapsed from the pain and was sent to a few hospitals, then to a nursing home. In that nursing facility, I insisted that the manager ask the doctor in charge to run some more tests because nothing was making sense. They finally did and after a simple X-ray, found something and sent her to Baptist Hospital, where they found a six-inch tumor on her spine. By then, it was too late for surgery, so I had no choice but to put her into hospice.

Looking back, maybe I could have gone to a third or fourth doctor, I could have made another call; however, I trusted the healthcare providers and the system. I trusted they would have done their best – but now I know that this is not the case. Maybe her insurance wouldn't have covered it, maybe the doctor did not care enough or did not see the point...but all I know is that my mother was in so much pain at the end of her life, that I wished it would end for her sake. That is not okay.

People deserve to be treated and treated well, no matter who they are or who they know. I have had M.R.I.'s denied from my insurance even when a doctor has suggested it. How does this happen? How are doctors spending so much time dealing with insurance that more and more doctors are not working with insurance anymore? Where is this system broken?"

Patients like Kerry, Cindy, Uva, and Erica represent the frustrations of so many out there, also trying to navigate our convoluted and cumbersome system. It is not difficult to listen to their story and easily point out two- to-three simple changes that could be made in their patient journey which would improve access, quality, and expediency, while diminishing cost. It will be the populace who grow weary of these stories and demand real change.

Chapter 10 – Opportunists Abound Cashing In On The System

If I do not violate this oath, may I enjoy life and art,
respected while I live and remembered with affection thereafter.
May I always act so as to preserve the finest traditions
of my calling and may I long experience the joy
of healing those who seek my help.

Rules are made to be broken. With respect to U.S. healthcare, too many people abide by this axiom. In its positive construct, entrepreneurs relish the opportunity to improve the status quo and make life better. But used in a negative and destructive manner, this cliché becomes the stuff of opportunists, as I will explore in this chapter. First, this saying is likely an abridged form of the famous line by General MacArthur, "Rules are mostly made to be broken and too often for the lazy to hide behind." His comments allude to the simple fact that for many, bureaucracy stifles innovation, often in large institutions such as government, insurance companies, and mammoth healthcare systems, where the guidelines and rulebooks prevail. It is not the stuff of progress.

I have already addressed this "same ole, same ole" mentality in previous chapters because it has truly constrained progress and efficiency in the delivery of healthcare. We have seen how relaxing certain groundless regulations during the 2020 COVID-19 pandemic has allowed more efficient delivery of care, and even saved lives. No need to beat a dead horse.

Instead, I now want to alert you to quite the opposite practice and its deleterious effects. Simply put, the abundance of rules and mindless protocols also encourages abuse and exploitation. When bureaucracy and large organizations focus on creating rulebooks, it allows the most cunning, and shameless, among us to "game the system," a pervasive phenomenon in society. When directed at healthcare, it hurts the most vulnerable, the sick, and retards the efforts of those trying to cure the ill. In many cases, society has turned the other cheek, but those of us who take an oath to heal are compelled to speak out and correct these injustices.

We do not have to look far to see that there are a whole host of cottage industries surrounding healthcare. Scant few of them contribute to the noble goal of healing. The legal field first comes to mind because it is easy to pick apart and deserves to be addressed and confronted (something I will do in a later chapter). Born out of a noble need to correct injustices and level the playing field in a civilized society, the legal profession's mission is perhaps nowhere more perverted than in the medical field. This encompasses so much more than the universe of medical malpractice, a distorted subject that my colleagues and I cover in detail in a later chapter. Clinicians of all types practically stumbled over each other to contribute their stories.

NEVER LET A CRISIS GO TO WASTE

Wikipedia defines opportunism as "the practice of taking advantage of circumstances – with little regard for principles or with what the consequences are for others. Opportunist actions are expedient actions guided primarily by self-interested motives. "Opportunism is much like the word notoriety. It falls slightly on the malicious side but with good intentions, it can be construed in a positive way.

Recent examples abound during what could be the most disruptive population health catastrophe the world has ever seen. The COVID-19 pandemic occurred during the last stages of compiling this book. One might even consider me "opportunist" at even making mention of it, but I cannot resist. COVID-19 can barely be mentioned in the same breath as the bubonic plague. The "Black Death" wiped out one-third of Europe, between 75 and 100 million, in a four-year period commencing in 1347. The difference is the rapid and widespread nature of this current Coronavirus, despite modern medicine and quarantine protocols that were not present in the barbaric 14th Century. What else is different? The spread of information, not just the virus.

Modern communication can be every bit as "infectious" as a pathogen because it enables the quick transmission of both good and bad information. While the SARS outbreak and H1N1 took place in the internet age, it was prior to the infiltration of social media. This has led to not only "fake news" and propagation of hysteria; it has facilitated opportunism. It may have led to the devastating effects on the economy, worldwide, as local newspapers and the evening news well know that "bad news sells". Recall that the 1968 Influenza A (H3N2) pandemic led to 100,000 deaths in the United States alone, predominantly in senior citizens. This did not disrupt Woodstock or other "60s" type behaviors, the antithesis of social distancing.

The constant media and web bombardment of information has led to a wave of COVID-19 associated cyber-scams that prey upon the public's fear of the disease and desire for more information. Scam robocalls and text messaging have offered everything from phony treatments to free viral test kits to health insurance peddling. My own social media and email boxes were filled with work-from-home opportunities, debt relief offers, and business funding loans.

As regrettable as this is, it pales in comparison to the malicious and unscrupulous peddling of PPE (personal protection equipment), worthless test kits, and ineffective remedies. The price gouging of masks (often inadequate) and other necessary materials is truly shameful. Many people have created businesses with fashionable masks, including personalization and branding. I imagine that most assume this will either be the "new normal," or they are at least banking on a prolonged period of continued isolation and distancing.

Excessive commercialization is nothing new but during this hypervigilant time, it is receiving more attention. COVID-19, as horrible as it is, will pass. However, the one constant that will soon resurface is the ongoing scams that obscure scientifically proven treatments and can even harm patients. Healthcare is a vital human need. Those who perpetrate opportunistic pursuits that endanger lives engage in heinous acts.

Access to PPE (personal protective equipment) created a hysteria in which many who know next-to-nothing about medicine or healthcare sought to capitalize on a desperate situation by selling even simple surgical masks at inflated prices. Such price gouging occurred amid many clinicians and healthcare workers "in the trenches," who were even dying in certain cases. They did not profit off the pandemic. That is eerily emblematic of what often happens to those who possess the expertise and provide care. For the first time that I can recall, many people called us heroes without capes.

Much like the business and legal strategies that hinder the delivery of care, harmful practices also often go unpunished or even acknowledged. One can only surmise that it is the inherent complexity of medical care and its science and processes that facilitate this behavior. After all, who is going to know if that pill or supplement is simply sugar and cellulose? This dangerous, costly practice is prevalent throughout society.

In 2015, Dr. Farid Fata, a hematologist-oncologist pleaded guilty and received a 45-year sentence, essentially life behind bars, for administering unnecessary cancer treatments to hundreds of patients in Eastern Michigan. Federal prosecutors called him the "most egregious fraudster in the history of this country." To Fata, "patients were not people. They were profit centers." This "doctor" profited off patients who, for the most part, were healthy, and made them ill from the aggressive regimens.

The opposite action occurred in 2001 in Kansas City, Missouri. Robert Courtney, a pharmacist, was sentenced to 30 years for diluting an estimated 100,000 prescriptions over a decade's time for profit, predominantly chemo-therapy medications. At sentencing, U.S. District Judge Ortrie Smith declared, "Your crimes are a shock to the conscience of a nation. You alone have changed the way a nation thinks… about pharmacists, the way the nation thinks about prescription medication, the way a nation thinks about those institutions we trusted blindly."

These extreme cases will live in infamy. What you may find equally shock-ing is the prevalence and penetration of lesser behaviors that permeate our system. While we often look the other way, we must confront these deeds that taint all clinicians who practice with ethics and compassion.

The burgeoning field of regenerative medicine is one that has caught the public's eye and revealed how innocent (and perhaps ignorant) the lay public can be. The broad term encompasses a wide range of disciplines and treat-ments, but as expected in an increasingly vain society, implies that we can be "rebuilt" and reverse aging.

The American Academy of Anti-Aging Medicine (A4M) was founded in 1993 by two osteopathic physicians who felt that a combination of hormones, diet, and even surgery could eradicate what has been termed the "grotesque disease" that is senescence (aging). Many scientific researchers interested in the scientific aspect of aging have distanced themselves from the organization and many of its members' views. Critics have pointed out that proponents of this growing field use extensive marketing to peddle often useless and expen-sive products and supplements, with occasional dangerous consequences. Dr. Tom Perls is one highly visible detractor, a principle researcher with the Na-tional Institute of Aging and author, who has fought against the destructive uses of growth hormone and anabolic steroids, often used to counter aging. Most scientists vehemently believe that there is no reliable therapy or inter-vention that can reverse, or even retard the normal aging process.

My cursory review of the A4M revealed a plethora of conferences and bus-iness meetings related to the field, including a wide range of certifications that cost a significant sum of money (of course), presumably to hang on the office wall to impress unwitting patients with your expertise in this area. For example, an endocrinology module costs a flat rate of $2,500. To put it in perspective, the annual two-day hand surgery course that I ran, including full cadaveric surgery lab, cost barely $1000. It was designed to cover costs, not be a profit center.

A search of members limited to only a five-mile radius of my home listed 59 clinicians, all members of A4M, meaning there are probably many more practitioners of this yet ill-defined and accepted discipline. Many members are not physicians, or even clearly certified clinicians, but some are former emergency physicians and even neurosurgeons. Of course, the hopeful layperson will likely shell out much more money for fancy treatment protocols than what a surgeon is reimbursed to remove a malignant brain tumor or replace the aortic valve, especially if under insurance. Most are likely well-meaning practitioners who have logically seized upon the public's desire for more individualized care and are willing to pay for it. The irony is that those same patients are often the ones who buck a copayment or want to negotiate a deductible from their more traditional physicians. When something is a luxury, not a necessity, people are more willing to pay for it. Think Prada or Louis Vuitton.

It has become quite fashionable to discount contemporary medical science. This attitude has given rise to an anti-aging philosophy partially helped by the rigors, cost, and complexity of obtaining traditional allopathic medical treatment. Furthermore, the increasingly absurd reimbursements within the traditional bounds of insured healthcare have encouraged even well-trained and ethical physicians to seek alternative models of care. Anything that is not reimbursed by insurance becomes highly touted by caregivers who seek to capitalize on the opportunity to provide care in a traditional fee-for-service model.

One significant component of the anti-aging pursuit is the growing field of regenerative medicine (RegMed). In this multi-disciplinary field, clinical applications and research seek to repair or replace certain cells, tissue types, and organs to treat disease, degeneration, and yes... aging. The field ranges from the most noble pursuit of transplanting *in vitro* grown organs to satisfy the narcissistic quest of avoiding wrinkles. The latter is so prevalent in Miami and other parts of the country and the world, that when a physician reveals his line of work to a new acquaintance, they inevitably ask, "Do you inject BOTOX®?"

Again, it often comes down to money. If covered by insurance, hopefully, a hip replacement or cholecystectomy (gall bladder resection) will reimburse more than a stem cell injection, but until then, many practitioners will exploit the fact that patients are willing to pay for this perceived luxury care. The irony is that they are much more eager to pay ridiculous amounts – as if that reflected clinical efficacy. Once more, reflect on luxury goods like jewelry or handbags. If you put a big sticker price on almost anything, there are people who will line up, along with people who will serve the demand.

The growth of these technologies, including stem cell and tissue engineering, was fueled by the financial world and a flurry of IPOs (initial public offering) in the mythical late 90s. Later, a political "injection" (pun intended) was provided when one individual largely funded a public effort to reverse policy on the use of embryonic stem cell research. Abuses within this RegMed field, caused mainly by money and desperation, have clouded the major advances that do promise therapies that halt or even reverse disease processes. One very significant area, obviously related to my specialty, is the field of Orthobiologics.

The role of various cell types and growth factors in ligament/tendon healing, joint cartilage regeneration, and bone creation is still under exploration. Many advances have been achieved, but again, the encroachment of poor science and economic pursuits has clouded the field.

The use of these agents to promote faster healing has also fueled interest and some successes in the sporting world. Little engenders more interest among the public than saying X professional athlete recovered faster and better using said biologic therapy. Patients often ask me, "Do you take care of the Miami Dolphins or operate on the Miami Marlins?" as if that signifies my worth and clinical acumen. It is simply a reflection of our constant exposure to this sector of pop culture and society. My answer, "No," is often followed by silence, or by my explanation of the politics involved, or offering how other athletes who flew in for my care, depending on my mood and how busy I was that day. No denying it, this is important to most people.

Recall I mentioned the "Tommy John Surgery," earlier. The reconstruction of the elbow ulnar collateral ligament became wildly popular due to his validation. The same is now occurring with Orthobiologics, which has the added value of avoiding dreaded surgery. This is a bit ironic since most orthopedic sports medicine surgery is done arthroscopically, with the insertion of a miniscule fiberoptic camera and instrumentation, via small portal holes that are rarely even visible once healed. The most successful MSC (mesenchymal stem cell) therapies require harvesting bone marrow from the posterior iliac crest – the back of the bony pelvis. Which would a patient rather have: an arthroscopic *surgery* or a stem cell *procedure*? Clearly, much of this is marketing, semantics, and perspective. I now often tell patients they are having a "procedure" when discussing their arthroscopic rotator cuff repair. I reassure them, "When I have to replace your shoulder with a metal/plastic implant, THAT is surgery!"

The intrusion of popular media hype and public perception greatly impacts the evolution of these scientific endeavors, sometimes for benefit, but often to detriment since unrealistic claims are made. Stem cells suffer from broad exposure since positive clinical outcomes are clouded by the abject nonsense in many communities and on the web. This is such a broad subject that I cannot amply cover it in this chapter or the book, but please heed my warning to assess and scrutinize claims with a critical eye.

Platelet rich plasma (PRP) is the component of blood which has a high concentration of platelets, the source of more than 30 growth factors that promote healing and certain tissue growth. The plasma is obtained by centrifuging the blood. This is a much easier process than obtaining autologous (self) stem cells, but it also invites a wide variety of concentrations and activation methods that make it challenging to compare techniques either clinically or in a research forum. If this is difficult for the sound clinician and molecular scientist, imagine the average layperson seeking pain relief. The potential for abuse is enormous. Conversely, be aware that it is illegal to inject PRP to a knee for arthritis, ligament, or tendinous pathology in the country of South Korea, based upon their perceived lack of clinical evidence in research trials. It seems we might seek a happy medium between our Korean friends and the current wild west climate of the U.S. Please note, I did not say North Korea, and remember the South Korean experience and protocols instituted during COVID-19.

Further challenges to objective science are the financial incentive to discount current successful treatments, such as rotator cuff repairs, compared to the less costly injection of biologics substances for orthopedic indications, also termed "Interventional Orthopedics." As I type this sentence, be aware I had an arthroscopic rotator cuff repair in my own right shoulder. I am very right-handed so I will confess that reaching for the mouse is a bit uncomfortable. However, it is nothing like what most of the lay public fear. Incidentally, my surgeon did inject PRP at the site of my repair, just like I do with my own shoulder cases. Beneficial adjuvant most likely but used alone it is not the panacea the public thinks.

A recent paper advocated this all-or-none approach regarding Orth biologics was written by a healthcare businessman seeking fellowship in the American College of Medical Practice Executives. Yes, you read that right. A non-clinician has the audacity or chutzpah to publish an article making clinical recommendations and how we (society or healthcare systems?) must train new physicians to administer such care, with the obvious suggestion that current surgical methodologies are not producing meaningful outcomes. The likely translation of his words? It is too expensive, and the profit margins are diminishing.

As this book is intended to illustrate issues and challenges via everyday anecdotes and stories, I will relate a discussion I had with a parent at my children's private elementary school. A group of us were seated in a barbecue restaurant, during one of those ubiquitous soccer tournaments, trying to distance ourselves from our screaming child athletes at the adjacent table. A fellow parent asked me, "Oh, you're an orthopedic surgeon. Do you do any stem cell or PRP injections?" I already can anticipate the onslaught.

I reply, "I do but I have strict clinical indications. I do think these Ortho-biologics are a valuable addition to our treatment armamentarium." I doubt I said it quite that way, but you get the picture. He went on to tell me that he had "stem cells" injected into his knee and that he "did great." "Wonderful," I answered. "What was your knee issue? A meniscal tear, early arthritis, or what?" He admitted he did not know; he was simply happy that it took his pain away. He then went on to tell me he wants to "inject everything" and that he believes it has anti-aging properties. Here we go. The conversation soon became surreal as he told me he wants to have his wrist injected soon since he has been having "some wrist pain." I had to bite my tongue.

Of course, he had no clue that I was renowned for solving wrist problems, having authored multiple articles on wrist arthroscopy, and he probably was not even clear on what hand surgeons do. Remember, we remove hand wrinkles. I could not bring myself to figure out if he had a TFCC tear, lunotriquetral instability, or perhaps Kienbock's disease. He was convinced that this injection by some doctor in Boca Raton, a town one hour away, could cure him. This is what we are dealing with and I am not sure how to remedy the problem. Remember that there are more than 50 certified anti-aging practitioners in my immediate area, minutes away, while there are barely 20 fully dedicated hand surgeons in our entire metropolitan county. My fellow hand specialists need to be available for the near 10 percent prevalence of hand injuries alone that present to a hospital emergency room. I will not even address the incidence of wrist, elbow, and shoulder pain that many of us treat on elective basis. But the mentality of my fellow school parent is what we are up against.

Opportunists would likely not be able to address his problem if he caught his hand in the treadmill gear, fell off his boat onto the dock, or developed a destructive giant cell tumor of the distal radius. I certainly would not be paid as well for any of those challenging scenarios as compared to a simple injection by my savvier colleague. One must present extreme examples to make a point.

The RegMed, anti-aging, and even OrthoBiologics world is emblematic of the bigger problem in U.S. healthcare where oftentimes the less expert clinician handles most of the care. I am not sure whether this represents opportunism or rather filling a void and serving a need. It is simply a pity that our convoluted system does not facilitate this process. Our OrthoNOW® challenge exposed that in stark terms.

For example, chiropractic doctors serve an important niche of treating mechanical low back pain, something that affects 80 percent of human beings at some point in their life. Their conservative measures truly bring relief to many sufferers, in addition to closely related issues, including some cervical spine issues. My mom, a loyal proponent of traditional allopathic medicine, does swear by her chiropractor.

During my fellowship year in Pittsburgh, I had the opportunity to work with (for) a chiropractor. He was an extremely charismatic clinician, with a large practice of mostly loyal and grateful patients. Keep in mind, much like primary care physicians, this is not episodic care but often a near lifetime of regular visits to keep them "adjusted" and feeling good. The model works, and I have no problem with it, given we respect our limitations. Accordingly, I have no business treating cervical spine problems even though many patients with shoulder pain, and certainly with numbness radiating down the upper extremity (radiculopathy) are due to neck issues. I simply rule out any primary upper extremity problem and refer them to the interventional pain management physician, spine surgeon, or even the chiropractor. I might order the cervical M.R.I. to begin the process but it usually stops there. Not so with many of my chiropractic colleagues. Not only do they often profess to have expertise in more medical issues, claiming G.I. or headache issues are related to "malalignment," they often continue treatment when a more aggressive approach is actually needed in the spine itself.

I recall an incident where an older gentleman came in for a follow-up manipulation. He had been involved in a car accident and I cannot recall if the insurance company or his attorney had referred him. Understand that I was brought in solely for the purpose of preparing a medical report that had to be done by a medical doctor, M.D. or D.O., and allowed the chiropractor to proceed with treatment but, importantly, bill for my services as a physician. Pretty smart for him AND me. Recall that I made a grand total of $25,000 my fellowship year in Pittsburgh. I was well over 30 years old and had been studying/training now for my fourteenth year, post high school. I was happy to make a few hundred bucks for some hours of work. It also provided some insight.

I remember looking at the lumbar spine series X-ray with my chiropractic colleague at my side, and we saw two different things. I also had the benefit of doing a more focused physical exam prior, using my orthopedic training and further knowledge gained during vascular surgery, neurosurgery, internal medicine rotations, and reading plain films for years. He was not trained in that, whatsoever. I noted that the patient not only had low back pain, but buttock pain, intermittent claudication, and improvement with lumbar flexion. The X-rays showed me disc space narrowing, subtle spondylolisthesis, and mild segmental instability with flexion/extension films. He saw some "malalignment," mild scoliosis, and some arthritic changes. I realized this 70-year-old man was suffering from severe spinal stenosis, and regardless of cause, had not responded to chiropractic or conservative treatment. He should at least be seen by a spine surgeon. This incident underscored our different skill sets and made me realize the importance of collaboration for the benefit of the patient.

This incident, and moreover, my entire experience with this sector of healthcare enlightened me to the potential dark side of medicine: what I term "the scavengers of healthcare." It is fascinating that the practice is rarely discussed openly, as if we must settle for the fact that lawyers are meant to sue, and patients will pursue free money. We might have to accept that – after all, lawyers make a living pursuing claims, even when questionable, and what beneficiary does not like money? Even more outrageous is that the entire be-hind-the-scenes network facilitates this travesty. Did I mention I was born in Cuba, despise communism, and fully embrace capitalism? The accident lia-bility racket? Not so much.

Take this excerpt from an article in the Detroit Free Press from May 2017. I did not select one of the hundreds of similar examples I could find in my beloved South Florida, known a bit for its opportunism. Call me a wimp, but I am already creating enough controversy in my hometown. Besides, I know some folks in the Motor City area who are not so ethical. Let us spread the love.

Detroit drivers face the highest average insurance rates for cars and other vehicles in the country. A car moving less than 5 m.p.h. bumped into a U-Haul van on a Detroit street. The driver of the car didn't even bother to stop. And none of the three men in the truck initially voiced any complaints of injury, according to deposition testimony. One filed a police report to show U-Haul, and within days, callers claiming to be lawyers contacted all three urging doctor visits and legal claims.

The U-Haul's driver said he wasn't hurt and hung up. A passenger also hung up on his caller, even after he was offered $600-$800 to see the call-er's doctor and file a claim.

But the second passenger got connected with a Southfield-based law firm and sued U-Haul's insurance company, claiming more than $25,000 in medical expenses under Michigan's no-fault auto insurance system. Those charges included $9,900 for MRIs and $3,200 for a transportation com-pany to shuttle him to appointments.

A Wayne County judge dismissed the case last year, after the man didn't show up for independent medical examinations of his alleged injuries.

But the lawsuit — and thousands like it filed each year in Wayne County Circuit Court, involving over tens of thousands of dollars in medical bills and in-home benefits — helps explain why Detroit drivers face the highest average auto insurance rates in the country, often more than $3,000 a year for a single vehicle.

This despicable case illustrates how perverse our legal system has become, now dragging our vital healthcare interests with it, and propping up a sub-culture of related services, all aimed at extracting money. I commented much earlier on integrity and how I taught my children to recognize it. That dis-cussion can barely be mentioned in the same breath.

As you read the numbers, it also sends the wrong messages to the public. They must think, "Wow, one can spend almost 10 Grand on M.R.I.s? Thirty-two hundred on transportation!?!" The appointments must have been in down-town Chicago...or were they by helicopter? Was the patient quadriplegic perhaps? I thought it was just a cervical "sprain."

Like my director of physical therapy says, "The transportation companies get paid better than we do to provide the actual therapy!" What kind of message does this send to your youngest and brightest contemplating a career in health-care, let alone physical therapy (PT)? I guess it is better to buy a used mini-van and stick a logo on it, as opposed to setting up a physical therapy unit with all the needed equipment, not to mention the expertise. While all the P.T. and O.T. (occupational therapy) readers are clapping by now, be aware that a whole host of "inner circle" denizens are questioning my every comment.

I can hear them now: "How do you know the injury was not that severe? *You are not a neurosurgeon. It costs money to pay these services. Injured folks have a right to the full spectrum of medical care.*" Yada, yada, yada...folks, remember I have been seeing patients (fortunately, not too many of this type) for the past 30 years. I may be wrong on occasion, but I think I, and most of my colleagues and staff, KNOW when somebody is full of shit. There I said it. Incredible how politically correct we have become. Frankly, if we were con-cerned with being correct, our system would not facilitate this travesty.

Think again. We live in a country where a celebrity former football player could get away with murder. Just hire the "right" legal team (whatever that means), and the system can allow you to get away with gaming it. At all of our expense. In fact, some of their children will become famous and wealthy just by free association, not anything they have actually done. Ask your teenage children.

The Detroit article only mentions how this disgusting practice affects the auto insurance premiums in that state. It does not discuss all the downstream liability that impacts the price of your car, the moving truck rental, the court system, and worst of all, the delivery of healthcare.

In my city, you cannot drive 500 yards on a highway without seeing a billboard that says "INJURED". I have noticed that this phenomenon is even worse in many small towns. This is indeed a puzzling spectacle given that I thought someone with an injury needed some type of clinician: a trauma surgeon, an E.R. physician, a skilled triage nurse. Why is any allusion to being injured immediately associated with a legal professional? I do not imagine that my image or our orthopedic walk-in center URL would appear on a blazing billboard – Being Sued??! Sounds ludicrous does it not? Imagine if you had spent years training at a trauma center like Bellevue, or Jackson Memorial, or Cook County Medical Center? We KNOW injured.........

Many of the billboards in Miami, and a litany of bus wraps, now display a large breasted woman in a provocative pose, pointing towards the name and website of one of these "injured" call centers. Does the public really respond to this type of branding? Understand it is these shady care networks who have the money – not the people who deliver care – to pepper the landscape with these tasteless ads.

Hence, in an ideal world, this type of expensive marketing and advertising would be reserved for someone who can treat you. It is a minimum $5,000 per month for a billboard in the Miami area. Let us analyze this: to make $5,000 when Blue Cross Blue Shield pays you $120 for a visit, my injury walk-in center (see- sounds weird) would have to see a minimum of 40 patients just to pay for the darn signage. It is not a level playing field. Not an even landscape at all. Many plaintiff lawyers seem to justify this expense judging by the fact that multiple law firms handling personal injury add up to a lot of billboards. They may still dominate the covers of the yellow pages phone directory (okay I am aging myself now), and a whole host of other community facing advertisements. Except for plastic aesthetic surgeons or large hospitals, you will see very few clinics announcing their services. I am not referring to elective practices, but rather walk-in facilities that truly handle emergencies. In other words, the people you really want when INJURED.

It is common knowledge that these shady practices occur. Perhaps our society will soon find some balance and a sense of priority with respect to these issues. The first step is recognizing them – no easy feat because our communities are inundated with this almost predatory network. It is challenging to even find data on the societal and monetary cost of the auto and personal injury conglomerate, since the first pages of Google are filled with ads from the law firms that service this sector. My colleagues abroad laugh at this practice and do not understand why it perpetuates. I tell them I don't either.

The auto injury is just one "specialty" and there are some law practices that literally focus on "slip and fall". Its listed in the services section, much like shoulder arthroscopy or diabetes management. However, no transaction occurs if your injury happens at home, although on second thought, you can maybe sue the rug manufacturer or the squeaky toy you stepped on. If you slipped at work, you might see a different legal specialist. We covered workers' comp ad nauseum.

There are people who make their living almost exclusively litigating ONLY slip and falls. For example, falls in the supermarket is a subspecialty and store videos have since been installed where they can capture people in the act, real or otherwise. I recall a video clip where a man intentionally slipped but apparently did not like his performance, so he stood up and did it again. The camera filmed the whole thing. Around the produce section, God forbid shit falls on the ground and things happen. I mean people do get injured, but those cases are clouded and obscured by the charlatans.

The medical issue related to these falls is that reimbursement takes on a whole new dimension, bringing in the supermarket insurer, both attorneys and even the patient's personal health insurance. All these hurdles to overcome to get paid for fixing an actual elbow fracture that occurred during this unfortunate incident. One must often wait several years before the case settles, or is litigated, and the clinician still doesn't know what his time and expertise investment will yield. Many of us simply will not do this kind of work. The surrounding drama is just too much not to mention delays in payment which disrupts your cashflow as a viable business.

You can imagine that people do slip and fall in the bathroom of a restaurant or airport, essentially heavily traveled restrooms in a public place. Double the traffic if it is a beer hall. Of course. Do we not want them to clean the bathroom after somebody sprays in there? Our legal system seems to suggest that. Clean means temporarily wet, folks. However, a wrist or elbow fracture is all the same to me. The mechanism of injury is inconsequential. Not so in our lovely legal system.

I painfully recall an incident where an entrepreneurial dermatologist from NY basically sued a very affluent South Beach restaurant because he slipped and fell in the bathroom. Of course- it was wet as it had just been cleaned for the 8th time that night. Thank goodness. But of course, somebody's got to be on the hook for that. He calls me at midnight, waking me up, and I direct him to the most time efficient hospital in the Miami area, well focused on orthopedics, although away from Miami Beach. I therefore save him a lot of time and he calls me with the x-ray findings, although I already suspected the result given his accurate description of his deformed wrist. At the time, OrthoNOW was not even a gleam in my eye. He is splinted promptly and comes over the next morning to now show me his X-ray. Telemedicine was near science fiction. After gifting me a bottle of vodka, he asks me what to do as he was returning to New York shortly. I suggested he stay as I have seen bad cases of flying after significant fractures including one NYU patient who died of fat embolus after a modest tibial fracture. He stays. I warn him that my practice can be a zoo. I was then in network and the volume was incredible, not to mention a flurry of walk-in cases every day like fingertip injuries and other fractures like his. He said no problem. Bad decision from me. He tormented my staff incessantly like Homer Simpson's kids shouting "Are we there yet" in the family car every 80 seconds.

I was in surgery at the old Miami Hand Center and in the middle of a typical 22-case day when he arrived and proceeded to wait. I should have given him one of those buzzer things like busy restaurants hand you when you are placed "on the list". At some point, I informed my frustrated staff that he was a "friend". He finally stormed through to the back to confront me. My so-called buddy then tells me he is leaving and flies back to NY the next day. He starts the entire process over but this time at a prestigious, but large orthopedic hospital. This is not a small outpatient facility, like mine despite the chaotic nature that day. Pretty foolish.

I do not think he grasped the fact that I was one of the wrist specialists who helped popularize the plating technique that is now standard of care. No matter. He, despite being a fellow physician, was focused on the long wait and wanted to make a statement. I wonder how he does on a busy day at Walt Disney World.

Fortunately, his wrist did well. A year later I was dragged into his lawsuit, despite my firm instructions to keep me out of his mess. I was asked some questions about whether he sounded inebriated when he called me that fateful night. "I was awakened from my own slumber", I told them quickly, to end to that nonsense line of questioning. I basically threw him a lifeline. Who knows what happened, but I am glad his surgery was successful, despite his torturing my office staff.

Ironically, he called me years later one lovely Sunday afternoon. Seems his girlfriend amputated the tip of her finger on his boat hatch. Bummer. I am not sure where I was, but I promptly referred him to the nearest hospital.

That whole lawsuit, the downstream effects, all those costs gets lumped into that almost three-quarters of a trillion dollars which INJURY costs the US economy. This represents the total lifetime medical and work loss expenditure from injury and violence in our US alone. Fatal injuries cost us $214 billion while nonfatal injuries accounted for $457 billion. This represents 2.5 million people who are hospitalized but the 26.9 million folks who are treated as outpatients, mostly in big, expensive emergency rooms has been my focus for the past decade. As you see, the time, money and energy our society puts into the legal aspect of physical injury (I mean INJURED?) will easily overshadow innovations that could alter the medical and convenience aspect via an orthopedic walk-in center concept. It's simply a matter of our priorities.

Sadly, the world-wide calamity of COVID-19 will not inject enough negativity in our world for some. The spate of upcoming lawsuits related to this tragedy will be further breeding ground for other opportunists, despite most of us fighting to simply move on.

Our television and internet are inundated by "snake oil" type products that are targeting people in pain with false promises. There are creams, supplements, braces, copper, this and that...all designed to generate hope that one of those remedies will finally cure your pain. It is a multi-billion-dollar industry and again, is amazing that they have the funds to embark upon this type of advertising, whether false or even based on some scant data. It is irrelevant. Let's take a critical look at where consumers choose to spend their dollars. Is it on a copper lined knee sleeve, or the copayment/deductible of a reputable knee specialist?

The complexity of rules and regulations has also spawned a bevy of cottage industries that in many cases earn more than the clinical services that they are intended to support, not overshadow. To be discussed further in the Moral Injury chapter, electronic health records has become a major drain on clinicians' psyche and pocketbook.

One study, assessing the cost and time associated with implementation in a primary care group of physicians, revealed an average of nearly $50,000 per provider and 134 hours per physician to train doctor, clinical and non-clinical staff. We have alluded to the modest net income most physicians now make due to these and other onerous cost centers. Despite this new intrusion placing serious demands on a practice's time and revenue, the healthcare system and practitioners continue to be inundated with new EHR (electronic health records) companies now totaling over 500 vendors. In a 2019 report by Business Intelligence, it was estimated to be a $30-billion-dollar global market, reaching $38.3 billion in 2025, coincidentally the same year many forecast that Medicare costs will reach unsustainable size. The number of companies alludes to the fact that there must be a lot of money to make and many still see opportunity. These figures are in stark contrast to the goal of a universal health record as put forth by President George W. Bush in 2004. The goal was to promote quality and reduce costs. Hardly. Few can deny that we would not want to return to the day of cumbersome patient charts that one has to spend hours often tracking on down on patient days or with a hospital transfer. However, given the number of systems, the humble goal of interoperability and a shared database has been lost to opportunistic players in the growing IT sector. Everyone thinks theirs is better, despite the fact that the three largest vendors, Epic, Cerner, and Allscripts, control approximately 50 percent of the combined market of hospital and outpatient EHRs.

Epic is privately held, charged $1.5 billion (yes B) dollars to the Mayo Clinic to implement and almost universally inspires groans from clinicians when discussing usability. Cerner eclipsed the Epic record by charging us taxpayers a whopping $10 billion for the V.A. contract which would also network with the DoD (Dept of Defense.). Allscripts has had a host of leadership challenges in recent years and perhaps represents the turbulent nature of this industry.

One thing is clear. The money being poured into the electronic part of healthcare, namely the documentation, often outshines the actual delivery. A theme increasingly evident. On an individual basis, the costs are daunting. As example, I am about to "upgrade" my PACS (picture archiving and communications system) which is essentially how we store and view diagnostic studies, mostly X-ray and MRI images. Pretty important for an Orthopod (orthopedic surgeon). A key point is that I simply don't want to. I am happy with my current system and functionality (well...somewhat). The problem is the industry gives you no choice. When one software, or perhaps operating system, has an upgrade, every program dependent upon that must fall in line- and it comes with a big bill. I originally purchased my entire EMR and Imaging system, hardware and PACS, from Stryker corporation, a huge orthopedic company. The ones who don't like "jungle parties". They simply white label it as their business is implants, not IT. You pay for the initial cost, implementation and then monthly fees which imply you had better be seeing patients and generating revenue. Then all the sudden, without warning or recourse, they sell that division to another company. You must pay more. Mind you, not a lot has changed, and you and your staff are already acclimated to the current system. Then Armageddon hits. They tell you "We can no longer service the software". Basically, it is IT talk for "You're shit out of luck." Now you need to find a whole new system. We did that. It takes a while, a LONG while, to catch up again. Patient care is no different, however. Shoulder pain or tennis elbow is the same. Treatment options may vary as our knowledge progresses. A new procedure may come to vogue and then you gradually change and adapt…grow. Not with EMR and PACS and your other IT solutions.

As I write, I am about to undergo yet another PACS upgrade which requires a nebulous amount of time and a dollar figure that is yet more ethereal to me as they could say just about anything. It certainly isn't that way with my charges. I am going to scope your wrist joint, place some pins and then the insurance company will pay whatever THEY deem "covered" and usually with some specific number, down to the cents. In other words, you get hit coming and going. The current charge is now $8,000 bucks. Just like that – a round number with no invoice unless I demand it. To put in perspective, that would mean eight shoulder replacements like I did on sweet Lew. The surgery, the post-op and follow-up visits, my time and expertise. Those eight reconstructions are equivalent in value to simply an upgrade of some software that some very smart folks wrote and some minor hardware changes. Incidentally, I consider myself lucky overall. The challenges are there. Omnipresent.

Now the hardware and software are in. There are other cottage industries that teach you how to maximize use, efficiency, and your reimbursement. The holy grail.

There is an entire industry that revolves around medical billing and coding. There are now bachelor's degrees awarded in that discipline and the BLS (Bureau of Labor Statistics) has estimated that employment will in that field will increase 11% in decades following 2018, adding 23,100 jobs. What does that signify about how many people in our workforce dedicate their lives to what somebody else does – provide healthcare? The fancy term is RCM (Revenue Cycle Management) and was barely a concept when I attended medical school. There is a host of certifications and exams for medical billers alone including CMRS, RHIA and CPB. I have no idea what they mean, and I am a doctor who generates work that they bill.

Why does this need an entire industry and is it any wonder it costs our country a half trillion dollars a year? Yes, I said the T-word, not the B-word. This is solely due to BIR (billing and insurance related) costs and is in addition to overall healthcare administrative costs which is more difficult to calculate. It's estimated that nearly half this number is wasteful and excessive, explaining why the U.S. spends twice as much per capita on healthcare as compared to other industrialized countries with similar type healthcare systems.

Recall that I have ten staff members for a solo surgical practice, and fortunately, out-of-network at that. My European colleagues typically have 3-4 staff members for equivalent type practice.

The reason is listed below. It takes a village to fulfill all these steps and this is mostly the economic and record keeping component. If I outsourced billing, which I did at one point and was disastrous for me, I might have 1-2 less staff members but then give up a lot of income. And direct control. So, what is there to do?

For starters:

Charge capture – converting a medical service into a billable charge.

Claim submission – sending that charge (bill) to insurance companies.

Coding – Properly coding diagnoses, modifiers, and procedures. People who have no medical education can become expert at this and certified.

Patient collections – determining what the patient owes and collecting payments. Good luck.

Preregistration – Collecting tons of demographic and insurance info to determine eligibility before any patient even arrives for medical care.

Registration – Collecting more information during actual registration to create a medical chart and fulfill multiple financial, regulatory, and yes, clinical requirements.

Remittance processing – Fancy term for handling payments versus rejections. There is a lot of the latter.

Third-party implementation – Trying to collect from a myriad of third party/ TPA insurers.

UR (Utilization review) – the part where an armchair clinician decides if the person treating the real patient really needed those pesky medical services.

Like any complex system, it is hard to backpedal. I am not sure how we can make it less complex at this point, but as they say, "It's above my pay scale." We will explore some ideas in the last chapter, but we have created an overarching, convoluted, complex system to simply pay for a service rendered. The restaurant analogy was good, but a longer thesis would be necessary if we assessed how a shopping mall gets paid, with its composite parts including the hapless restaurant.

Now that we have such a complex, convoluted system merely to get paid for what is a relatively straightforward service, we must master it. I am not suggesting healthcare is easy, but it is not a hard concept to grasp what I do. I take this busted bone and put this metal thing in there to fix it, and my colleagues help you get back to using your arm again. Pretty clear. Not so with "management consultants" or "industry analysts" of which I still don't know what they actually do. Collecting payment for my clear-cut bone-fixing service requires a bevy of outside consultants and trainers who provide initial and ongoing training, a myriad of courses, and manuals all of which have a cost of course. I get these emails EVERY day, not to mention hundreds of LinkedIn invitations which are usually coming from Asia. For American healthcare delivery. You have to pay to get paid.

The worst part for me regarding EHRs is not even the complexity, cumbersome prices, or cost, albeit onerous for clinicians earning less and less. It is the quality of medical documentation seen in the EMR (electronic medical record). My first EMR when going into practice, that I purchased from Stryker, who again just put their name on it, was essentially a document filing program. All the notes were mine, dictated in detail, and I did have some simple template notes that document a simple post-op carpal tunnel visit, or maybe a corticosteroid injection for a trigger finger. It did simplify the more repetitive actions. However, a patient experience and medical condition is not a template. The notes these days are appalling. The longer they get, the less useful information. It is gravely concerning and worse, we are coerced into going along with this behavior.

Healthcare may not be as simple as ordering the blue plate special, or buying that new laptop, but there is no question that the complexity of the transaction should be mostly centered around the actual clinical care. We must refocus our priorities and energies.

Due to the high cost of medical equipment, a cottage industry of lending capital to physicians has been spawned in recent decades. This can be a very good option since the application process is more streamlined, funds are more readily available and you may not need collateral, important for young clinicians who spent much of their young adult years in education or training. The drawbacks are often much higher interest rates, lower financing amounts, and sometimes, questionable ethics.

These companies know full well that most physicians are reliable people with good standing and are not going to skip out of town. The loans are typically for equipment of high value that will be used to provide patient care for many years. Frankly, it is a good deal for those companies, and let's be clear. Their ONLY aim is to make money. They are not providing a service such as legal or accounting advice, let alone taking out your gall bladder or rebuilding your transmission. Essentially, it is a social, and financial, contract where they make money by simply having money. No criticism, it's the American way – credit access fuels growth.

My problem is with how predatory some of the companies can be. The financial contract component is understood. However, the social component and how sympathetic they are to physician challenges has been disappointing to me and other colleagues who have related similar issues. I present this as a warning to those who seek capital for the noble cause of caring for patients. This sector may not be so noble.

When I built Badia Hand to Shoulder, it was a major undertaking as I related in section one, but I did not take a loan for my office buildout. I was already inundated with the commercial real estate loans due to the magnitude of the project. Often, and clearly to my detriment, I was to learn that I have little risk adversity. This can be a pitfall for entrepreneurs. Regardless, I pushed on and decided to invest in THE most state-of-the art digital X-ray machine, no regrets there, and an in-office MRI. This was before OrthoNOW®

so the machine was not optimal for spine and hip but sufficed for the upper extremity. These are not inexpensive for a solo practitioner.

Based upon the recommendation of a healthcare businessman, I was engaged by a Midwestern capital lending company called Baytree. As physicians, we do not understand the concept of networks, kickbacks, and loaded referrals. We must comply with rigorous laws against fee splitting, anti-kickback, and the whole gamut of Stark, which we address in the moral injury and government chapter. Remember, we can barely have someone buy us a New York strip steak, let alone hold a party at "The Jungle." It is not a level playing field.

I certainly realize some of the pitfalls but be very wary of more devious behaviors that a harried clinician may not recognize or even think of. In the case of Baytree, my then office manager came to me and said, "Dr. B, I hate to share this with you, but are you aware our capital leasing company has been charging you $200 late fees every month?" I was surprised considering I knew that she was fastidious in paying bills and keeping the books. Apparently not enough. "Well, I just realized this has been going on for over two years and we do pay every month, like clockwork, but I pay most bills around the 6th of the month so we have clearer idea of the books by then". We called thinking there must be some mistake. Apparently, we had to pay by the 2nd, if I recall, and even though we were very regular, we technically were late, and they simply neglected to inform us. Thinking this was not human oversight, we held payment for one month to schedule a discussion and come up with an equitable solution. Fat chance. Baytree clerical staff, sounding quite robotic, immediately telephoned us inquiring about that month's payment as it was the first time we had ever missed. It induced a dialogue – really quick. When explaining the late fee issue and asking if we could be refunded for most of those months where we were never informed, she simply echoed the policy. Of course, technically they had us, but the human component is missing, something most caregivers do NOT understand.

The oversight by my office manager cost me over $4,000 on top of the very hefty interest rate payments they were receiving. No matter. It's a technicality in their favor and the odds of any human sympathetic action is near nil, akin to an aggressive attorney's action capitalizing on your oversight or misstep.

A non-medical example is my first and only apartment in Miami, in Brickell Key. I did many nights of trauma surgery when I first got to town, as related in Chapter 3, so mail would often pile up. Simply due to being late with a condo maintenance payment for a second month triggered a nasty letter threatening a lien on my property. Naively, I telephoned the law firm that handles the account and the barrage of cold-hearted policies that the attorney fired at me took me aback. I remember being in the surgeon's lounge at Doctors Hospital and realizing what different jobs we had. I told you real estate was a jungle. I learned that day to never be late with a payment and engaged my own sister to help me in this task. I learned my lesson, but I also swore I would never live in a condominium again where I pay the bills for the staff to berate me. I guess he did his job but at what price? In essence, a late payment or possible DNA tainting at a murder scene will trigger what the law dictates, not what is right. It is a different code of honor and as clinicians, we need to be vigilant.

You would think I would learn. Well, in some cases, responsibility to handle these issues is handed off to someone on your team. In my case, I am horrible at reviewing contracts and picking up on potential pitfall clauses.

During our early years at OrthoNOW®, we were approached by a very colorful salesman that wanted to show me a medical device for rehab and pain control. Realize that subject alone, pain is a breeding ground for opportunists in the medical field. Naturally, we all want our patients to not have pain. There are literally dozens of electrical, laser, ultrasound, radiofrequency devices that all have different efficacies and it is up to the clinician to sift through the technology, and data if even available. It is a field rife with opportunists. We discussed that issue in the opioid crisis, where a greedy pharmaceutical company leveraged new, and senseless, government guidelines to ensure our patients do not have pain.

The ARP device was simply another version of a neuromuscular stimulator, with a series of specific, and powerful, protocols that facilitate rehabilitation and diminish pain simultaneously. I met the cofounder who was also a very charismatic, almost evangelistic, man with a background in exercise physiology. He was not a physician nor a therapist, but he could sell snow to an Eskimo. The long and short of it is that he managed to convince my OrthoNOW®, rehab and recovery room team that we should be using it on many of our patients, therefore requiring more units. The price was well over $20,000 which should have been a red flag, but nevertheless, the clinical results were indeed quite impressive. No regrets there. It is the economics of the situation where we were sold a bag of goods.

To finance the presence of multiple machines, we engaged another capital leasing company. Big mistake. I should have worked out an arrangement with the neurotherapy vendor where I simply paid him monthly for leasing them, and could return them if need be, or eventually pay them off. What is amazing is that I am one of the first reputable orthopedists who brought some credibility to the device, not to mention opened all sorts of international contacts for them. I asked for nothing in return. Well, let us just say they took advantage of a busy surgeon and since we do not anticipate any malice from people, they recommend a capital lending company. Sounds like my first experience. This time, we did make our payments on time, but the machine had a well-designed feature that allowed the inventor/owner to remotely turn off its function, since we decided to seek less expensive options. Well, despite having a functionless machine, we were still on the ropes for the exorbitant cost of the device and the capital leasing company didn't care. Naturally. While we figured out the best way to come to an equitable compromise, even sending back the machine, since after all it's worth $20,000 + bucks, the calendar kept ticking. In the end, Ascentium Capital ran up a legal bill that was more than the price of the machine, if that is even possible. Telephone calls to them were met with the same gruff answer and unsympathetic ear that the previous lender, Baytree, displaced and our condo association bulldog property attorney. I will say I am a bit envious. To make that much money and be able to turn your phone off at 5 PM, not have to produce something of substance, and leverage the money you already have to make more of it is a panacea of sorts. However, I quickly reflect on what I tell my children about integrity.

Lending can have high moral values, however. One person, who is now an accomplished author and helped advise me about this book, made a major impact in this field. Alex Counts is a Cornell fraternity brother of mine who spent five years in Bangladesh under the tutelage of Mohammed Yunus, the Nobel Prize winning financial pioneer who founded the Grameen Bank, revolutionizing micro-lending. Alex went on to create the Grameen Foundation, a Washington D.C. non-profit that is committed to ending world poverty via microfinance.

I relate the contrasting story of Grameen Bank because most healthcare professionals would have much more affinity to this concept, and its benevolent culture, but it's not realistic in the context of first world healthcare. Major capital is needed to purchase real estate, fund high tech medical buildouts, and finance equipment as discussed. I urge clinicians at all levels to be very wary of this necessary, but risky, sector of healthcare delivery.

Since physicians have little background in finance or business, it does lead to many of these problems, compounded by the fact that our altruism makes us an easy target. It is hard to become expert in business matters when one is focused on biochemistry, later internal medicine, and dealing with hospital call schedules once in practice. I made this abundantly clear in section 1 and I am certainly no exception. The unfortunate thing is the gradual erosion of trust when others more versed, take advantage of that fact. This will also be discussed in the moral injury chapter.

I would caution many clinicians to thoroughly research investment opportunities, particularly when brought forth by healthcare related professionals, but not clinicians. They better understand our naivety and may prey upon that coupled with the understanding that you might even be able to contribute primarily, or peripherally, to the investment.

I was fortunate in that my first, no second investment was based upon working knowledge of the landscape. I had used the product, helped even develop the concept, and was confident that my then partner would act honorably, despite later conflicts that led to the group's dissolution. The other investment was with my other partner and I would chalk that up to bad luck. I have no real regrets.

Some years later, I was given an opportunity to invest in a spine company, knowing full well that this was not my area of expertise, but I trusted in the company who enlisted me. For years there was scant information, even though my review of spine company revenues and transactions gave me hope. After FDA approvals and significant growth in revenues, they were purchased by a large orthopedic company that wanted to expand its portfolio into this sector. I thought for sure that I would be made whole again at the very least. There was no fine print. Simply put, the largest investors were repaid first, even though I came in early, and the remainder was to service debt. Too bad. What recourse does one have?

It reminds me of a hedge fund investment I made, ironically via a friend who was one of the fund managers. The fund was sailing during wall street heydays but soon began to tank. The information was inconsistent, and it soon became apparent that they were putting our money into toxic investments. I was certainly willing to take a major loss, but the fund actually had the audacity to bring the NAV (fancy term Net Asset Value) to 40% of my investment, then suddenly Nothing. I can't say zero as they never even gave me THAT figure. Just nothing. I even travelled to the Cayman Islands, not once but twice, to meet with their monetary authority and discuss options. This was set up by former finance ministers AND prime ministers who had all been patients of mine in Miami! Further phone calls and inquiries by interested friends, and even patients, led to double speak by the fund people who turfed the issue off to another company. It is a shell game. Many of us have seen the series Billions on Showtime TV. Would you invest in those people? Be wary of these investments, particularly when they are based in small, obscure island countries.

Similar issues, albeit less scandalous, occur with many of my colleagues who invest in medical device companies or even healthcare ventures, such as ACOs (accountable care organizations), specialty hospitals, or physician groups. One of my colleagues in New Jersey was in a very busy ASC (ambulatory surgery center) that had incredible case volume, week after week. They had been purchased by a large, national ASC company, managed to further grow their caseload, and he shared with me that "the docs" barely receive any distributions. That is what we are called. The surgeons who spent a decade and a half preparing to then make money for others.

A few years ago, a large group of Miami surgeons invested considerable sums with a midwestern hospital company to rebuild a local, outdated facility that had closed years prior. There were promises of big future dividends, even though much of the money went towards truly spectacular infrastructure for a state-of-the-art hospital. This is of little use to orthopedists like me who rarely have a need for a hospital. These same surgeons consequently did not have funds to invest elsewhere, in more prudent investments better aligned with their specialty. Such as an ASC or rehab facility, or even a walk-in center that would feed them relevant patients. So, where did the money go? Call it "fuzzy math" but Ross Perot had a point. Unless you are one of the principals, or the founder, anything outside your wheelhouse is a risk you must ponder carefully, and you could soon hear a "giant sucking sound." It might just be your money, Doctor.

Chapter 11 – Medical Malpractice, Trial Lawyers, & Tort Reform

"If I do not violate this oath, may I enjoy life and art,
respected while I live and remembered with affection thereafter.
May I always act so as to preserve the finest traditions
of my calling and may I long experience the joy of healing
those who seek my help."

No discussion of skyrocketing healthcare costs is complete without a thorough examination of the 300-pound elephant in the room: medical malpractice, trial lawyers, and tort reform.

Does everyone remember the infamous McDonald's coffee case from 1992? 79-year-old Stella Liebeck bought a cup of coffee from a McDonald's drive-through in Albuquerque New Mexico, spilled it on her lap, suffered third-degree burns, sued the company, and was awarded nearly $3 million in punitive damages from a jury. While people to this day still debate the merits of the case, a friend of mine who defends doctors for a living shared this perspective: in these types of cases, and particularly in medical malpractice suits, it is the ridiculous pain and suffering settlements that drive up costs.

There is little disagreement that the punitive pain and suffering awards are often absurd and even sensationalistic, hence the media feeding frenzy after something as headline grabbing as the coffee case. However, to be fair, and that is indeed the intent of our jurisprudence system, we must have all the information before even passing judgement. The McDonald's coffee case has several rarely discussed caveats that should not make this symbolic of the medical profession's battle against unjust malpractice.

Mrs. Liebeck was not driving or even in the drive-through lane when she placed the cup in between her thighs, while in her car, and indeed suffered 3rd degree burns. Apparently, McDonalds, a multi-billion dollar (and billions of burgers) had received more than 700 prior complaints about the near nuclear temperature of its coffee, yet never bothered to make simple changes. The media seized upon the $3 million-dollar figure, not reporting that the claimant was willing to settle for a mere $20 grand to cover costs of her inner thigh skin grafts. They also did not widely report that the final judgement was later diminished to $640,000 and the plaintiff did not even get that sum. A later undisclosed settlement occurred to avoid yet another appeal and court time.

While this case was politicized, offered as example of frivolous lawsuits, and widely distorted, it did serve to engender a national debate on real tort reform. I wish we had a similar case in the malpractice realm to bring public awareness to the debacle that continues to occur. A medical "Stella Liebeck" is needed, not to scandalize some outrageous pain and suffering judgement, but rather to fully bring to light the actual mental, and often economic, pain the defendant, usually a well-meaning clinician, must endure during the process. You see, it is not the final verdict, or even the amount, that pains the physician. It is the assault on our values and noble intentions that causes the real pain. A strong component of moral injury, this does deserve its own analysis.

The reality is that barely a quarter of malpractice suits proceeding to litigation end with a judgement against the doctor anyway. That is not the matter. The issue is the mental anguish of going through that process, not to mention time/energy disruption which erodes into what our prime purpose is: to help our fellow man. Even the defensive medicine posture is secondary as is the anxiety I experience every time I pick up a scalpel. Although it is rarely discussed, it eclipses all other sources of stress that contribute to what we will explore in a subsequent chapter on moral injury in the medical profession.

Let us imagine that the plaintiff is a patient who lost his hand in a devastating work injury and despite his orthopedic surgeon's diligence, training, and skills, there was no way to reattach it. That is a tragedy both for the patient and the surgeon who wanted nothing more than for the operation to be a success. Alas, life is not perfect. Next, this patient seeks out an attorney, sues his doctor, and shows up in court with a missing hand, which elicits sympathy from the jury as they listen to the details of his case. Aside from the obvious negative impact to his body and mind, there is a significant work-related economic impact because he cannot do his job anymore. For his monetary compensation, you could calculate his lost wages by multiplying his current salary by the amount of years he would have continued to work to arrive at a fair settlement. It is only right to pay that out because he can no longer perform his job duties. But in a case like this, juries tend to get highly emotional about the poor plaintiff who must go through life with a missing hand; therefore, they award excessive amounts of money for pain and suffering—to the tune of $50 million.

Pain and suffering compensation increase the number of lawsuits people can bring. And there is no downside because there is no cost to sue. Attorney ads for free consultations run at 3 a.m. when someone is sitting at home stewing over an accident or an injury they have suffered. They see the commercial, make the call, and meet up with the personal injury attorney. Of course, lawyers are excellent at screening the good cases from the bad. They know what they can make money with, so the potential plaintiff who walks into their office is either S.O.L. or about to strike pay dirt (at least that is the goal). Yet the person hiring a lawyer to defend them does not pay a single red cent. Whether their lawsuit is deemed frivolous or not, that person should have some skin the game. If they want to file a lawsuit, there should be some cost associated with it that is commensurate with their income. This is my counter argument to those who argue that if poor people could not obtain free representation, they would never have their day in court. There are ways to adjust for that to make it fair. This alone would solve a lot of problems and I am not referring to the economics. I am referring to diminishing the anguish practitioners must endure when we receive that dreaded letter on our desk, often a few years later. The person bringing the claim has almost no downside to do that while the plaintiff attorney must carefully weigh the risks of filing – thank god.

In October 2009, Jackson Healthcare conducted a national survey of physicians that found that defensive medicine was an issue that physicians constantly brought up as a primary cause of increasing healthcare costs. Participants reported that they ordered medically unnecessary diagnostic tests and treatment services to avoid lawsuits. Board-Certified Emergency Room physician Laurent Dreyfuss, concurs:

> "Many of healthcare costs are driven high because there is so much redundancy, meaning a few people consume most of the resources. They tend to be patients who are coping with chronic medical issues such as pain and opiate addiction. Of course, they deserve the utmost in care, but they do a lot of "shopping" from hospital to hospital, which increases healthcare costs.
>
> "E.R. physicians are particularly liable. Because our environment is so litigious, we spend more time ruling out things, rather than using our medical knowledge to prove and diagnose a patient's condition. When people come into the E.R. with a complicated medical history, we get a good hunch that their visit could have an ulterior motive, like a desire for pain

medication. We spend a significant amount of money to appease the patient and ensure that we diagnose and treat their medical problem.

"Physicians in the E.R. are held to a high standard of perfection. Although many patients tend to shop different hospitals, these hospitals do not share medical records. By the time someone sees me in the emergency room, they do not have their most recent studies with them. Since I cannot confirm or review the tests they have already had at the other facilities, I have no choice but to order *more* tests. And they are expensive.

"The patients who consume the most healthcare resources generally do not share the financial burden. For example, with a family of four, I pay $1,800 dollars a month for healthcare insurance. And I am a doctor. I can only imagine how hard it must be for the average family of four to pay for their health insurance coverage. Yet their premiums mostly cover other patients who take advantage of the system.

"Many people use the E.R. as their primary care doctor because an E.R. cannot turn anybody away. Yes, we could say, "This is not an emergency," and refuse to see a patient, but who is going to do that? We cannot turn away a two-year-old with a fever even though they look fine, simply because their parents did not give them Tylenol at three o'clock in the morning. We are going to take care of that child and educate the parents. We will not turn away a 19-year-old pregnant woman who wants us to examine her baby because she has no prenatal care, even though it does not appear to be an emergency. Of course, we will examine that patient and assure her that everything is going to be okay. On the other hand, healthcare consumers who pay their insurance premiums do not run to the emergency room for every little malady. Instead, they make an appointment with their doctor, even if they must wait an extra week to see them.

"Furthermore, insurance companies do not deny tests ordered in the emergency department, the way they sometimes do when a patient receives a referral to a specialist from their primary care doctor. The E.R. physician is obliged to diagnose and treat the patient; the insurance companies do not have time to deny claims from the E.R. by telling us, "Oh, this is the fifth CAT scan this person had this month." For example, if I am dealing with a patient who has a history of heart disease, I need to figure out if she is having a real or perceived problem, and I can only do that by ordering the appropriate tests. At that point, it is hard for the insurance company to say 'no.' I do not encounter resistance or blowback from insurance companies in terms of authorizing tests; however, ordering multiple tests adds to the ever-increasing cost of healthcare."

According to PolicyMed.com, a 2018 study conducted by authors from Harvard University and the University of Melbourne estimated that defensive medicine is costing America $45.6 billion annually (in 2008 dollars), accounting for more than 80 percent of the $55.6 billion total yearly cost of the medical liability system. And this number did not "attempt to estimate social costs or benefits of the malpractice system, such as damage to physicians' reputations or any deterrent effect it may provide."

Michelle Mello, one of the study authors and a professor of law and public health at the Harvard School of Public Health, explains that the study includes estimates of defensive medicine costs both for hospitals ($38.8 billion) and for physicians ($6.8 billion). These estimates were calculated by looking at costs in high- and low-liability environments, and the authors reasoned "that the difference represents spending due to fear of being sued — i.e. defensive medicine."

As I mentioned earlier, many years ago I was involved in the effort to achieve tort reform in Florida. At one point, I had the District 2 seat on the Dade County Medical Association, the kind of organized medicine that protects our profession and ultimately, patients. To be honest, I did not enjoy it because I often found that we were not often effective and had little support from area colleagues. However, I learned a lot. Our crowning achievement was the passage of the Florida Medical Liability Compensation Amendment, also known as Amendment 3, in 2004, which limited the amount of the payouts a jury could award a plaintiff for pain and suffering.

Unfortunately, since the amendment expired in 2017, the lawsuits have been flying. Dr. Dreyfuss notes,

"Everybody wants to see if they can make their quick million. I did not get sued for 17 years. In my seventeenth year I got sued, ironically after tort reform expired. It is a money grab. Somebody must pay. The problem for E.R. physicians is that we carry expensive malpractice policies, compared to other physicians who might carry a lot less liability. As the E.R. doc, you have the deepest pockets next to the hospital, so you always get thrown in.

"Then, these attorneys think, 'Alright, that is just the cherry on top. We can hit him for 10 percent. He is not really the primary, but he must pay for something.' They all agree among themselves that the physicians must pay. This is how they speak about our lives, our licenses, and our pride about everything we put into our profession. 'He didn't make the main mistake; he gets 10 percent or 30 percent.' This is how they talk.

"The public regards doctors with little pity. In their eyes, we are the ones making the money. We drive nice cars, send our kids to private school, and live in beautiful homes. Yes, we do well; I take no issue with that. At the same time, the public sees no problem with rock/pop stars like Taylor Swift, athletes like LeBron James, and various entertainers – whether it's music or sports or celebrity chefs – making millions and millions of dollars, driving luxury cars, and living in expensive mansions."

We will talk more about public perceptions of doctors in the next chapter.

"GOING BARE" IN THE SUNSHINE STATE

In the last few years, I have been shielded from malpractice lawsuits because my practice is mostly comprised of workers' comp patients. When they suffer an injury, they sue the employer, not the treating doctor. By contrast, my international patients come in with a mindset of "I just want to get better." Most of them do well and even if they do not have the perfect outcome, they are not looking to sue. They realize nothing in medicine comes with a 100-percent guarantee. You can go to the best oncologist in the world, but still die of pancreatic cancer, along with many other people who are battling that insidious disease. It does not mean that their doctor committed malpractice and deserves to be sued.

Due to the threat of lawsuits, I stopped taking hand calls. There was a time when I used to cover emergencies. The E.R. would wake me up to tell me they were sending a patient to my office with a little metacarpal fracture after getting into a fight in a bar. That is a routine injury, one they could just send to me for follow-up. Well, no, now the E.R. and everyone involved is covering their ass so much that they must call and wake me up simply to tell me they are referring this patient. Please understand, I do not mind being awakened in the middle of the night for severe injuries. But they started calling me about nonsense that did not require my skills – certainly not at that time. Little by little, I began to pull back from some of the hand calls, but the final straw for me involved the tragic case of a profoundly retarded, epileptic, 60-something year old man. He lived with his sister, who brought him to the E.R. at Hialeah Hospital one night, where my colleague Dr. Jose Lamas, General and Vascular Surgeon, was Chairman of Surgery.

While the patient came in for routine abdominal pain, he also suffered from a seizure disorder. His attending nurse put an IV into his hand and infused Dilantin, an anti-convulsant. Well, it extravasated. The vein popped and the IV catheter released a gush of this toxic chemical into the dorsum of his hand. It is well accepted that this class of drugs should be infused by a large bore IV into a major vein, such as antecubital area, not the dorsum of the hand with its tiny, fragile veins. They called me *three days* later and at that point, there was nothing I could do. I told them I might eventually do a skin graft, but we now must await "demarcation" and see how it goes. It turned out they had called another hand guy who did not want to come in. I was covering for my hand group and they tried to make it seem as if I had to come in, even though I could not have done anything. I remember the plaintiff's lawyer, a young pretty gal looking right out of law school, described me as "cavalier" when reciting the medical record. While a romantic notion, I do not think any colleagues or staff would EVER describe me with that term. Other choice words… perhaps. But not cavalier.

This patient's sister sued the hospital, the E.R. doctor, the vascular surgeon, neurologist, everybody. Some of these people, including Dr. Lamas, did not even have malpractice insurance because in Florida, many of us "go bare" (which is not an option for other doctors in states like Pennsylvania). Everyone who was sued had to pay a lawyer to defend them, whether from their own pocket, or via their malpractice insurance company which likely increased the following year's premiums. After a year and a half, the hospital finally settled for about $400,000. Why didn't they settle beforehand and protect their doctors? Nobody has ever explained this to me or the physicians who do *their* work for them.

Instead, they put me (and others) through this mill. I met with the lawyer more times than I can count to go over this B.S. of something I did not do wrong, while the hospital left us to twist in the wind. Guess what happened? I stopped taking calls at the hospital. This hostile climate of malpractice made me, a guy who did whatever he needed to do for any patient, stop taking E.R. calls over six years ago. None. Now the community does not have the benefit of someone with experience because the system itself made me realize, "Hey, I'm not Mother Teresa here. Why am I doing this if they're going to screw me?"

Dr. Lamas recalls,

"This case created tremendous pain and suffering for me. I am BARE and do not have malpractice insurance. At $153,000 per year for a 250/750 policy, it was not affordable – and I am talking about 15 years ago. With that type of policy, my lawyer's fees come off the 250, so the longer the case takes, the less money available to settle, which is what the lawyers want because it is easy money. The hard work is taking a case to trial, where they stand a high chance of losing. This is a multi-million-dollar business that is abusive to both patients and doctors. The medical malpractice system needs fixing, but the big organizations that are supposed to protect and defend us do not – they continue to delay the monumental task of reform.

"With respect to the case of the retarded, epileptic patient, none of us ordered a Dilantin peripheral IV infusion that infiltrated into the subcutaneous tissues of the hand, causing what is known as Purple Glove Syndrome secondary to tissue ischemic necrosis. There was nothing to do except conservative management and allow demarcation for amputation. I even ordered a vascular arterial doppler study that demonstrated unobstructed flow to the hand. Eventually, I was dismissed but I paid the price of lawyers' fees to defend myself and endured the daily torture of pain, suffering, and agony until it was over. The reason why lawyers now get as many doctors and institutions early in the case is to make sure they do not end up with the Fabre "empty chair" defense. Named for the 1993 Florida case Fabre v. Marin, the empty chair defense seeks to apportion blame to someone who is not a party to the litigation. Or, to put it another way, the defendant is either not brought to the case or let go early after the process of discovery, thereby rendering the plaintiff and their attorney unable to collect. Lawyers I know tell me not to get mad at them because if not for prostitute doctors who sign affidavits stating that there was substandard care in exchange for money, they would not be able to bring a case to litigation.

"It is my firm conviction that healthcare delivery is not any better nowadays. E.M.R. robs a doctor's time from the bedside care of the patient, but lawyers and insurance companies love it because it allows them to pinpoint notes, dates, and times from healthcare professionals, with no penmanship issues. Speaking of healthcare professionals, years ago the doctor and the nurse team assumed full responsibility for the patient. Now there is fragmentation into PCP (primary care physician), hospitalist, intensivist, ARNP (advanced registered nurse practitioner), PA (physician's assistant), AA (anesthesiologist's assistant)...all with different levels of training and experience that cut both ways in the care of the patient in the new millennial practice of medicine. To protect against litigation, doctors order many studies with little touching of the patient in a practice we used to call a physical exam. I guess in the future, advances in technology and artificial intelligence may diagnose a medical condition for a patient, but as surgeons we are safe today since our knowledge and ability in the operating room has no substitution."

As Dr. Lamas notes, the lawsuit was ridiculous for everyone involved. I did not put the IV in. The hospital did not call me right away. I contacted one of my friends at the Indiana Hand Center who wrote one the few articles about Dilantin toxicity to tell him they were suing me and six other doctors. I am grateful for his testimony, but it cost me money. Thank goodness I am active in academia, otherwise I might not personally know him and get him to stick his neck out this way. We had to endure unnecessary stress over a protracted period because the hospital refused to settle right away over what was clearly a medical error, a nursing error in fact. They did not have their doctors' backs. And that same scenario is happening all over the country, not just in Florida or Miami-Dade County.

Thanks to our litigious society and medical malpractice, there was a time when no neurosurgeon was taking any E.R. call in Palm Beach County. If somebody had a head injury and they needed burr holes, there was no brain surgeon to take acute emergency room calls for fear of being sued. They had to be transferred to another institution in a neighboring county. Think about this for just one minute. Furthermore, why was the Palm Beach Post not sounding the alarm? It is amazing what we prioritize in terms of information to the clueless public.

At the beginning of this book, I included the Hippocratic Oath. *Why?* To emphasize that most physicians abide by a centuries-old code of ethics. We want to do the right thing and to the best of my knowledge, few professions other than first responders (who also deal with life and death) take one. A lawyer, for example, could never uphold a similar oath in their profession. In general, every time there's litigation, somebody is in the right and somebody' is in the wrong. Even in a high-profile murder case involving a famous athlete or actor, either the prosecutor is full of shit and hiding exculpatory evidence that would prove their innocence, or the defense lawyer is hiding things that might show their client is guilty. For lawyers, the point is to win the case, regardless of the truth or justice. And in medicine, that perspective does not exist. I cannot think of a single scenario where you would bury the evidence and lab tests of a certain X-ray. The worst that you might do is not tell the patient they have a malignancy, like in the old days when that was common practice at the distraught family's urging. Even now that rarely occurs.

Despite the long hours and the integrity of most physicians, we work and live under the constant threat of lawsuits. I do not think about it much anymore because I put myself in a strategic position where it is highly unlikely to happen. A lot of physicians still worry about malpractice suits, but my practice has evolved to the point where my main goal is to serve international patients and work related injuries which transfer that risk to the employers, which is almost as unfair, unless of course the work environment is devoid of safety measures. Consequently, I do not have to worry as much about the "liability lottery" issue. My international patients do not have an agenda. In other words, nobody is flying over here to get their problem fixed if they are upset with their employer or they have a chip on their shoulder about something. However, for many of my colleagues, practicing medicine under the relentless threat of legal action is a reality they face every day with every patient. Read their stories for a new perspective and understanding of the scourge of malpractice on physicians, patients, communities, and the skyrocketing costs of healthcare.

A LANDMARK MALPRACTICE "CASE" FOR A
PHILLY GENERAL AND VASCULAR SURGEON, 1979

Dr. A.J. Di Giovanni recalls,

"It was the second patient that had brought a lawsuit against me. The man had fallen 30 feet from the top of a scaffold in a junkyard where he had tried to fix a steam shovel. He landed on concrete instead of metal; otherwise, he probably would have died from the fall, his body severed from the metal scraps below. When he arrived at the hospital, he was admitted on someone else's service. However, because of my expertise in trauma, the chief of surgery asked me to take care of him.

"This man had chest problems: multiple rib fractures and segmental rib fractures and fractures of both upper and lower extremities. Furthermore, he had blood coming out of his urine and a small amount of blood on each side of the chest.

"When I first saw him, I did not have to put him on a respirator because he was able to ventilate. But I advised the resident who was watching over him that if the patient had any change in the character of his vital signs, or breathing difficulties, to give him the heparin that was set aside for him in the event of a pulmonary embolism. Due to the multiple sites of trauma and blood in his chest and in his urine, I did not want to give him heparin right away because it would have augmented those issues. When he developed signs of a pulmonary embolism, I instructed the resident to give him heparin – a decision I made between a rock and a hard place. Sadly, the patient died.

"A lawsuit was brought against me, which led to a trial of great proportions. A witness testified against me who campaigned as an 'expert' in trauma surgery – a claim that my defense counsel Jim Griffith exploited. A magnificent lawyer, he dismantled the testimony given by witnesses, especially this alleged trauma expert, who had no surgical experience at all. On the stand, he admitted that the only thing he did was assisted surgery for six months; he had never been trained as a surgeon and had never done surgery of his own.

"In all, it took eight full days of testimony. It was a landmark case in medical malpractice and set a standard from that point forward that the expert witness must have surgical experience. We won the case – which was awarded in 20 minutes – on the basis that the testimony the so-called expert witness offered was inappropriate and that what I had done was correct. I met the standards of the medical community.

"But it was an emotional and difficult problem, not only for me but for my wife and children. Seeing them distraught over what was being done to their husband and father added another layer of anguish. I did not want them to feel as if they had to suffer and did my best to put on a brave face. I wanted to minimize their pain as much as possible.

"From the beginning Jim Griffith advised me that he could outline the legal process, but if I wanted to win that case, I had to do it on my own. He told me that I had to be an actor, not in the Hollywood sense, but an actor who could portray a positive image to people on a jury who had no medical experience, so that they could believe I was sincere, capable, and well-trained. If I did that, I would win. If I did not, I would lose. I admire Jim for the kind of support he gave me as my legal representative.

"As I moved forward in my career, I never knew the attitudes and motivations of patients. Would they sue me? Some of the nicest people seem to be the ones that want to victimize you with a malpractice suit. I had a couple of other suits against me which we won without difficulty because they were based on poor evidence and dubious expertise. I had a respectable and honorable surgical career and met the standards I was supposed to meet in a professional way."

"The first thing we do, let's kill all the lawyers."
~ William Shakespeare

Dr. ROGER KHOURI ON THE SORRY STATE OF MEDICINE

"The crisis in medicine is due to multiple factors. In his play Henry VI, William Shakespeare famously wrote, "The first thing we do, let's kill all the lawyers." And he did not even know *our* lawyers! If Shakespeare were alive today to see our lawyers, my God he would be upset.

"The one thing I blame our past president for is the Affordable Care Act, otherwise known as "Obamacare." Although I believe it was well intentioned, in his multi-thousand-page report, there was not a single line about probably the most expensive item that increases medical costs more than anything else: frivolous suits and malpractice. There are two bad aspects. One is the parasitic industry of the malpractice lawyers and the malpractice insurance companies. They play good cop, bad cop. It is a huge, multi-billion-dollar industry. Anybody can sue anybody. It is like going to court with a loaded gun and playing roulette because even if you have the tightest case, the best case in the world, you still have a 20 percent chance of losing.

"Lawyers know that, and they willingly play. They know that they may not win, but they hope most cases settle for at least $100,000 to $200,000. And it is easy. It takes a few days, they are in court for a few minutes, and they make some money. If you look at all the fancy offices in those beautiful skyscrapers in downtown Miami, they are all lawyers' offices. Doctors cannot afford an office there. That is one aspect of tort reform that should be addressed. Make it like the rest of the civilized world, where a jury of your peers determines if there is malpractice. In the United States legal system, I am not judged by my peers. As a matter of fact, if any of my peers are in a jury pool, they are pulled out because the last thing lawyers want is a doctor or nurse on the jury. Therefore, even though the United States Constitution upholds my right to a jury of my peers, I do not get that. Yet, my medical peers could determine if it is something (malpractice) or nothing (meaning, I met the standards of the medical community).

"In the rest of the civilized world, malpractice suits are rare, because any perceived potential of malpractice is brought to the Board of Medicine or whatever governmental institution is part of the justice system. The members are chosen by the judicial system, the Board of Medicine, the legislature, or the governor to review and judge cases – they do not have a bunch of paid *prostitutes* come to court to say you did something wrong so they can cash in.

"That is right. You can always find a – forgive my word – *whore* doctor. I hate to call them that, but that is what they are. Even if they have been stripped of their title, if they once practiced as an M.D. they qualify as a professional, expert witness. And for thousands of dollars, they will say anything to convince a jury that you have done something wrong. Some of them are fantastic actors who can play the game well and convince an uneducated jury. That is one major aspect of malpractice and the tort reform.

"The other big factor is the defensive medicine doctors play. If you go to an emergency room, you are going to get a thousand remote tests that have nothing to do with what might be wrong with you, but they're ordering them just to cover their ass. Even if there is a one in one- thousand chance that the patient may have a certain problem, would you, the physician, take the risk of not ordering that test? Because you stand to lose your livelihood and your home – *yes, they can take your home* – and everything you have if you miss that diagnosis. I would not take that risk; I would order the tests. And to go along with that, hospitals hire physicians precisely for that reason. They pay these physicians a decent salary, much more money than they are worth, because they know they are going to order all these tests to be performed in the hospital, and these tests will be covered by insurance. What happens? Insurance costs escalate.

"Not too long ago, one of my patients who had surgery with me a few weeks before, went to the emergency room for abdominal pain. After spending just 23 hours in the hospital, his bill was $320,000! *$320,000*. There is not a test in the book they did not do. He had three scans, all the lab tests possible, all the things back and forth – and it cost $320,000 for less than a 24-hour stay. In the end, he was discharged with simple gastroenteritis. Throughout this whole admission, not a single doctor touched his abdomen or examined him.

"Hospitalists often tend to be second-rate physicians who could not make it in the real world, so they work full time for the hospital. Their only role is to order tests. You do not miss anything if you order 500 tests, right?

"Whereas, if you are a good clinician, you examine the patient, touch their abdomen, talk to them, feel what's going on, and you probably would not need any tests to make a gastroenteritis diagnosis. The whole process costs maybe $200 instead of $320,000. The hospitals love defensive medicine because the insurance companies pay for the tests the doctor orders. I refer to it as "second-rate medicine" because you do not have the best doctors working for the hospitals.

"Furthermore, hospitals have now become giants invading the entire city with tentacles all over the place – E.R.'s, urgent care, etc. They capture everything, then they dictate the rules and the cost. They put themselves at the best places in town, with hospitalists working on their payroll ordering tests that must be reimbursed by insurance. **Insurance reimburses those tests because by law, if you order them within 24 hours, you do not have to get authorization.**

"Think about this: I pay $60,000 a year for malpractice insurance. Now a busy surgeon would have done 600 operations a year. That means the first $100 of every operation I do goes toward my malpractice. My bread-and-butter operation, my most common operation as a hand surgeon is carpal tunnel release. When Medicare gives me $300 for this operation, the first $100 goes right back to the lawyers and the insurance companies.

"Recently I had to go to court for case with a history that makes me sick. Thirteen years ago, the eight-year-old patient was left alone to play with the sprocket of a Moped, which completely chewed up his thumb. He showed up at the emergency room, where I saved his thumb by doing a flap and cover, instead of rongeuring the bone and thereby shortening it, then closing the wound. He had an exposed, fractured bone and I saved his growth plate. For some reason, his family had been told that in America, you can make money with malpractice. So, they went to see one of those whore doctors who sent them to a lawyer. Fortunately, the first lawyer realized there was nothing to the case and turned it down.

"Undeterred, the family consulted with another lawyer, who declined the case after doing a little exploration. Next, the family found a *third* lawyer, one of the bottom-dwellers, who took it on, believing it would result in a big pay day for him. Then, they found an opportunistic surgeon who agreed to be their 'expert' witness. We estimate that this surgeon made anywhere from $60,000 to $100,000 on that deal. For over a decade, my malpractice insurance has spent more than $350,000 defending this case. When we went to trial, I lost two weeks of my practice, and I still had to pay my employees, my mortgage, my insurance, my overhead...everything. My staff sat idle during that time because I could not do anything. I was in court every day. It was fortunate that the jury ruled in my favor. The plaintiff's lawyer, hoping he would win the lottery, asked the jury for four-and-a-half million dollars in compensation. Luckily for me, I had an excellent lawyer and doctor who agreed to be expert witnesses in my favor. Dr. Badia appeared because he had been asked to do an independent evaluation that also went in my favor, and I won the case. But you know, I could have lost, which would have meant I would have paid a few million dollars.

"And I *saved* the kid's thumb. Thanks to my operation, he has one. Yet I am still sued for that. There is no oversight about what you can sue for. All you need is a sellout doctor to say, 'Yes, I'm willing, for $60,000, to come to court and play the roulette.'

"Malpractice is one factor. Defensive medicine is another. All the ramifications of defensive medicine are tremendous, due to the multitude of tests mediocre physicians order to protect themselves. A good physician would know there is no need to order a certain test. For example, E.R. physicians will order an MRI for a fingertip, when you do not need an MRI to diagnose a tendon laceration. But they order MRIs out of ignorance to protect themselves.

"As I said, my biggest beef with Obamacare is that there was not a single line about malpractice or tort reform in the entire legislation. Of course, he was a lawyer protecting his cronies. Lawyers protect lawyers, a problem the brilliant bard Shakespeare recognized five centuries ago. As brilliant and insightful as he was, I do not think even he could have foreseen the avaricious nature of many lawyers today and the havoc they wreak on our healthcare system.

"These are the big frustrations we're facing with healthcare: excess paperwork; defensive medicine; big hospitals controlling everything and hiring less-than-stellar doctors to run up the bills by ordering excessive tests; and the loss of touch and interaction with the patient. And I do not see it getting better. It is getting worse and worse."

Dr. Mark Rekant on Medical Malpractice Insurance Costs & Other Hidden Healthcare Costs

"Number one, the cost of malpractice insurance gets passed along in some way to patients, like every other cost in business. And if my malpractice insurance is $60,000 a year, I think that equates to a fair amount of cost to each patient. The first two months of the year, my practice basically covers malpractice insurance. Do the math. Take the $60,000 and divide it by the number of patients I see each week – which is an average of 200 – times the course of the whole year, it adds up to about 10,000 patients a year. Each one's cost increases by six to 10 dollars.

364 · ALEJANDRO BADIA, M.D., F.A.C.S.

"With a lower malpractice cost, we could offer a discount on every patient's copay, which could be $10 less. I mention this to help people understand how high the costs really are. Then there are the hidden costs associated with all the excess testing that is done because physicians fear poor outcomes and malpractice lawsuits. These tests include M.R.I.'s and X-rays. To put it into perspective, in the United States there are 3,000 hand surgeons. If everyone orders one M.R.I. more than we need, that equals about $3 million a day. Crazy. But that is one major component of out-of-control healthcare costs.

"In my world, I have faced three egregious malpractice lawsuits. First, a patient sued me for causing a stroke he suffered two and a half years *after* the surgery to his wrist and after the statute of limitations expired, without a letter of medical necessity, which is mandatory per state law. And of course, he sued me for something that had nothing to do with his wrist surgery. He was in his late 70s and he had a stroke.

"It obviously did not last long. He did not have an attorney; he did it on his own by filling out a piece of paper, something referred to in the legal Latin term as 'proceeding pro se'. Still it cost me about a month of my energy, not to mention the cost of paying for an attorney, along with my malpractice insurance rates, etc. for a frivolous lawsuit. I think any reader would be shocked that a physician can get sued for something that happens two and a half years after the fact and is completely unrelated to the surgical procedure.

"The second lawsuit involved a patient who claimed that I didn't appreciate that he ended up with a post-operative infection snag. He failed to mention that he did not come to my office for post-operative evaluation. And I think it is extremely difficult for a physician to diagnose a problem when the patient does not come to the office. Well, that case ultimately went on for settlement agreement because a hospital was involved. And the way the system is set up, for me to fight that case would have been too expensive. The lawyers told me I was going to have to sit in court for perhaps three or four weeks, which means time not working and getting paid, not to mention the frustration of sitting in court doing nothing. This is not productive. On advice of counsel, I was told to settle without admitting defeat and without admitting fault. I just paid the guy off, in effect, so I would not have to spend all day in the courtroom while the lawyers make money because that is the way the system is set up. I did not really lose any money because it came from the insurance company, whereas if I had taken time out of my practice to fight a frivolous lawsuit, the money would have come out of my pocket.

"And then the third case, which still puzzles me to this day, was a fantastic surgery I performed. It went so well that my hand fellow and ortho resident took pictures. The patient claimed that I did not have consent to do a portion of the procedure. And the judge, after seeing the pictures, indicated that I did not need consent to do this portion of the procedure because it was implied and *yet the litigation was NOT immediately thrown out.* To this day, I still do not understand why. But the message that I have gotten from the attorneys on both sides is that our society is lenient towards giving people their day in court, so to speak.

"In yet another frivolous case, one of my partners was sued for failure to diagnose and treat properly for a condition that is treated without surgery, by a patient who did not get better when they had surgery at an outside institution. Although the medical literature supports non-operative management for this specific condition, the patient found a surgeon to operate for reasons that astound both my partner and me. Of course, the patient did not improve after having surgery for something that did not require surgery. Yet he still sued one of my partners. As you would expect, the case was ultimately dismissed."

The cases we have discussed should shock, or even offend you. How can some of them even be accepted within "the system?" Obviously, the system is flawed, although not completely broken. The reason I say that is there is a mechanism to bring a hopefully legitimate and well-founded grievance, to seek recourse in a court of law in the United States. The goal should not only be to compensate that patient for harm suffered, and the attorney working to represent them, but to also institute changes that can minimize it from happening again. I have always felt the latter should be a major aim of the medical malpractice arrangement. Much like product liability, it does not seem to achieve the latter goal. It ends up being too much about the money which is a pity. I mentioned the McDonald's coffee case because it turns out that the powerful restaurant franchise never did lower the temperature of its coffee, which continues to be served at about 180 degrees Fahrenheit, nearly 30 degrees hotter than needed.

I recall a case where the wife of prominent cardiologist was killed when a boat ferry struck their small boat, reportedly because the doctor did not clearly see the approaching ferry due to poor navigation lights until it was too late. I am an avid boater in Miami. The lighting has not changed from what I can tell, and I am profoundly nervous whenever I navigate in that section of the cut at night. Was the litigation not about seeking to remedy a clear problem? Whether about hot coffee or poor illumination for safety, we should not be focusing solely on the money. Perhaps I am naïve.

Medical malpractice should be about protecting patients and having a set of controls to ensure the practitioners are qualified and not practicing medicine far outside the medical standards. Even the latter can be construed in many ways and therefore, we should have an objective tribunal system of specialty specific medical experts to screen cases before they clog up our already overburdened court systems. Should this not be the role of our medical societies amongst other charges?

The case of Dr. Christopher Duntsch, aka Dr. Death, brings a chill to our spine, pun intended, and points out the occasional holes in our system. Our malpractice system SHOULD have stopped Dr. Duntsch from maiming, or even killing, the number of people that he did. Furthermore, our hospital review boards, and state societies should intervene soon after even the first lawsuit was brought forward.

Chris Duntsch, a recently trained neurosurgeon, began to perform surgery in Dallas at Baylor Plano hospital in 2010, before moving to several other hospitals within a short time. Within two years he had only operated on 37 spines yet had maimed 33 of them, including two deaths. How could this happen?

A series of precautions and administrative hurdles are designed to ensure that patients are not harmed by doctors, beginning at the department, hospital, county, and state level. There is even a National Practitioner Data Bank in place, but consumer studies have shown nearly half of U.S. hospitals have never reported a physician to this entity. The unbelievable case of Dr. Death demonstrates how these checks and balances can fail, even in the most heinous of cases.

Multiple physicians, and obviously Duntsch's own patients, made every attempt to get hospitals to fire him, and later for the state to pull his medical license. These people, along with the attorneys from both sides of the criminal case brought against Duntsch, felt his extreme case would alter how the system polices its own.

Hospitals administrators told Duntsch he would no longer operate at Dallas Medical Center. But, as had happened at Baylor-Plano, Duntsch was permitted to resign and the hospital did not notify the National Practitioner Data

Bank (NPDB). Amazingly, they are under no obligation to report the incompetent doctor since he technically resigned. The healthcare systems are also afraid of litigation since a report could lead to a lawsuit from the beleaguered physician. See, even the hospitals are afraid of our legal system, and consequently, patients are harmed.

The Texas neurosurgeon case is so egregious, so unbelievable that there is a widely viewed podcast on the story, and an upcoming Hollywood film. Dr. Death is currently serving a life sentence for the intentional maiming of one of his last patients, not even for the two deaths that he caused. He is not eligible for parole until 2045. It is one of the only cases where a doctor has been sentenced to jail for intentional harm committed during a surgical procedure. The challenge for the prosecutors is that there was no precedent.

How does our system fail our patients in this manner? I mentioned how fear of litigation can have the opposite effect of what the malpractice code is supposed to do: protect patients. A patient should be able to bring a justifiable action against a clinician when they clearly fall outside the standard of care, and the healthcare system, and even colleagues, should be able to report that person BEFORE they harm somebody, leading to a suit. It seems the money is the priority. On both sides.

I recall two incidents where I was in early stage of my career and witnessed two elbow operations, one that I was assisting in, another that I observed, with the clear conviction that the surgeon had no place handling that case.

The first was at a community hospital in Queens, New York. As orthopedic residents at NYU, we had the opportunity to moonlight in night shifts where we covered the orthopedic service, including any emergency room admissions. It was a sweet deal for the attending surgeons who didn't have to run in to reduce or splint every fracture, could have us take care of any inpatients on the ortho ward, and even assist them in surgery for add-on cases. I considered it a better deal for us as I could make some money doing what I liked and receive further training at reasonable compensation. I remember thinking, "Why is this ankle sprain or wrist fracture sitting in a hospital emergency room for hours and hours?" It was the first inkling of an OrthoNOW® concept.

One night I admitted a complex intra-articular (into joint) elbow fracture in an elderly female. These intra-condylar distal humerus fractures are relatively common in busy emergency rooms with a high volume of older patients; however, they are complex injuries. I already had interest in the upper limb and recall assisting one of the general orthopedists with the case, late at night.

I recall sweating as he "dug around" the ulnar nerve, what laypeople term the funny bone of the elbow. It is a highly sensitive nerve and he was certainly not dissecting it free with the precise care of a hand or peripheral nerve surgeon. What was I to do? I could push him out of the way, take over, and tell him I had done a bunch of these at Bellevue, or perhaps call in my mentor, Dr. Lamont. I was to do neither. I was a peon resident assisting an attending surgeon who was simply terrible at complex elbow pathology, which was nothing surprising. If there was an anonymous reporting board, it would have been ideal. Once that system receives several complaints about same surgeon, they could investigate. Call me an idealist. I do not consider myself a whistleblower.

A similar case occurred in my first few months in Miami, in private practice, but still wet behind the ears. I was waiting for a gunshot wound of the hand to be prepared for me in one O.R. and I decided to stroll around the O.R. and meet some of the other surgeons. After all, I was "the new kid in town." I sauntered into a room adjacent to me where the surgeon was clearly operating on an elbow. I thought "Perfect, this is my gig." I introduced myself to the much older surgeon, elderly in fact, and noted his patient had a huge muscular arm. On closer inspection, he was evidently a young, African American male, perhaps an athlete of some type with a simply humongous tricep muscle. I noticed the surgeon was preparing to pass some wires, percutaneously (through skin), to address the fracture. I then made the mistake of looking at the X-ray board and my heart sank. The young man had a complex articular elbow fracture, a similar pattern to the old lady's that I had seen in New York. However, this was a much different clinical setting. The anesthesiologist must have noticed my puzzled expression because he gave me that shrug of helpless resignation, likely familiar with the surgeon's work. I said something like, "Hey, Dr. X, tough fracture, huh? I kinda like to open these, do an olecranon osteotomy, put 90-90 recon plates on the fracture and move 'em early. What are ya thinking of doing?" I tried to play it low key and not sound too authoritative. Certainly, I had to right to be, but I KNEW how to handle that case. He responded, "Nah. I am just going to get the best reduction I can and shoot some big K-wires in there as it will turn into a mess if I open this. He's a young, strong guy and should heal fine". *Nothing could be farther from the truth,* I thought. *What to do?* I had just arrived in a new city. How would they react to an arrogant upstart making waves at their hospital? A hospital I had never even been in. I still often wonder how that kid did.

You can see how things can be sticky. I do not have a solution for this, but the case of Dr. Death is indeed egregious. We should have an online system where questionable care can be reported anonymously, prompting more thorough investigation. Yes, that can certainly lead to abuse, particularly among the more jealous of colleagues, or those with an axe to grind, but something must be done.

The legal system has a responsibility to keep society in line. Whether doctors, therapists, hospitals, or other attorneys, we must have a system of recourse to ensure any sector of society is behaving appropriately. I cannot think of anything more important than ensuring safe and appropriate medical care.

The current system, however, has providers running scared, expending too many resources with a "cover your ass" approach and even avoiding participation by good clinicians who have become risk adverse. "I only want the easy cases," is a logical reaction. I have not been that jaded and enjoy addressing the most challenging pathology, even with a revision case treated elsewhere. However, I will not put myself out there any longer with the catch-all hospitals and I am also careful not to disparage a colleague since the "You had to be there" mentality is often true. One cannot second guess a fellow professional with sound training and reputation. However, policing each other remains a challenge to be addressed. Like in Texas.

I have been fortunate to only have two cases brought against me in my quarter century of practice and I related one earlier in the chapter. That was an absurd odyssey where multiple doctors were dragged into a mess that was innocently set in motion by one hapless nurse. The other involves one of the most common adult fractures, the metacarpal of the hand. Many occur during drunken bouts or angry fits where the wall usually wins, but nevertheless, they usually do quite well with either closed or operative treatment when indicated.

My patient came to me, nearly 20 years ago now, with a displaced, shortened ring finger metacarpal fracture. Apparently to my demise, I explained that there was a newer method of metacarpal fixation, intramedullary, which my partners and I had devised and begun to popularize. The procedure is not difficult for either patient or surgeon, is minimally invasive with barely a stitch, and a newer instrumentation was used that would further simplify it. Great. *Wrong.* Anything that the attorney could deem "experimental" was simply another notch in their belt against me. The fracture had collapsed a bit over the nail, leading to minor shortening that was barely perceptible in examining his flexed knuckles and certainly there was no functional deficit. I feel he may have stressed the hand prematurely, but no matter, it had no real bearing on his outcome. Well, a slightly shortened bone on X-ray led to the cavalcade of legal steps, meetings, depositions, and processes that would only serve to annoy me for the subsequent 18 months. If he prevailed, what was that worth? Certainly, my time was enough.

"Your honor, my client has this slightly ugly X-ray (here is the problem by the way...) and I think it's worth, um, eh, say 100 Grand!! Deal?? See my point. What was the purpose of all that? Granted the kid did not have his act together and might have fallen off the ladder inebriated, but who cared? It did not prevent him from working; however, the lottery mentality sets in. Shame on the attorney who took his case. Well, he eventually got his as you will see. My friend, a coauthor of a major book in hand fractures, reviewed the case and opined that the case fell WELL within the standard of care. Regardless, he proceeded.

I remember clearly meeting with my attorneys to discuss strategy, as if deciding to kick on the 4th down. I met the "litigator" for the first time. Until then, my defense attorney, hired by my malpractice insurance (enough said), was the only person I had met. While she was very competent and reassuring, she was not the professional who does the talking at trial. I remember shaking his hand, an older, distinguished man with salt and pepper Princeton haircut, who exuded calm and confidence. I said, "*This is my guy...*"

Well, the trial never happened. The female attorney thought the jury would like me "because I was kind of cute," and we had even picked my tie. A sedate red, not a lackluster blue or power yellow. Everything had its strategy, but I would never don the tie...well, not for trial anyway. Reportedly, the plaintiff kid marched into his attorney's office, day before trial, and said, "Ah, I don't really want to go tomorrow. I am not interested in pursuing this anymore". I really wonder how his attorney held himself from breaking his other metacarpal. I guess he too is afraid of his colleagues. Remember why sharks do not attack lawyers? Professional courtesy.

I did not have my day in court, but the damage was done as I had cancelled an entire week of patients, elective surgeries, and other professional activities because I was to sit in a courtroom...over a metacarpal fracture. *Your honor, I am sorry I used an innovative, minimally invasive technique on the plaintiff. My bad.* Not quite, "Dr. Barnard, why did you do this heart transplant on your victim patient with the crap heart? You do realize this has never been done before. Shame on you." I think I made my point. At that time, I truly wish the trial had proceeded. I often see life as a collection of positive and adverse experiences; it certainly would have been surreal, if not comical. At least I can *still* say I have never been the defendant surgeon in a malpractice trial. Lucky, I guess....

Fear of malpractice or litigation of any kind, stifles innovative and efficient care while driving up costs. There is no recourse for the victim, ***the doctors***, since they (Khouri, Rekant, Lamas, me, etc.) could not earn a single penny while they were confined to those four wooden paneled walls. Worse, there are a multitude of patients who could not receive the care we are trained for. I think of the elbow fractures I have discussed, which I know without a doubt that I could have done a better job than some of my colleagues, while others are much better than me at other clinical challenges. If we are confined to a courtroom, a different kind of trench, the human consequence will never be fully known.

Dr. Robert Terrill

"I remember a lawsuit from about seven years ago when I was on call. And there was nothing I could do because the problems predated me. They sort of called me in at the 11th hour and they sued everybody in the world. And it has been going on for seven years. I'm thinking, 'What the hell is this? I mean there is nothing to this case. For example, if you cut the wrong 'X,' there is no argument. If somebody had a heart attack after surgery, while I do not view that as a complication of a procedure, you could make an argument. However, in this case there was absolutely nothing. It has been incredibly frustrating for me because I am sitting here wondering what is going on. We did the deposition two years ago and I have not heard anything.

"One of our experts, a prominent hand surgeon, reviewed it and told me, 'I have never even heard of this. I do not think there is anything you could have done. That made me feel better. However, you are simply left up in the air because any time you are on call it could happen. That is why doctors are saying, 'Screw this.' A hand surgery colleague in L.A. said, 'You know it's gonna happen every 10 years.' That is wrong. If something has been done incorrectly, that is another issue entirely. For example, I took care of two patients after another doctor missed something and I got stuff cleaned up. It is like a fact witness. In both cases, it probably was malpractice: they missed a significant injury, and it resulted in significant problem. Okay.

"But this other nonsense is too much. One lady sued me, claiming I had 'guaranteed' a perfect result. I thought, 'What are you smoking? No, I did not. No doctor can guarantee anything.' Patients must understand that medicine is not a perfect science."

ANOTHER VOICE FROM THE TRENCHES: A PENNSYLVANIA MEDICAL MALPRACTICE DEFENSE ATTORNEY ON THE TANGIBLE AND INTANGIBLE TOLL OF LITIGATION ON U.S. HEALTHCARE

"Having been fascinated by the practice of medicine from listening to stories from my surgeon father, my intention was to attend medical school and follow in his footsteps. Then my world came to a screeching halt when my dad, a devoted and excellent surgeon, was sued in a frivolous medical malpractice case which literally tore him apart. With a demand of $7 million dollars and insurance coverage of only $1.2 million dollars, the fear of the unknown was overwhelming. Consumed by the anxiety of possibly losing our home and being unable to provide for five children, his self-esteem and worthiness as a husband and father were destroyed. I never saw my father cry until he broke down and sobbed like a baby at the dinner table in front of all of us. As a family we supported him wholeheartedly and told him to stand strong on principle, with all of us by his side.

The injuries caused by a traumatic fall from a scaffold left this man's life hanging in the balance upon arrival to the emergency room. It would take a miracle to save his life and unfortunately his injuries took his life. His wife, while understandably distraught, was looking for someone to blame. As a high school student, I attended the trial in Philadelphia every day and watched the so-called justice system at work. At that point I had a revelation. I wanted to aspire to be the type of attorney who represented my father: smart, articulate, compassionate, and determined that the truth be told by my father. For me, this trial was a life-changing event. In this career path I got the best of both worlds. I could learn medicine and at the same time, defend physicians. And so, my career began.

I have now been defending doctors, hospitals, and nurses for over 35 years. It has been the most rewarding experience of my life. Every day, I can look myself in the mirror and know that I can live with my conscience. Daily, these heroes deal with life and death issues unlike any other profession. What the public fails to understand is that they took an oath to do no harm and go to work every day trying to do their best. There are two important facts the public chooses to ignore or simply fails to acknow-ledge: first, these people are human and secondly, medicine is not an exact science. However, people expect a perfect result every time and although the providers do the best that they can, every procedure carries risks and sometimes the patient is the reason for the outcome.

Patients need to take responsibility for their own actions. The physician-patient relationship is a two-way street. When a doctor makes a recom-mendation, that patient with autonomy over their body, has the right to accept or reject it. However, when they choose to reject it, that is their decision. Yet all too often in medical malpractice cases, patients who defy medical advice and get an unwanted outcome sue their doctors. Such be-havior is not only unfair but increases the cost of healthcare. The amount of money that it takes to defend a single case is significant: the medical malpractice insurer hires the law firm and the longer the case goes on, the more expensive it is. That does not account for all the time, money, and patient care the physician loses when defending themself against often frivolous lawsuits.

Then there is the intangible cost which many do not see but I witnessed at a young age. A medical malpractice suit weighs on the physician's con-science, causes disruption to what they were trained to do, and is a source of much anxiety and stress. In Pennsylvania, fortunately through tort re-form, starting with the Healthcare Malpractice Services Act in 1979, later superseded by the MCare Act of 2002, plaintiffs' lawyers must first file a Certificate of Merit from a qualified expert to support their case within 60 days of filing their Complaint. Long gone are the days of simply filing the lawsuit, trying to extort money, and never really having a qualified expert to testify. MCare requires on standard of care that the expert must be in the same medical specialty as the defendant physician (for which there is one exception if they have received training in a similar medical field such that they would be knowledgeable of the standard of care). This has resulted in a significant decrease in the number of malpractice cases filed."

SECTION III

OPIUM FOR THE MASSES: HOW POLITICS, POP CULTURE AND THE MEDIA CONTRIBUTE TO PROBLEMS IN U.S. HEALTHCARE

Chapter 12 – Moral Injury and the Future of Medicine

"The moral injury of healthcare is not the offense of killing another human being in the context of war. It is being unable to provide high-quality care and healing in the context of healthcare."

Simon G. Talbot, M.D. and Wendy Dean, M.D.

The term "burnout" has become almost a cliché amongst physicians in recent years. When a term has been overused, such as "social distancing" it most often implies there is a pervasive problem that demands our attention. If you do a Google search for "physician burnout," you will get over seven million results.

My search yielded a paid ad at the top of the page from some type of service that "offers proactive resources to reduce burnout in physicians. We are passionate about helping physicians become their best selves." The site encourages you to download a copy of their "Physician & Advanced Practitioner Well Being Solutions Survey Report *now to save yourself the headache and cost of onboarding a new physician.* I am not kidding when I tell you I read the ad three times to ensure I was seeing it right. This organization, which I am sure charges a fee, has taken the initiative to save organizations from us troubled doctors, stressed clinicians, and wayward children.

They warn organizations that any failure to provide preventive or therapeutic solutions can result in the dreaded physician turnover. *Oooooooooooh.* Who are the clients? A cadre of healthcare systems who likely employ lots o' docs. Gee, perhaps *that* is the problem. Funny how this company can afford to be at the top of a search on such a timely issue affecting professionals who are supposed to be well compensated. The subliminal message: get your spoiled medical "providers" help before they commit suicide or worse, lead to you having to spend more money in recruiting and onboarding new doctors. Mind you, the help clinicians need to manage their "burnout" is provided by other clinicians: psychiatrists, psychologists, clinical social workers, and counselors. Who is going to manage their stress then? Others? It reminds me of the blind man and his seeing eye dog from New York City, I discussed in chapter two, who were both run over, resulting in the same handicap for both. In this case, should we get a seeing eye cat for the poor doggie? Marcus Welby, M.D. is probably rolling in his grave.

Now, there is an entire initiative from the AHRQ (Agency for Healthcare Research and Quality), another government agency paid by you, the taxpayer, that is tasked with *"improving the safety and quality of America's health care system."* For the past 20 years, the agency has invested major resources in projects that "examine the effects of working conditions on health care professionals' ability to keep patients safe while providing high-quality care." As the lead federal agency charged with this task, the AHRQ develops the knowledge, tools, and data needed to improve the healthcare system and help Americans, healthcare professionals, and policymakers make informed health decisions. It a noble and necessary cause. The question is, how does this agency achieve its objective of improved healthcare?

This research is part of the agency's ongoing efforts to develop evidence-based information aimed at bettering the quality of the U.S. healthcare system by making care safer for patients and improving working conditions for clinicians. Now patients must be protected from us *stressed out, bad doctors?!?*

How do they define burnout, per the government and the myriad of organizations that somehow feel that the public and for-profit healthcare companies need to be rescued from our foibles and stress reactions?

Let me quote straight from the agency's website: *"The health care environment—with its packed workdays, demanding pace, time pressures, and emotional intensity—can put physicians and other clinicians at high risk for burnout. Burnout is a long-term stress reaction marked by emotional exhaustion, depersonalization, and a lack of sense of personal accomplishment."*

The consensus is that a combination of chaotic environment, family responsibilities, time pressure, the dreaded E.H.R. (electronic health record) and "low control of pace" were the culprits responsible for this so-called physician burnout. I can save our system a tremendous amount of time, money, and mental wrangling: it is the lack of control that leads directly to our compounded frustrations that result in what they have termed "burnout."

What happens when one is frustrated – especially a high-performing, conscientious, and motivated individual? They lose faith in the process and their work and become melancholy, which diminishes the energy they need to perform a task. That is what is happening, and the solution is simple: GET OUT OF OUR WAY and let us care for patients. Whether a physician, nurse, therapist, or technician, we *know* what to do. We simply seek support and collaboration for our required tasks, not obstacles. Can you imagine a neurosurgeon trying to approve, advise, deny, or set guidelines about a forensic accountant's calculations? It is ludicrous. The accountant might fall into depression, and by nature they are not exactly the life of the party as it is. Sorry, guys but stereotypes abound during this discussion.

From a clinical point of view, the term "burnout" has 142 different meanings. As you will see, most of us do not even agree on the word or its implications. We do, however, agree on the cause of the problem – our frustration with a fragmented medical system in which the traditional steward of that system, the physician, is now beholden and subservient to a non-clinician.

An AMA article from 2018 pointed to an excess of bureaucratic tasks as the leading cause, although abusive hours, lack of respect, insufficient reimbursement and excess computerization were high on the list as well. Robert Pearl, M.D., a physician, educator, and healthcare C.E.O., offers a different and more nuanced perspective. In his opinion, the current physician dissatisfaction is due to two major conflicts:

1. The emergence of clinical guidelines that relegate many physicians, chiefly primary care doctors, to practicing cookbook medicine.

2. The intensifying sense of competition that comparative performance reports spur by ranking doctors on their clinical outcomes and data points.

The obsession with outcomes data and performance measurement has further alienated physicians and brought us back to the college days of organic chemistry, where our unhealthy competition started. I am quite convinced that the business and insurance interests in healthcare have spawned this culture and are its prime beneficiaries. One thing is certain, it is not our patients or our own mental health.

These metric issues are most amplified in large, behemoth healthcare settings from which Dr. Pearl hails. It still does not explain the frustration many of us feel from the daily grind of private practice, even in the most independent, idyllic setting that I am fortunate enough to enjoy. I am completely outside any organized healthcare system, have direct access to all the modalities of treatment necessary under one roof, and am even "out of network" with commercial insurance companies. So why would I experience any frustration or so-called burnout?

Lack of full control.

The restaurant analogy hits home for many clinicians who read it, with irritated nods intermixed with chuckles (although less laughter). As you read the piece, you feel for the restauranteur. The hoops they must jump through, the hurdles they must leap, as well as the struggle to even cover their costs to make a profit in a vital business: feeding their customers. Imagine the same experience every day, in the art and practice of medicine.

Due to this lack of control in the profession, most physicians do not even encourage their children to follow in their footsteps any longer as compared to some decades ago.

Recent studies have shown that nearly 90 percent of physicians are unwilling to recommend medicine as a profession.

Dr. Roger Khouri agrees. "I have five kids. Two of them are in medicine, and I can tell you they are the two most miserable and hardworking compared to the others, who are in business, law, and engineering. Three of my kids are enjoying their lives and traveling all the time. Compare that to my doctor daughter, who cannot even come to her brother's wedding because she is on call. These guys and girls make a tremendous sacrifice to get to where they are and yet the public looks upon them as people who should not make money. That is fine. Most of us did not go into medicine to make money; otherwise we would be doing something else. This is not a profession where you make money, but if you happen to make a lot of money, you are looked upon as a crook."

Tragic. In my case, up until only a few years ago I did not feel that way. At one point my daughter seemed to show interest in medicine, but she is entering the tumultuous teen years. My son, who is slightly younger, now says he wants to be a scientist *and* an engineer. When you get right down to it, he is interested in what I do but as he grows older and notes my frustration, the long hours and the challenges, he may pursue a scientific career outside of healthcare. I am not sure I would encourage medicine, based upon my own experiences, but I would not dissuade it, either.

It is widely quoted that physicians have the highest death rate of any profession. The reality is that a truly conclusive study has never been done, largely due to the fact that statistics are state administered and gathering that data would be a monumental task. Regardless, the number is much higher than it should be given the direct access to professional support and the simple fact that most health professions are fulfilling vocations. However, the use of drugs and alcohol, the "impaired physician", is a sign of troubling issues, although it has not been determined if it is job-related. On the other hand, there is little question that current stressors are exacerbating this unfortunate trend.

The first and only orthopedist to ever serve as president of the AMA, Dr. Andrew Gurman, focused on the topic of physician burnout during his acceptance speech back in 2016. I am honored to say that he is not only a fellow orthopedic surgeon, but a hand surgeon and someone that I can call a trusted friend and colleague. His inaugural address is about 13 minutes long and touches on the long road and challenges to become a physician and surgeon. The video is a delight as our mutual colleague friends, Dr. Peter Amadeo of the Mayo Clinic, and Dr. Bill Seitz of the Cleveland Clinic, emblematic premier surgeons from prestigious institutions, are seated behind him. This reminded me of a Presidential State of the Union Address, where the Speaker of the House and the Vice President, a la Tip O'Neill and George Bush Sr. sat behind the President as they listened with intent.

The primary theme that Dr. Gurman speaks about is physician burnout. He quotes that 60 percent of physicians are burned out, meaning, they are so frustrated with the profession that they are abandoning their vocation and retiring early. He attributes this to "being unsupported by administrators, dogged by unnecessary regulations, stressed by the pace of their jobs, and mired in mountains of paperwork."

Many criteria define physician burnout, but certainly one of them is a sense of helplessness. That helplessness translates into an attitude of, "Well, fine. Why try to advance care when blocked and encumbered and nobody seems to care?" Apathy and frustration abound because you realize there is nothing you can do to change or even impact a certain situation. Dr. Gurman feels we can counter this by encouraging physician advocacy and participation in organized medicine. This book represents one of several efforts to address the challenges we face in medicine, yet even these have been muted by my colleagues' perplexing apathy. Furthermore, there exists a palpable disinterest in our community and society beyond…unless, of course, it is *their* kid who gets hurt. I think of my kids' school, soccer team, municipality, and our business associations.

I have experienced this disinterest for a decade via our OrthoNOW® contribution. The overall system simply does not care. We will touch on what our society seems to better value in the chapter on physicians and money. However, I would not necessarily call it burnout, which is considered an occupational phenomenon, not a medical or psychological condition. Strangely enough, it is included in the ICD-11 (International Classification of Diseases) book and listed as a reason that people might seek health services. You see, it is due to outside forces – many of which I have described, reiterated, and brought to light within this book.

The WHO (World Health Organization), now increasingly relevant due to our COVID-19 pandemic, simply states that the syndrome is due to chronic workplace stress that is not being appropriately managed. It is not due to home issues or problems with the kids, although those can certainly exacerbate the problem.

They define burnout as being characterized by these 3 criteria:

1. Feelings of energy depletion or exhaustion;

2. Increased mental distance from one's job, or feelings of negativism or cynicism related to one's job; and

3. Reduced professional efficacy.

I am certain that many of us reading this book may have experienced all three symptoms during a job experience. There are solutions: resign and change employers or your firm, or even your career choice.

Physicians do not have this luxury. We took an oath. Caring for patients is the integral component of that charge, no matter the setting. I would argue that physicians are some of the most motivated, resilient, and driven individuals in our society. Did Section I of this book not resonate? In my case alone, I devoted 14 years of education, exams, and training in which I sacrificed my third decade of life – with no regrets. When the dreaded Bell Commission decreased our work hours, did physicians celebrate or it argue against it, making a case for continuity of care and the hours needed to fully grasp the skills needed for clinical excellence?

It is tough to "exhaust" us. Furthermore, how dare anybody suggest that we are negative or cynical about our job? We know what we want to do with our lives and how this affects others, whether compensated or not. Read the insurance chapter once again. We are engaged with our patients, often to a fault. Just ask a physician's spouse, significant other, or their children. Professional efficacy is vital to us. We know what we know, and we know what we do not know. I do not label our sentiments as "burnout" since the only validating criteria is the final one: lack of efficacy, brought on by diminishing lack of control. That is the central theme.

Just like I know I am unqualified (and disinterested) to read a legal contract thoroughly, or fully elucidate a P&L statement, I know that the peripheral elements in healthcare are not at all trained for actual patient care. When the latter occurs, whether by authorizations, "peer" reviews or unending obstacles placed by those interfering with my vocation and passion, I might experience what some call burnout.

However, I prefer to call this "moral injury" a concept first brought forward via an opinion article by Dean and Talbot in 2018. They equated this to serving on the front lines of war, like combat soldiers. Yes, in the trenches. The term "moral injury" was first coined in a Clinical Psychology Review article in 2009, "*Moral Injury and Moral Repair in War Veterans: a Preliminary Model and Intervention Strategy.*"

This emerging concept of moral injury epitomized the feelings clinicians experience when their convictions and deeply held moral beliefs are violated by witnessing and participating in acts that run contrary to the professional oath they swore to uphold. Soldiers, too, often witness unspeakable acts, and are forced to participate in missions they may profoundly disagree with. There are many parallels. We have now seen this exposed through the Coronavirus pandemic where even the public equates it to war and finally sees the beleaguered and embattled clinician as somebody who deserves our respect. What physicians seek is not respect, but rather support, and to eliminate all interference in our noble and needed tasks.

The simple fact that our healthcare system is interfering with our ability to practice sound and ethical medicine is damaging enough. Add to this the additional stress of work hours, bureaucracy, and even litigation against us, the caregiver, is enough to push any individual, however resilient, over the edge. If you needed further proof, look at all the physicians who are now writing articles and books about the healthcare challenge. That is testament enough. For the past 25 years, I have written articles, reviews, and book chapters on a litany of subjects all within my chosen field – surgery of the hand. The mere fact that I decided to compose this book, despite limited free time, makes a bold statement.

Physician frustration and moral injury stems from the increasing lack of control in several forms, as I have already outlined. One is, of course, the dreaded and inane authorization process. Add to that the cumbersome and time-consuming nature of EMRs (electronic medical records). Then there is the constant specter of litigation hanging over your head. And the final nail in the coffin: because most physicians have a philanthropic and altruistic nature, we are taken advantage of by multiple outside forces. The unending figurative roadblocks to delivering care: that is what frustrates physicians.

As Dr. Khouri observes, "If you look at college, the most competitive kids are the pre-med kids. The hardest working students in college are pre-med, and it is only the beginning of the road for them. As I mentioned, despite my best attempts to convince them otherwise, two of my kids became doctors. Despite the difficulties, they wanted to go into medicine. With the internet these days, we are constantly exposed to bad news and fake news. And terrible stories travel much faster and further than the good ones. That is part of the tainted image of doctors, which I must admit started with the Clinton Administration in the 1990s, in a deliberate move. In her failed attempt to overhaul healthcare, Hillary started the whole thing.

"That is when there was a deliberate attempt to tarnish the reputation and social standing of doctors. They just had all kinds of bad stories about them. It used to be that the doctor was the medicine man; he was the respectable guy, the guy who was caring for and curing people. That image has been tarnished. Most of us went into medicine because we wanted to help people because we love people. We wanted to help and be good to humanity.

"And we still do. I love taking care of patients. I love operating. But it gets tougher and tougher to wait for authorization, protect yourself from malpractice, spend time on the computers, and fight the system every day, instead of just taking care of patients. But nothing is perfect. I still think we have one of the best systems in the world. It is all part of the growing pains.

"I am convinced there are too many lawyers and middlemen taking money out of medicine. All the guys who make billions from medicine run insurance companies. It is the business of medicine that makes money, not the doctors. It is the executive of GM who makes the money, not the poor workers assembling the cars. You walk in the corridors of the hospitals now, the CEO and all his cronies – the executives – make salaries in the millions. Never mind that it is supposed to be a nonprofit hospital, the CEO takes home $6 million a year and the vice-CEO makes $5 million a year. They spend their time collecting money and donations. Baptist Hospital, for example, holds all kinds of affairs and fundraisers for donations yet combined, their executives make close to $100 million dollars.

"There are more people doing the non-medical B.S., including lower-level employees. The bureaucracy and regulations pile up. The regulation feeds itself: more regulation requires more regulation and regulators that must justify their salaries and jobs by creating more regulations. And it feeds itself. It is a vicious cycle. There is no control over the stuff they regulate, and these guys have no clue.

"Somebody informed me the other day that nurses control hospital regulation. Doctors have lost that territory. We are not in charge of anything anymore in the hospitals. Our nurses decide how to practice medicine. By the way, these nurses do not practice medicine; they are business nurses who have jobs as administrators. The last time they laid their hands on a patient was probably two decades ago, yet they make the rules about what doctors can and cannot do. For instance, if you want to open an O.R. for minor cases, you must have laminar air flow all the way that goes up and down, but there is no science behind it. Yet the regulations get bigger, more complex, and more onerous every month and every year. Why? They must justify their existence."

Just "Google" Us

In the internet age, another interesting phenomenon has arisen that now permeates healthcare: online reviews. Today, patients log onto their computers and give a board-certified fellowship trained surgeon, a simple star rating – from one to five – about their experience. Their reviews often have nothing to do with the quality of medical care they received. Rather, they tend to focus on the time they had to wait to see the doctor, which was longer than they had hoped after a stressful day at work or dealing with the kids. Or maybe a staff member was a tad curt with them, or worse, God forbid they had to pay a copay – as if the treating physician and his office have anything to do with the inner workings of their insurance plans. The worst part is, disgruntled patients almost never post a balanced review, where they highlight some positives and negatives, then give an overall 3 or 4 rating because they weren't completely satisfied. No, it is always a one.

Yes, happy patients publish 5-star reviews – bravo! Fantastic! But unhappy patients go to the opposite extreme, which is ludicrous. It is a well-known fact that folks who have an axe to grind will devote much more energy to disparaging a doctor than happy patients. Sadly, it is human nature.

The online review system has become so silly that a well-known restaurant in San Francisco, Botto Bistro, pursued an interesting strategy out of frustration. It seems Botto Bistro finally got fed up with the numerous bad reviews they were receiving on Yelp, in addition to seeing many excellent reviews taken down in a form of marketing extortion. Keep in mind, many negative reviews were based on frivolous reasons and restauranteurs were becoming slaves to their Yelp rating.

So, what did the owners do? They decided to promote the fact that they were getting multiple bad reviews and encouraged 1-star ratings by providing major food discounts. They drove their average down to something like 1.5 – and the demand for the restaurant shot through the roof!

This real-world example proves that the online review system lacks validity. Kudos to the restauranteurs who realized the ridiculousness of the whole thing. I mean, what is more personal than food preferences? Of course, not everyone is going to walk away satisfied, which is why it is a mistake to base your judgment on someone else's singular experience…someone with a different palate and preferences than you. I like almost everything except lima beans. God knows why. You get the point.

Healthcare works the same way. You may not have chemistry with your internist or your sub-specialized surgeon, whose sole purpose is to remove a tumor from the base of your brain. If that surgeon does their job well, based on their years of education, training, and experience, isn't that what truly matters? Who cares if there is a long wait, or the bathroom ran out of soap; what relevance does that have to your loved one's glioblastoma?? It seems that few people truly complain about waiting nearly two hours in Disney World to ride the three-minute Dumbo ride, yet God forbid a physician gets backed up and patients must wait. It is not like the doctor has his feet up on his desk, smoking a cigar, right?

Keep in mind, this comes from a staunchly pro-customer service physician. Furthermore, books such as "The Endangered Customer" and "Beyond Bedside Manner" are required reading in my hand practice, and serve as guidelines for OrthoNOW® center practices. In a case like this, reviews are probably not that important. But because they are so prevalent now with Google and other search engines, I wanted to call it out. For any patients reading this, I encourage you to be a little more research-focused when choosing your doctor or specialist. Put less emphasis on the "Kim Kardashian dress" rating and more emphasis on competence and skill.

Bread, Circuses, Celebrities and Athletes

During my kids' spring break last year, I took them to the Miami Open. As I was watching a bit of tennis, Petra Kvitova was featured prominently. Her claim to fame is coming back to the sport at a high level after being assaulted with a knife in a home invasion. A guy posed as a boiler repair man to get into her home, and when her back was turned, he held a knife to her throat. In fighting him off, she instinctively grabbed the knife and cut several tendons and the sensory nerves in her hand. This is the kind of procedure I used to do every other day. I do not do it as often now, but these procedures are not uncommon for a hand surgeon. Obviously, a skilled hand surgeon repaired the damage for her.

And yet, all I heard from the media was, "Oh, what a comeback!" We never heard the name of the doctor who saved her hand, even though that doctor is partly responsible for her amazing return to tennis. As a colleague, I would like to celebrate the hand surgeon who should get much of the credit, because there aren't many people out there who know how to do that.

Why is it that every time I read about a baseball player getting the Tommy John surgery, there is no mention of Frank Jobe, the orthopedic surgeon who invented it? Instead, it is named after Major League Baseball pitcher Tommy John, the first patient to have the surgery. Yet as Wikipedia notes, "Jobe made sports medicine history on September 25, 1974 when he performed the first reconstruction of the ulnar collateral ligament of the elbow (UCL), using a revolutionary procedure he devised." Dr. Jobe reconstructed the ligament by taking the Palmaris longus tendon from the forearm. He told Tommy John that the surgery would allow him to throw a slider with 100 pounds of torque. Years later, I met Tommy John with another hand surgeon who used to treat athletes in New York.

In 1997, Patrick Ewing, one of the best centers to ever play basketball, suffered one of the hardest wrist injuries to recover from – whether you are a professional athlete or perform manual labor for a living. When he crashed to the floor during a game and used his wrist to break his fall, the force caused a high-speed, high-impact injury typically suffered by NFL linemen. He sustained a wrist dislocation (perilunate injury) implying severely torn ligaments. After surgery, he "rebounded," if you will, and played in the NBA again.

But all you ever read in the paper was some generic throwaway line about "doctors repairing it." Always plural in the press. The truth is, for a surgery of this kind, it is ONE doctor. It is not as if it is a team of surgeons who participate in a huge organ transplant surgery on a patient, or to separate Siamese twins. In Ewing's case, if anything, there might have been a P.A., or orthopedic resident, assisting the doctor. That is it. In fact, I believe it was done by my initial hand surgery mentor, Dr. Charlie Melone, but it is not common knowledge. It just incenses me that his surgeon did not receive the credit he deserved, yet it is symbolic of our society. The public just expects doctors to do these things; therefore, there is no praise or congratulations. It's like, "You're a doctor. You're supposed to perform miracles."

I experienced this in similar manner on one of my own high-profile patients, wide receiver T.O. (Terrell Owens) as I previously discussed. His agent, Drew Rosenhaus, mentioned the surgery I did live on ESPN, so it is technically public knowledge. I recall being a bit surprised to hear my name as one almost never hears the treating surgeon mentioned in the media. Why is that?

Several years ago, there was a high-profile fireworks hand injury on another pro football player. I received the call at well past midnight but remember being indisposed to be able to address it. Besides, he was in a local hospital and I am no longer on staff at the hospitals partly due to the reason I mentioned in the malpractice chapter. See the consequence? Well, I understand the athlete received excellent care from a colleague, but it did take me some months to finally learn WHO had performed the definitive surgery. Yet the case was all over the news, the athlete was widely celebrated for being able to return to a linebacker position, sans 1.5 fingers, and…ZERO mention of the surgeon who was able to restore enough function to allow that near miracle to occur.

It certainly is a moral injury when an excellent medical outcome by a skilled clinician is trumped by the patient's recovery to return to his livelihood. Physicians don't want a medal but it's a basic human need to be recognized or at least acknowledged.

The irony, of course, it that nowadays when you do not deliver that miracle (because medical science, like life, is not perfect), you will be forced to "lawyer up" down the road. It will not be immediate; it will take two years or more before you get slapped with a lawsuit out of the blue. One day, you receive a letter and you think, "Who is the patient?" Then you go back to chart to find that patient who came to see you two years ago. You realize there was some minor issue, but it does not matter. *Why?* We live in a country where all they have to say is they do not like your tie, or the fact that they must pay a copay, or that they had to wait in your waiting room an hour longer than they wanted. And, after all that, they did not get a perfect resolution because again, medicine is not a perfect science. So, they might sue you.

Another NFL player caused a decade of grief for his well-intentioned surgeon who at the time was the team doctor for the illustrious Miami Dolphins. It seems that O.J. McDuffie, or rather his lawyers, felt that mismanagement of a "toe injury" led to a premature ending of his career. Given the outrageous salaries these athletes garner, the jurors awarded Mr. McDuffie 11.5 million dollars. Just like that. No matter that the team doctor often has to work in collaboration with the coaches and training staff because many elements come into play when you speak about a pro athlete and their role in their team's success. It is simple common knowledge that team physicians, consulting orthopedic surgeons, and athletic trainers will all use a wide variety of modalities, including corticosteroid injections, to keep a player on the field, more so when in playoff contention. It is a high-stakes, big money world. It certainly ain't grassroots medicine.

Fast forward ten years (much like what happened to my colleague, Dr. Khouri) and the case again went to trial on appeal, fortunately exonerating Dr. John Uribe, the treating surgeon. He simply indicated that the athlete could continue to play after half-time assessment of a toe injury sustained earlier in the game. To pay such a price for that decision, someone of impeccable credentials and stature in the sports medicine world, it is truly a devastating moral injury. I wonder if Mr. McDuffie might consider directing his anger to the 300-pound beast who probably caused the injury, but then again, that's football. The fact that an athlete playing a known and accepted violent sport, such as American Football, can transfer fault for a game-related common injury to an appropriately credentialed physician is simply a travesty. You don't want to get hurt, take up chess.

There are some bright spots, however. In late 2014, popular Tonight Show host, Jimmy Fallon, sustained a horrific injury termed a ring avulsion type amputation. This typically occurs in a fall where the person catches their ring, typically fourth finger, on a firm object, effectively ripping it off. The finger was salvaged, thanks to microsurgical techniques and the skill of the treating surgeon, Dr. David Chiu. I know the drill since the celebrity took a cab ride to Beth Israel Hospital, New York City, where they promptly told him they could not help him because it required a microsurgeon with a specialized team and equipment that was not available there. It may come as a surprise to many patients, but not every hospital can resolve every problem. Much like my four-finger amputation patient, Joe, Jimmy was whisked away to another facility, this time eight blocks up 1st Avenue to Bellevue Hospital, my ole stompin' grounds.

Jimmy tells the humorous anecdote, hilarious as he is, via multiple media news sources, including his own TV show. Most importantly, people connect to him. "Really, this is like microsurgery. This is like a thing. I was at Beth Israel. I had to go over to Bellevue Hospital. This amazing doctor, Dr. David Chiu, comes in. He has a bowtie and cowboy boots. That's my doctor! That's my guy! I knew it when he walked in."

Well, Dr. Chiu is an Asian-American surgeon who does, in fact, wear cowboy boots. Like many surgeons, he wears a bowtie to prevent his tie from becoming a fashionable petri dish every time he bends over a patient to examine them. Jimmy Fallon gave credit to the surgeon who did the work, along with the entire staff, but more importantly, he educated the public. He explained what a ring avulsion injury is, how wearing rings can be somewhat risky, and the general concept and existence of microsurgery. It is not "small incision surgery" or even arthroscopy, but rather the use of a high-powered operating microscope that allows us to suture together (anastomose) high-powered arteries, veins, and nerves often less than one millimeter in diameter! It truly is an amazing thing and thanks to a beloved entertainer, folks better understand its existence, lest they ever need it. His celebrity even encouraged further discussion among less experienced surgeons in that area. Another surgeon on the team, Dr. Anup Patel, was able to bring attention to an important social cause via the media exposure regarding Jimmy's hand injury.

I had similar experience, although not newsworthy, when my colleague and now friend, Dr. Andy Gurman called me, many years before he gave that illustrious address I shared on burnout to the AMA. It was in the evening while I was still doing elective cases at our old Miami Hand Center. Dr. Gurman informed me that his friend, a dentist, had just sustained a ring avulsion injury in the Florida Keys. Seems he was on a dive trip with his son from Pennsylvania, when he rolled back off the boat for his 2nd tank dive and caught his ring on a metal prominence at the edge of the hull. The rest you can imagine. He was transferred to one of the Miami hospitals at my direction, where I could call in the microsurgery team. During that interval, I finished my elective surgeries and then went to the hospital where I spent all night revascularizing the finger using a micro vein graft from the palmar forearm surface, not the foot as in Jimmy's case. It was successful and the dentist went back to his work with full function. He sent me a follow up video clip from his office a decade later, when I was asked to speak about Jimmy Fallon's case, and ring avulsions in general, on Univision – a Spanish speaking network. Sadly, it requires a celebrity, ala Enrique Iglesias, to bring attention to the work we do. Many people in Miami asked me with excitement, "Did you fix the Latin crooner's hand?" It is only a slight moral injury but does lay bare the priorities in our society.

Surgeons like Dr. Chiu are doing this work around the world, largely unheralded. The economic component is another issue (see next chapter) but the gratification comes from seeing his patient, every night on TV now, with an intact and functioning ring finger. I know that this is his priority and the priority of nearly every clinician: to restore a patient back to good function and health.

David and I spent a wonderful hour at lunch during a Hawaii microsurgery congress with Story Musgrave, the astronaut who has spent the most time in space, who also happens to be a trained surgeon (and engineer, physicist, pilot…aargh). Like a wide-eyed wondrous schoolchild, I got to ask Dr. Musgrave what it felt like to blast off, seeing the fire roaring below amid the incredible vibration seconds before lift-off. He simply said, "I looked out the port window below and realized I shouldn't have done that." However, the conversation, surreal as it was, went back to the care of patients. It often does with physicians, a fact that often causes my father, Cristobal, a brilliant electrical engineer and math whiz, to exclaim, "I hate having drinks with your doctor friends, Alex. You guys always talk about medicine." He is right. Its perhaps the reason we suffer so much from moral injury. Thank you, Jimmy Fallon.

The challenges that physicians face within the healthcare world and even with our fellow man is not restricted to the United States by any means. I often commiserate with colleagues from abroad, particularly in Europe and South America, who describe the same constant challenges in the ongoing fight against insurance companies and the healthcare infrastructure of their countries to be treated fairly and compensated according to their importance in society. Much of the responsibility comes from the public, who now seem to be holding clinicians in greater stead given the current worldwide viral pandemic.

The issue of moral injury may rest on how greater society views us. It begins at the individual patient level. Our patient interactions are increasingly demonstrating that the healthcare challenges we face are misunderstood by the lay public, and we as the "providers" bear the brunt of this angst. A great example is a local community website that provides useful information to folks within a geographic area, neighborhood, or specific zip code. Well before the COVID-19 crisis, my neighbors were well connected and informed on the site Nextdoor, a public facing site with no fee to join. I have found a property manager, plumber, and boat mechanic all via the site – folks who make money for their valuable services. They are not advertising per se, but people are able to share their name and contact info as they need help. There is a section for actual advertising where complete services, website, and hours can be posted.

Many people, however, make helpful recommendations for a variety of services. You would think it would work the same for healthcare services. Not so. On occasion I have seen a flurry of clinician names posted by members when another asks for a great dentist or chiropractor. I am not sure if those folks were reprimanded, but this occurred when a former patient of ours and a fellow Cornellian acquaintance, posted her recommendation regarding the availability of convenient orthopedic walk-in care services. She had gone several times to the hospital for a femur fracture – definitely hospital indicated! However, during the aftermath of some minor bicycle spills and to assess routine back pain, she felt the time and cost-efficiency of the nearby center, OrthoNOW® warranted a mention to her neighbors. She was spanked and later told me about the incident. I was not aware she had done this till after the fact. I related to her that I TOO had been scolded by the "Nextdoor administrator" for this action, as if I was selling real estate or yoga mats. It was amazing to me, but moreover, gave me insight as to the public's mentality of healthcare. I doubt a hospital administrator would be berated in this manner, because of the perception that the "saintly" hospital serves the "public good." Oh, yeah, and they are also "non-profit". Well we dissected that myth already.

It is clear that medical services, even outside of aesthetic surgery, are seen as businesses that should not be "promoted" despite our struggles to actually be reimbursed by the nefarious insurance industry, rarely the subject of true consumer angst, or the public themselves. It is a curious dichotomy that emblemizes many of our challenges and adds to moral injury.

All of us who provide care in various forms can share a multitude of stories that demonstrate that our patients, the people we serve, often do not "get it." The problems of healthcare delivery cost and inefficiencies are rarely the fault of the providers or the work we do. On the contrary. As patients increasingly bear the burden of their own care, the clinicians also suffer, because people do not place sufficient value on their own medical care. Therefore, they do not want to pay for it with their own money.

My fellow contributors and I could fill this book with amazing anecdotes of how our own patients, grateful as they may be (or not), contribute to the problem and our ongoing detriment. This insider account is designed to illustrate the problem by anecdotes that expose issues the public is not aware of in the hope of inspiring solutions. I have hundreds of stories, many of them related by my staff who are truly "in the trenches." They are the ones who must schedule appointments, inform patients of the complexities of their insurance, and reveal to them their financial responsibility. It is perhaps medical office workers who best understand the challenges; therefore, they tend to be grateful consumers of healthcare.

My staff has told me on more than one occasion that even fellow parents at my children's private school tend to be the worst offenders in terms of resisting payment for services. Why is that? They send their kids to an expensive school, drive the best cars, and enjoy a privileged role in society. Their attitude is probably due to a multitude of factors; however, I suspect the primary cause is their grave misunderstanding of our own healthcare system. Like most people, they do not realize that insurance companies have adjudicated financial responsibility to the healthcare consumer over time: the days of paying premiums and receiving full coverage are over. Who pays the price? For one, the orthopedic walk-in clinic that still struggles to make ends meet, not the large hospitals where those same parents accept the long waits and high copayments in exchange for what is often NOT real treatment – just the application of ice, a Rx, and a referral to someone like me.

A recently departed executive for this innovative delivery system, OrthoNOW®, even took for granted my own services. He had complained of left shoulder pain since the time he came to work for us, blaming an old high school football injury. The pain became acute during a fall on ice at his ski house in Colorado. You get the sense that he has the resources to pay for healthcare in the field that he himself is invested in, right? I scoped his shoulder and did a combined repair of his labrum (type II SLAP tear) and his rotator cuff. It was an acute on chronic injury and I was more than pleased to help him. He did beautifully and did not miss a beat at work. When I went to visit him the evening of the surgery, he was wearing his sling as he stood in the kitchen with one leg up on a stool while answering (presumably) work emails from his smartphone. It was amazing to see.

Despite his choice to limit his rehab sessions, I observed his recovery as he regained full function within months. He boasted that he NEVER had pain, thanks to the combination of innovative use of EXPAREL®, a new regional anesthetic. Furthermore, efficient surgical intervention led to an unremarkable post-op course. I even inserted a bovine collagen patch, Regeneten® in his shoulder to augment healing, a practice that allows these patients to experience less pain and a faster recovery. It is carte blanche care.

Remarkably, months later, after he accepted a higher paying job in his primary area of expertise, he ignored all requests for his payment responsibility of his sizeable deductible. This speaks volumes about our healthcare system. When the CEO of an innovative healthcare delivery model in orthopedics shirks his own financial responsibility for care in same discipline, it signals a greater problem than simply his own lack of character or ethics. He continues to pay high premiums to an insurance company that has NO idea how to provide care, let alone perform a complex shoulder surgery, but my practice must simply eat it. *Zero* payment for high level services rendered. This is a pervasive problem. It is not burnout but rather moral injury.

My colleague and former hand fellow recounts below that moral injury is not a uniquely American phenomenon. He and other physicians in Spain face formidable challenges for even bare bones compensation for the work that we all do.

Dr. Juan Manuel Rios Ruh on Physician Compensation

"There is an interesting aspect of my upbringing. I was born and raised in Latin America, where the healthcare system has major failures, due to corruption. It was it was quite a challenge for me to help people with minimal financial means, even though there were major oil resources in my native country of Venezuela. We should be a rich country for the people, but instead all our wealth was lost to the corrupt 'middleman'.

"Once I came here to Europe, I realized the history is quite different. Here, you do have a lot more resources to treat patients, but there are other problems. In Spain, medical doctors receive extremely low payments due to some government decisions that sometimes punish us. If a medical doctor has a private practice, they earn less in the hospital because they have a private practice on the side. The government punishes that activity. And we deal with a lot of exploitation from insurance companies that sometimes pay as little as five Euros for seeing a patient – even for a complicated case where you spend an hour with that patient and use all your knowledge and experience to explain the complications of surgery to them. Even for a visit like that, they will only pay you 5 Euros...which amounts to about $5.50 in U.S. dollars.

"And this really works against the quality of attention a doctor can give a patient because a doctor – and this may come as a surprise – must also pay for things like their rent, car loans, clothes, and food. To make ends meet, they will see as many patients as they can in the shortest amount of time, trying to reach a decent compensation level.

"I have had exposure to the American healthcare system, thanks to my American colleagues. Even though it is portrayed as an ideal in the movies or in sitcoms, the reality is quite different. When we see the American hospitals, we assume patients receive excellent medical attention, but when you visit some of them, you notice a rampant misuse of resources. Whether it is the government or an insurance company, there is too much interference by people who are not medically trained.

"It is frustrating to see that, once you become a physician and you are the one who's providing value to the user (the patient), you are NOT the one who's receiving the deserved benefit. Between your education, knowledge, the amount of work you provide, and everything you do for patients, you get this minimal amount of money. The big money goes to middle managers who don't know what the patient is dealing with, nor have any idea what to do for them. Yet they are in a position where they can deny resources to the physician and their patient. Regarding healthcare, the fact that I have been in contact with different models in various countries gives me a comprehensive perspective to analyze it objectively.

"This interference from non-medical people creates problems. The system does not account for the importance and relevance of medical decisions, and where and when they must be made in society. Physicians are being left out, yet we are the ones who clearly see what needs to be done in both the public and private arenas. We detect a lot of trouble in healthcare. We can offer solutions that could solve many of the problems, not just for physicians but also patients. The image society has about doctors, even here in Europe, is that if you are a doctor you must be a millionaire. Or, if you are a doctor, you should not be charging to see patients because it is your vocation and you love what you do.

"Well, it is the same with an architect or an engineer. We all love what we do. But doctors work hard and take on a tremendous amount of responsibility and our compensation should reflect that. We should be paid at least as much as other professions."

A Surgeon/Attorney/Legislator's Perspective of U.S. Healthcare Challenges

Dr. Julio Gonzalez, my fellow practicing orthopedic surgeon in Florida who weighed in earlier about self-pay patients versus insured patients, brings a unique qualification to the moral and economic injury we continue to suffer in our profession:

"The issue of insurance paying me in a timely manner has decreased considerably except for area of workers' comp. Some workers' comp providers have been extremely problematic. Reimbursements used to be a huge problem with Medicare private payers, but not so much anymore, due to the passage of laws regarding prior authorizations and things of that nature. So, it really has diminished to rare occasions. However, about a year ago, I dealt with a situation with an insurance company that was not convinced I was doing the work I had claimed that I had been doing. To be specific, I am talking about charging a level five for a consult.

"For example, there is a 9924 series that goes from 99421 to 99242 to 99243, 99244, and 99245. Code 99245 is reserved for the most complicated, most high-risk patients. And maybe six or seven times in a row, I went to the hospital under the coverage of this one insurance company. Every time, it was an elderly patient with a hip fracture and multiple medical problems, who needed to go to the operating room as soon as possible. It was high risk in every way you can conceive.

"The insurance company started holding my payments because they wanted to see if I really was doing 99245-level work. What is interesting is that they were not questioning whether I was laying my stethoscope on the patient, getting their blood pressure and vital signs, or doing whatever else was needed to prepare the patient for the O.R. They were questioning whether I was really engaging in high-risk interactions with a patient, which is absurd. These were elderly patients with multiple medical problems and a few fractures that required major surgery: you cannot get more high risk than that.

"Yet I got held back for about a year and a half, while they reviewed every subsequent case I did for its appropriateness. I remember I called the physician liaison and talked to him about the ridiculousness of the whole thing. It took a year to finally resolve – and more than a year of withholding my sizable payments for consults I did in the hospital, plus the rather big surgeries. In the end, the insurance company reinstated me, but I know for a fact that this is a recurring problem. They do this to all sorts of other providers. I hate to use the word 'routine' because some of these cases rarely are, but when things go smoothly, the insurance companies have been reimbursing me in relatively quick manner. However, they use a lot of techniques to either slow down the reimbursement or force the reimbursement to be less than the work that you did.

"Instead of honoring your 99245 they'll tell you why you only did a 99243. "We're going to pay you for your 99243," which is a difference of about $75 to $250. Then you must fight for that, and most of the time, you lose. More often, they challenge your coding to try to pay you less than the work you completed. In general, the decision-maker is somebody sitting behind a desk whose main role is to save the insurance company money.

"It is a stall tactic, but also a nickel-and-dime tactic. They know that if they can cut you 50 bucks, you are less apt to fight over it than a full denial. Whether they stall or not, they are still going to nickel and dime you into submission. The decision-makers tend not to be your colleagues or your peers. They go by algorithms on their computer software and by their policy; they will outsource the review of your case to another physician, who they will underpay to review the case. I know because I did that for a while. Then if you are going to have a peer-to-peer, they will call you back to tell you, "We're denying your procedure."

"Prospectively, they can also deny your procedure, because they don't think you met the criteria to proceed with that next step in a patient's care. If you contest their decision, they will put you with a peer to peer who generally has a funny accent who argues literature with you. Most of the time, it is not an orthopedic surgeon. Often it is not a doctor. And even when it is, it is not a practicing American physician, nor is it someone who shares your specialty.

"The whole process steals a lot of time from my schedule. For example, if they ask me to get on a peer to peer, I must stop what I'm doing, call the number, dial the code they gave me, and connect with somebody after the phone rings a number of times. After I give them the case number, I must wait while they put me on hold to find a doctor I can talk to.

"Sometimes he will rule in my favor; sometimes he will not. But when he does not, you do not get the answer right away. It takes a couple of weeks. Peer to peers are mostly a waste of time, which is why I stopped doing them. Instead, I tell my patient, 'You can call the insurance company and tell them this is what I'm recommending. Let them know they are interfering.' Oftentimes that works well, but it places the burden on somebody else. I tell my patients that the insurance companies are one of the few organizations we pay to support them in *not* doing their job. Because what they are doing behind the scenes is trying to figure out ways that they can escape the responsibility of paying for the service. And again, nine out of 10 times it goes well, but when you really need them, it becomes a bear."

The struggles to be appropriately compensated, valued, and even respected for the unique skillset that physicians possess has led to a moral injury, exacerbated by the constant hurdles and obstacles placed in our path to heal our fellow man. It is a good thing most physicians are resilient and not focused on money as we are about to explore.

Chapter 13 –Doctors and Money: The Great Divide

"It's not the employer who pays the wages.
Employers only handle the money.
It's the customer who pays the wages."
– Henry Ford

To use a cliché, "Perception is reality." Well, let me tell you, the public perception of doctors and their compensation is far from reality. In fact, it is a huge *misperception*. By now, I hope the many real-life examples of physician altruism I have shared throughout this book have resonated with you and given you a newfound understanding that our inherent desire to help our fellow man has been exploited by health insurance companies and others for their own gain.

While we work endless hours caring for patients and expanding our knowledge, we deal with the moral injury of the loss of control that has been imposed upon us by outside forces. We do our jobs with the threat of lawsuits hanging over our heads. And those of us in private practice must maintain high overhead in the form of administrative staff just get some reimbursement for the important and lifesaving work we do.

Yet despite our multiple years of education, sacrifice, and training, it is taboo in our society for a medical doctor to earn a six- or seven-figure salary. Celebrities? Sure. Athletes. Absolutely. Doctors? No way. While I am not diminishing the ability to cry on demand or to throw a 60-yard touchdown pass (both of which require skill and training), I am pointing out that our priorities as a society are mostly upside down.

For me (as I suspect for most of my colleagues) the decade of my twenties – when most of my friends were partying – remains a blur. I have no regrets about sacrificing those years to achieve my goal of becoming an orthopedic surgeon; I am simply saying that these efforts have intrinsic value. In my case, I trained for 14 years. What I do is important. Yet the public begrudges my colleagues and me for making a good living – if only their perception of our take-home pay matched the truth. Consider this: for the first time in years, I had a month where I did not *break even*. I worked 30 days as a busy surgeon with a thriving practice and I still did not make enough money to pay my bills. That is astounding. Do other professionals and business-owners fail to break even in their respective areas of expertise?

Let us draw a comparison between the physicians in the medical profession and leaders in other businesses and professions, starting with healthcare CEOs. In 2017, Mark Bertolini, CEO of Aetna, Inc., earned $59 million. Was there any public outcry over this excessive payday? What does a health insurance CEO do every day? And where does the money come from?

As Dr. Mark Rekant points out, health insurance companies "have these huge infrastructures, large buildings in Chicago and throughout the Northeast, so everyone's health insurance premiums increase. My health insurance costs about $25,000 per year with a $6,000 deductible. The average person with Obamacare has a $5,000 deductible, which means the first $5,000 of their healthcare is on them, anyway. It would be better for them to just save the money for themselves in the form of a mandated health savings account in which their employer sets money aside for them. It would be a big improvement over our current system."

I tried to convey this concept in the chapter on insurance. Furthermore, I tried to eliminate the health insurance money pit within my own practice. I told my staff that I would place the same amount of money I pay monthly, and then some, in an interest-bearing account for any "what if." Do they need to go to the OB GYN? We offer a reasonable consult fee that would likely make the doctor's office leap for joy. Same with their kids' pediatricians. What if something major happens? Then I negotiate a total care package with the local hospital who also likes to get paid immediately by credit card. My staff rejected my offer, proving how entrenched we are in our current system. But that could still change.

Dr. Rekant continues, "If you argue that physicians make too much money, then we need to pay our medical students and residents commensurately with their 23-to-25-year-old peers. For example, if I graduate college and enroll in medical school while my peers become vice presidents making $80,000 at whatever job they're in, as a medical student or resident, I should be paid in kind, instead of coming out of medical school $300,000 in debt. If we want physician reimbursements to go down, then medical school costs must go down. Residency salaries must go up, and then everything can be neutral like it is in Europe. The European trainees get paid more than the United States trainees. Does that make sense? Our residents get paid about half of what their European peers get paid. In Europe, once they become physicians, they do not make as much money as U.S. physicians but as far as I know, they are not crippled by debt either.

"It is a tough thing to change because the system is an embedded behemoth. How do you do it? I do not know. If you pay someone, all the sudden their medical school costs come down and those medical students realize that their reimbursement is now going to go down. We would end up with a two-tiered system of reimbursement and would have to eventually ramp up to one system. It is doable, but it would be painful at first."

The spiraling cost of medical education has certainly been blamed on the perceived glut of specialists. The accepted mantra is that specialists make much more money, therefore, the students who are saddled with debt, most these days, will lean towards a subspecialty to have less financial hardship. This thinking assumes that specialists *always* make much more money, which is often true, and assumes that someone as driven as a medical student, profiled in Section I, will decide their vocation solely upon perceived financial gains.

Despite physician grumbling, we are making more money overall, as per Medscape Physician Compensation Report, than in previous years. The reimbursement for specific procedures or evaluations is not keeping up with inflation, but due to increasing volume and productivity, doctors are earning more. Good. The issue with most physicians and many allied health professions, is that the bureaucracy and "busy work" has become overwhelming. As discussed in the Moral Injury chapter, we resent the amount of free work that we often perform, coupled with the progressive lack of control. Despite public misconception, for most physicians, money was not a primary motivator in their choice to enter the medical field. The same is also true for the decision to embark upon a specialty. In addition, personality types may influence earnings: the type A, hyper-driven types that enter surgical specialties might have earned more if they pursued internal medicine, traditionally a cerebral specialty. The nature of psychiatry, for example, would tend to reimburse less overall as most psychiatrists are not working all night long or running to the hospital in the wee hours. They are simply different fields with different commensurate earning potentials.

Overall, a primary care physician (P.C.P.) earned $237,000 dollars in 2019 as compared to the average specialist, at $341,000. While a sizeable difference, the P.C.P. often starts earning income three- to- four years before the specialist due to length of training. Many specialists earn their income based on surgical or medical procedures, while the P.C.P. is much more focused on the highbrow approach to long term management and prevention of disease. The latter pursuit deserves greater compensation. Various approaches to reach that goal are being considered.

Regardless of what specialty a physician chooses, the cost of medical education in the U.S., especially, has become exorbitant and deserves assessment. I found it ironic that my own medical school alma mater, N.Y.U. became the first private allopathic medical school to offer free tuition for all. This represents nearly $60,000, not including room and board expenses, and is four times the amount I paid when I attended in the late 80s. I can assure you the cost of living has not quadrupled in that time. Medical school education became unaffordable for most. It overburdens students with debt that adds to the already tremendous stress and expense of starting a medical practice. It is little wonder that most enter a fully employed position after completing graduate medical education (residency). Since it has a startling effect on how healthcare is delivered in the U.S., we must question this trend. N.Y.U.'s decision may reverse It by encouraging other universities to follow suit. If this happens, it will allow young physicians to consider the pursuit of a traditional private practice in the field of their choice. See, it is not all doom and gloom.

The CEOs of health insurance companies are not the only ones taking home an enormous paycheck (excessive as they may be). The collective salaries of such a huge workforce leads to a massive drain of real healthcare dollars. Money that could be spent on actual care -- not administrating or managing money, which is what insurance companies really do. A recent Google search, for example, reveals that United Healthcare, another big player in the market, currently employs 320,000 people. That is a significant number of paychecks. Even if you calculated a conservative estimate of costs using the average hourly rate of $16.95 for a patient services rep and excluded higher paying positions within United Healthcare, $16.95 per hour equals an annual salary of $32,544 for one full-time employee. If we multiplied that by 320,000 it amounts to a "conservative" estimate of $1.04 billion dollars. Ironically, as advertised on the employment website Indeed.com, the job titles "primary care physician" and "physician" come with an annual salary of $154,222 and $162,938, respectively. What was United Healthcare CEO David Wichmann's annual compensation in 2018? $21.5 million.

Now let us look at my "favorite" health insurance company, Blue Cross Blue Shield. According to the Detroit Free Press, their President and CEO

Daniel Lopp's salary "tumbled" from $19.2 million in 2018 to $12.1 million in 2019. I wonder how he will ever survive.

While I have no doubt that CEOs like Bertolini, Wichmann, and Lopp are smart, savvy guys who can probably read a P&L statement very well, does that justify these exorbitant salaries? I am certain none of them could perform a life-saving surgery or repair a rotator cuff, yet there is little, if any public outrage about it. On the other hand, most patients think doctors are "rich." Some, as I have described in earlier chapters, have no problem skipping out on their payments after the limb or life-saving procedure has been done. I already mentioned a CEO who worked for me and did just that. Wonder if he knows the guys above?

Now let me be candid. I have done well for myself. However, my economic successes are largely due to some good business decisions, not my prowess in the surgical suite. While my team can tell you that I do not read a financial statement very well, or cannot decipher a contract like an expert, I do have vision for what is needed in the marketplace. I have capitalized on that hunch while also exhibiting little risk adversity. Most physicians are wary about investing. Understandably so, since we feel we should make money based upon our unique clinical skills and the vital role we serve in the community. Sadly, that vital skill and knowledge is not rewarded as it should be. Those who venture out and provide a superior approach to healthcare delivery *may* be rewarded. While this has been true in the still evolving A.S.C. space, it has not crystallized in the orthopedic walk in center arena, which remains a novel and poorly compensated healthcare solution. Although many of my colleagues would not stick it out, as a reluctant healthcare entrepreneur I am confident that the marketplace will catch up. If that fails to occur, it would not be my first error in judgement.

Therefore, risk is often rewarded and steady adherence to traditional medical care is, sadly, not. That is why many younger physicians are now obtaining their M.B.A. Is that what we want as a society? I would guess most patients prefer that their doctor focus on keeping up with the scientific literature and attending conferences, not spending time with their executive team and predicting trends. However, *that* is what is rewarded in our society; therefore, each clinician must judge for themselves how entrenched they will be with the business of healthcare. I, for one, learned that actual healthcare delivery will struggle to evolve if I do not contribute to its betterment. I am not complaining at all about my own finances; rather, I want to advocate for rewarding clinicians for what they do best: care for their patients.

The inclusion of sound business practices and even marketing principles, is strangely out of grasp for most physicians. Again, we all have our strengths and weaknesses, but you would hope we could leverage our collective strengths with simple dialogue. As I explained in the chapter on collaboration, it remains a formidable challenge in our profession, one that continues to haunt us. Speak to any practice administrator or health system executive, and they all chuckle with recognition at the "herding cats" analogy. Our individuality and stubborn single-mindedness are the stuff of folklore in healthcare corporate boardrooms, pharma summits, and my own orthopedic industry meetings.

Clinicians can evolve, adapt and put our virtues together to emerge from moral injury and better serve our patients. The ongoing challenges I face within my own humble medical infrastructure is emblematic of the problem. We built a one-stop shop for orthopedic care yet cannot find synergy in pooling our resources for the greater collective good. The insurance companies take full advantage of our division, along with out altruism, as previously discussed.

But the great divide between doctors and money is not limited to the health insurance industry. The other night I had an awful experience. I could not sleep because I was distraught about a communication I received from a lawyer regarding a property I own – a nasty, boilerplate letter fired off by a secretary that got me to thinking about the inequities of pay for physicians and the valuable work they do.

The lawyer's letter informed me that I owed a fee of $580. *Fine.* If I am late on a payment, which can happen, then I can add a late fee or penalty to the total, something most of us accept and understand in contemporary society. The possibility of late fees dissuades the lackadaisical and provides a major deterrent to anyone who even entertains the idea of not paying. However, the "courteous" letter informed me that I now owed about $1,200 – more than double the original fee. It encompassed a bunch of little charges from the law office that represents the condo association. The association told their attorneys, "Oh, we have a deadbeat apartment owner who hasn't paid X additional charge." Yet because nobody called me, I was not even aware of it.

The list included items that no physician, including me, gets to charge: management fees, a letter of preparation fee ($250), copying fees, and even a courier fee – as if the good ole U.S.P.S. (United States Post Office) was not good enough. The nasty form letter concluded with the threat that if I did not pay in 30 days, they would put a lien on my apartment. I thought to myself, "God, what a difference in professions. If I do not pay in 30 days, this major event will be set in motion. Yet, no physician is paid within 30 days for just about **anything**, unless it is a plastic surgeon doing aesthetic work for cash in the form of surgeries and procedures."

In our profession, physicians are expected to accept that it may take six months to get paid, with most cases taking about 45- to- 60 days. There are fancy words for this, but it does not excuse the fact that in ANY other profession or trade such a practice would result in major penalties. And nastiness. When the doctor's office calls to try and make a payment arrangement, we are treated with hostility. Wait a second, *who owes whom?*

Furthermore, when doctors use a collections service, they DO add a percentage as late fees; otherwise, in most cases the patient would surely not pay. Remember, they did not pay in the first place – a third party, their insurance company, paid a portion of the responsibility (maybe). Yet when they call the office manager irate and yelling (funny, they never get mad at their insurance company for putting most of the burden on them), we placate them. The words "write off" and "discount" are almost endemic in healthcare. One of the few times I asked one of my dozen or so attorneys for a discount, due to a huge bill for "Asset Protection," (more irony), he smiled and said he would be happy to extend a five percent discount. Yes, *five percent.* Ask any clinician, whether a dentist, physician, or therapist if they have EVER given that number as a discount. It is closer to 20 or 30, or…free. Yes, sometimes we completely write off any patient responsibility to fulfill our primary goal of keeping our patients happy. Meanwhile, the insurance escaped much responsibility, the patient received the care they needed, and the "rich" doctor must figure out how to make up for it somehow…by seeing even more patients.

To put in perspective, that $250 fee for some stupid legal form letter, is equivalent to three new patient consultations at the Florida workers' compensation fee schedule. Each of those patients requires time, knowledge, and interpretation of diagnostic studies, and physical examination. THEN we must "memorialize" it by creating a consultation note for the medical record, the increasingly complex steps of E.M.R. input. There is ZERO payment for that time. If not done, however, the actual time assessing, thinking about, and treating the patient is for naught. It is the ethereal medical note that matters and nothing else, in terms of the payors. For a typical work comp patient presenting with say, severe shoulder pain, or a saw injury to the forearm, my services are only valued at $82 dollars to include the documentation and phone calls to colleagues, the therapist, the family, or even the "peer" review physician at the insurance company that is supposed to pay you. Something is gravely wrong with this setup.

Let us recap the solid work ethic of physicians, especially those in specialties required to work all hours. When you call a doctor like an OB/GYN in the middle of the night, he or she will typically answer in a prompt manner. Who else does that? Yet these specialists, along with others like trauma and critical care surgeons had not slept much during residency. If you want to get an earful, tell them they are suffering from "burnout." If you are a patient about to have a baby, the last thing you want is a doctor who is not used to sleep deprivation and responds to ringing phone at 3 a.m. with the thought, "No, no, no, this can wait until 6 a.m." During those three hours, the woman might experience preeclampsia or some other life-threatening problem. While not perfect (none of us are), the OB/GYN uses their best judgement to decide the next course of action – which often involves jumping out of bed and running to the hospital.

Now consider this: the patient's phone call, the disruption of sleep, the time, the stress, and the drivetime to the hospital is totally uncompensated for that doctor. We can apply the same scenario to the poor pediatricians who deal with screaming babies and hysterical mothers at 4 a.m., forcing them to practice late night veterinary medicine from afar since the kid does not speak …yet.

As our South Florida pediatrician relates:

"As a child, I was interested in veterinary school. My school counselor discouraged me, but I knew I wanted a career in medicine. I chose general pediatrics – straightforward, primary care. I could see a case and find a cure or a healing quickly.

"The healthcare system is not properly run. We do not have one system, but three: a socialized system, a fee-for-service system, and an insurance system. When physicians complain, they get no empathy from a public that does not see them as sympathetic as compared to their peers like C.P.A.'s, attorneys, etc. Yet physicians face more obstacles than their peers, especially in primary care when it comes to compensation and reimbursement for work. Much of our work is NOT reimbursed.

"I agree with Dr. Badia that the healthcare business takes advantage of doctors' altruism. An attorney bills for everything, but a doctor cannot.

The day is not over when the last patient leaves. At that point, it is on to emails, calls, and education of patients. But we do not get paid for this. Patients do not realize how much it costs to run a practice. They complain about a co-pay because they have insurance. Yet the doctor only gets a fraction of the cost of the visit. Medicine is the only profession that works this way. Yet someone is getting the profits, for example, insurance CEOs and executives. The middleman (insurance) makes it hard for patients to appreciate the value of something like a doctor visit.

"I am part of a three-woman practice with an office manager and an assistant who works with insurance issues to get the maximum reimbursement. Our office generates $400,000 in overhead – more than 50 percent of our expenses. The cost to run the practice is MORE than our take-home pay. Diagnostic and educational services cannot be billed to insurance because they are not procedural. The minimum reimbursement is $50 to $100 dollars for things like taking wax out of a baby's ear or the cauterization of an umbilical hernia. From one colleague to another, I wish I were reimbursed for my time. I see anywhere from 24 to 36 patients a day, four to five patients per hour, and that includes sick visits and well child visits. During lunch, I use my time to answer calls, respond to emails, and finish charting while I eat.

"Although I give free advice to parents (for example if a child has diarrhea or has not had a bowel movement in several days) over the phone, it's deemed inappropriate to charge for them. Sometimes the calls are as lengthy as 15 minutes, which means the person should have just come into the office with their child. On an average day, I am on the phone for 30 to 60 minutes. On a great day, it is 10 to 15 minutes.

"There is less acuity with emails because they are non-urgent issues; the problem is high volume. They flow in constantly because with technology these days it is so easy. People abuse it. It is not an emergency and it could have waited until the next visit, but it is free and easy, and people want answers NOW. It is free medical advice. There should be a way to incorporate costs into an insurance-run practice, but it is expected of us to do it. And we do. Patients do not think for a moment that it is inappropriate to talk for five minutes on the phone or send an email. Due to the sheer volume, one to two hours of my day is not reimbursed.

"I'm 49 years old and I plan to work another decade. My husband is a surgeon and we could live on his income, but I want to have a profession. I believe medicine is a noble profession. Even though my paycheck is shitty it is still a great profession. We practice great care. Not all practices return calls and emails. We even have an on-call doctor for emergencies that is abused. My profession is charity. When I come home, I do not have energy for my kids and it is because of the two extra hours I spend at the office. My children tell me, 'We're never going to be doctors!' Despite the problems, I like helping people and the profession. I like using my brain in the care and wellbeing of children."

The Culture of Free Work

Physicians have a solid work ethic. I do not know if the public really understands it, but it plays into the whole compensation aspect. When I got the lawyer letter, it elicited strong feelings within me, like "Jesus, I don't know a single profession where we are worked this hard and then a lot of what we do isn't paid." I mean, this lawyer did not do much for that $250. But if you get a lawyer on the phone, you will receive a bill in the mail within 48 hours. They are great at tracking their billable hours and invoicing their clients for them. Contrast that with that OB/GYN who gets up at 3 a.m. to care for a patient: they will probably get some flat fee from the patient's insurance carrier to deliver that baby, but they will not be compensated for the early morning call and the required decision-making skills to care for their patient based on years of experience and study. Not one red cent.

When you consider the amount of decision-making involved, it is staggering. This is real work that requires expertise. As a doctor, you have a responsibility to decide what is best for your patient based on your years of education. And you give that away for *free* because that is how the system works.

While there is a little bit of rebellion among physicians, it has not reached what Tony Robbins, a popular motivational public figure and author, would term "threshold." Many physicians (mostly primary care doctors), have forged concierge service practices where cash-paying patients can register to have more direct access to them. Patients may pay an annual set fee with additional payments for specific encounters at an agreed upon fee schedule. An alternate arrangement is for lower annual fees where the physician continues to bill insurance at contracted or OON (out of network) rates because they are providing added value, including direct access, in many cases. The final model is a throwback to traditional fee-for-service where the patient pays all fees at time of care, but then submits claims to their carrier for reimbursement, with the understanding that the insurance company will probably not pay for much of the care rendered.

The latter is a cruel twist on the old "taste of your own medicine" adage and permits the patient to fully understand what their healthcare professionals have been dealing with for decades. There is a burgeoning movement to require patients to bear a significant component of their care costs, but this only works if their insurance premiums go down, assuming that their employer pays less, and then passes along that savings to their employees. As you might expect in our litigious society, there are legal pitfalls for delivering this type of excellent and attentive care since it can be claimed that other patients are being "abandoned". Naturally, anything the physician does will be highly scrutinized and even distorted. It is par for the course in our profession.

With respect to specialists, we do not yet have a robust concierge approach to care, although several companies have been trying to formulate a model with limited market penetration. I have devoted significant time and man hours to create accessibility for patients via my website, well before it was common practice to even have a URL address. I felt the direct access to me, although not by traditional telephone, would help me grow my practice while providing a significant service to the community. Furthermore, I enjoy patient education, especially in the arena of dispelling myths, and an informative website is the ideal forum for this mission.

I soon learned that a subset of patients would often draw me into long back and forth discussions about their condition, without benefit of their history or an examination, abusing my good will and even putting me at risk of liability since this is perceived as indirect medical advice by a professional. At this juncture, I try not to spend a lot of time answering questions, as I previously did, but I do feel the easy access to a specialist is valuable. I pride myself on that. I would often send a wealth of information, but most of those patients would not even respond, let alone schedule an appointment for a proper consultation. For that, I never received any compensation. Now, my own office staff would admonish me for that kind of behavior, knowing full well what my time and expertise is worth. These days, I direct patients to a telemedicine visit, something I was doing years before the COVID-19 pandemic. Prior to the pandemic, which necessitated more flexibility, there existed a plethora of regulatory and legal hurdles that slowed adoption of this methodology. Ironic that it took a destructive virus to allow physicians to provide care with less interference.

Most patients do not even answer the phone when we call them after *their* email inquiry. They submit a question, or even request a consultation via my practice website, I *personally* respond at whatever hour I see their message, and it curiously stops there. This is the public responsibility I talk about if we are going to change healthcare. If you do not value a clinician's time, do not email them, call the office, or schedule an appointment that you will not show up for. For that behavior and oversight, I am charged a full fee by my hair-cutter, yet there is outrage when my staff tried to do the same when a patient "no-shows" for a consultation – or worse, an hour-long intense physical therapy session. What should that therapist do with the time allocated to the inconsiderate patient? Cut hair? We ALL must do our part.

For my telemedicine consults, I recently termed #teleorthopedics, my staff charges a flat fee which patients can pay with a simple credit card transaction like PayPal. In return, the patient in need receives my undivided attention, one-on-one. They get to see me while I impart my expertise, address all their questions, assisted by screen sharing that enables me to show them animation of a procedure or explain the relevant anatomy. Amazingly, I get paid in a good old-fashioned way: at time of service, without delay, at what both parties consider a fair rate. There is no insurance carrier, T.P.A. or extraneous facility to skim off my work, knowledge, and clinical experience. Sure, it is still much less than what a high-priced lawyer makes, and I still have my high overhead, due to robust staffing and infrastructure for the majority of my patients whom I must palpate, examine, or cast.

Dr. Robert Terrill

"People think physicians are rolling in it. That is not true. There is a significant number of nurses here at my hospital that make more than the doctors. I think it is a lack of respect. Athletes are entertainers, and if not for their athletic gifts, probably many of them would be in jail. For example, Roger Clemens was obviously a gifted pitcher, but he also had some skeletons in the closet. When I was a resident, I was part of the team of doctors for the Red Sox many years, so I speak from experience. I can also tell you that some of the players were down to earth.

"But in terms of public perception of doctors there is a disconnection. Let us revisit the CEO position, this time the CEO of a hospital. I am generalizing a bit but there is not a CEO of a single hospital who is making less than one million dollars per year, and many of them make significantly more money than that. I did some stuff in Pittsburgh where U.P.M.C. is a "nonprofit" and the CEO earned $8.54 million in 2019. The CEO of the

University of Pennsylvania Health Systems, another nonprofit, made over $2.5 million in 2016. And you think, 'Wait a minute, what is that? How are they doing that?' You know, Philadelphia is getting reamed because they cannot tax all of that 'nonprofit' property but oh, by the way, the CEO is making millions in profit.

"I don't argue that the healthcare should be a right. It is why I lean more towards a universal system like England's – be it good or bad – because everybody gets base care. If you choose to purchase above that, you can. In the United States, Americans are in for a rude an awakening with the brain drain that will take place in medicine over the next five to eight years. Patients will not have access. It is going to be, "Now serving #107 and you will not have a relationship with your physician. I mean, I would not want to practice the way the multi-specialty group at my hospital does, where the surgeons often do not see the patient before surgery. It is bizarre. I know because my office manager's mother-in-law had some arthritis surgery and she met the surgeon in the holding area. She had been cared for by the nurse practitioner since day one with medicine injection therapy, braces, and this and that. And she met him in the holding area. He did the surgery and never saw her again.

"But that is what's happening. I would not be surprised if that is what some of the total joint surgeons are doing. That is not why I went into medicine. I went into medicine because I want to help people. I want to work with them together to get better. If I wanted to be a surgical technician, then I would be a surgical technician. I would not be interacting with the patient at all. Yet this is kind of the new model. That is what is being taught to the residents. You cannot be in practice, you must have a P.A. You do the surgery, then the P.A. sees the patient post-op. Patients want personal contact with their doctor, but I think it is going to disappear.

"Getting back to the single payer system, think of the amount of money that could be saved when you are not spending 30 percent of your premium dollar in overhead to cover the salaries of all these different middle managers. How much more care can a doctor provide? Could you save some money? Could you provide care to more people that are not getting care right now?

"My son works in Jacksonville Florida at the Nemours Clinic as a pediatric orthopedic P.A. He loves taking care of patients, but he said, 'Dad, for me to be where you started, it would take me 10 years and I'd be a half a million dollars in debt.' My mom left me some money that I put it in a trust for the kids. It paid for his P.A. school and living expenses, so he graduated without any debt. Medical schools recognize the problem, which is why N.Y.U. just had a huge capital campaign. They raised enough money that if you are accepted to the school, you will not be paying.

"I think they need to. I was at a meeting this past Saturday for the History of Medicine Committee for the Worcester District Medical Society. We had a lecture by a historian about the history of medicine in the 17th, 18th, and into the 19th centuries. It was interesting, talking about the difference in healthcare between now and then. In the late 1800s, 80 or 90 percent of care was provided in your home. And the only people who went to the hospital were the people who did not have any money.

"And it is the reverse now. It is a fascinating difference because I am also a third-generation healthcare provider. My great-grandfather was a general practitioner in Maine, from around 1892 to 1931. My dad was a general and thoracic surgeon in the military. And then myself and my son James. I have some of my great grandfather's stuff. I have some of his old books, his old glasses, and a print of a painting that used to hang over his desk. I am grateful to have some of that neat history.

"I am looking at some of the old stuff he did, like the poultices (cataplasm) and decoction. That is what they were doing. It was unusual to have specialists. He would go to Boston to see what the surgeons were doing. And he did basic orthopedics. I think probably part of what got my dad interested in medicine is that he was living with his grandparents one summer when he was around six years old, and my great grandfather was called to an accident where a guy had broken his leg and he had to straighten it.

"He had to put the guy under anesthesia to reduce it. Since they did not have a hospital, he had my dad at six years old dripping ether for this guy, obviously under his close monitoring, until he was sufficiently sedated. Then he was able to straighten the leg and put it in a cast. And of course, if you are a six-year-old, you are like, 'Man, this is cool. Yeah, I want to do that.' I am sure that is what got my dad interested.

"I never realized, for example, Arthur Shaw, my great grandfather, went to the med school at Bowdoin College in Brunswick, Maine, where I attended undergrad. Bowdoin also had the sixth med school in the country. This past summer, I had my 40th college reunion. I went to the archives, contacted them, and I was able to look at my great grandfather's thesis. They have a signature book, so I looked at my great grandfather's, my father's, and my signature (when you could actually read it), along with my wife's signature. I am in the process of collecting stuff for ancestry. And one of the things I did not understand was my great grandfather had written his thesis on acute articular rheumatism. I said, 'Wow, that's kind of weird. His great grandson is an orthopedic surgeon who takes care of rheumatoid arthritis.'

"As I researched, I found out that his father had been in the Civil War and developed rheumatic fever, followed by acute articular rheumatism, and was mustered out of the Union Army. He was disabled, but in those days, we did not have anything like Social Security. He became a farmer in rural Maine. And his son wrote this thesis later and then, you know, 100 years later or more, the great grandson read it. That is the part I love. I am glad my son is doing medicine. He and I have been on five medical missions. We started going about a year after my wife passed, and we were looking around for things we could do. It has been wonderful. It is the purest healthcare: you are not dealing with insurance companies, and you have people who are truly motivated to get better. You are not necessarily solving all the problems in the world, but you are helping them. If you can teach some of the local orthopedic surgeons some of these techniques, maybe that will help future patients because they will know more what to do. We have been once to Africa, and four times to the Dominican Republic. I was going to go to Tanzania this summer, but the trip would have been two-and-a-half weeks, and I would be getting married two weeks after I got back. It was just a little bit too close together, so I declined.

"And then somebody called me and wanted me to go down to Honduras. They were getting back the day before I was getting married. I said, "I think my wife's going to kill me if I don't show up to my wedding." But I will continue to do medical missions. I was talking to Dr. Badia about that. I think he was over in Africa with some with some colleagues. I mean, physicians in general love to serve. And it is something the hand society has encouraged, starting with the former president of ASSH, Dr. Scott H. Kozin. It is something I will continue to do. If I can do some with my son, that would be great. Either way, I want to keep going to these places. The one in Tanzania sounded cool because it is a medical school and a big hospital at the base of Mount Kilimanjaro in a town called Moshi. You would do lectures, teaching the residents, make rounds, and perform some surgeries. A mix of things. That would be fun."

It is obvious what moves Dr. Terrill and so many of us. You can almost feel his beaming emotion as he describes serving others. This is the essence of being a physician. I plan to recruit him for Ghana perhaps, but more likely Ecuador, Quito specifically, as I was tasked with developing the Latin American program for Groupe International Chirurgiens Amis de la Main (GICAM). It would be an honor to serve others – together.

INSURING TELEMEDICINE

Post COVID-19, it appears that many insurance companies will reimburse for telemedicine services, which brings us back to the same problem with delayed payments and partial reimbursement. Their compensation will probably amount to much less than a patient is willing to pay me out of their own pocket. Of course, the for-profit health insurance companies want to make money, even though they are not the ones answering the questions and addressing the pathology. Their transition will be slow and arduous, oddly enough. I feel a bit vindicated because to me, it makes the simple but profound statement: "My time is valuable." That has been overlooked, which is grossly unfair to our entire profession. This is my small way of making up for the injustice.

The insurance companies have gotten away with seizing upon our altruism because most physicians are generous. You heard Dr. Terrill's account of how he prefers to spend his time and utilize his knowledge. I can tell you that over the years I would suck it up because I knew this was what the patient needed. Now, I work by specific guidelines to ensure that when I see patients, there will not be interference – as opposed to an "open door" policy, because once I see them, I feel obligated to them. After I have developed a doctor-patient relationship with them, I feel I must take care of them. However, if I allowed this to become the norm, my practice would go under.

My colleagues and I deserve to make an excellent living. I am not ashamed to say it. I have no regrets about sacrificing my late-teens and the decade of my 20s to my intense education and training, but it has a certain value. The work I do is important and vital. Yet in our society, there is no outrage when other professionals charge an excessive amount. We simply accept it.

For example, I hired a diesel mechanic to assess engine issues on my boat. Guess how much his company invoiced me just to do an assessment? $1,200. Yes, I understand a boat is a luxury, but we somehow tolerate these excesses. Many times, a skilled tradesman will charge for "travel time." What is the message here? That the client is responsible for the location of their home office or what other job they took so that their drivetime, which I cannot even verify, amounts to X? I could just imagine if I charged a patient – forget a third-party payor – for my "drive time". Oh yeah, the 30 minutes it took to drive at 2 a.m. to reattach that ring avulsion injury? Then, if I am lucky, to go back home since I was sometimes up all night and would go straight to the office to see patients. Imagine charging for all that. Push doctors enough and that MAY just happen.

In the aftermath of Hurricane Katrina, followed by Hurricane Norma in Miami, I remember the opportunists that came out in droves to cut away my destroyed landscaping for thousands of dollars. Some crews came from as far away as Alabama. Like the COVID-19 scavengers, they saw a way to gouge for profit. Thank goodness the medical profession does not operate (pun intended) that way. Gee, you REALLY need medical care in the aftermath of that hurricane or earthquake. Now we are going to stick it to you. See, you cannot even comprehend that coming from a caregiver. Physician, nurse, therapist, etc.

Following the hurricane, I consulted with a tree surgeon because my gumbo limbo tree, a gorgeous specimen with brown velvet appearing bark, cracked at the base. He stuck his arm up along the trunk base roots, all the while uttering "Hmm, umm, eh," like Bugs Bunny playing a doctor. No joke. I am not making this up. After literally three minutes, he announced, "Can't save her." While I was not devastated, I was bummed because it was my favorite tree. Then came the $350 bill. Okay, I get it: the tree surgeon possesses specific expertise. I wonder what would have happened if insurance had to pay the bill? Oh right…windstorm covers none of that. The ultimate irony is that the tree surgeon gave me an erroneous opinion because I soon learned that the Gumbo Limbo has amazing regenerative properties. We could have harvested a large branch and stuck it into the ground and salvaged part of it. Should I have sued for malpractice? I mean, it was my favorite tree. You get the point.

All professions and trades have intrinsic value. Reimbursement should be commensurate with that value, along with the amount of time and effort to prepare for and pursue that line of work. It is a logical conclusion. When youth read the absurd multi-million-dollar contracts a pro athlete gets, it distorts the value of traditional professions that require years of study and effort. The same goes for today's entertainers and certainly the emerging "job" of social media influencers or even You-Tubers whom the younger generation worships. Our children take notice.

Although most of us do not have regrets about our extensive education and training, our compensation must be considered, given the critical fountain of knowledge we possess. Compared to other professions, our role is vital, and it must be cherished. Somehow, we have lost sight of that as a society, even though people still esteem physicians. However, while a certain aura of respect for the profession remains, it is not commensurate anymore with our compensation, compared to many other disciplines. One silver lining to the COVID-19 pandemic could be a paradigm shift among the public towards physicians and other clinicians, but that remains to be seen.

Chapter 14 – Where do we go from here? Healthcare 3.0

"The best way to predict the future is to create it."
– Abraham Lincoln

What definitive solutions can I offer for the U.S. healthcare crisis? I do not know. Truly.

Outlining a solution or a series of firm recommendations was not the intent of my book. There are already some truly enlightening works on this subject, some of which are listed in my references. I have read most of them and certainly have my own thoughts. However, change will not come from me or any other practitioner. It must come from the end-user of healthcare: the patient.

My goal was for you, the reader, to understand our challenges via a series of stories, anecdotes, and vignettes that clearly illustrate the hurdles to practicing high quality, cost-effective medicine. I am sure by now that the reader has some of their own ideas, formulated as you read some of the outrageous occurrences that continue to plague us every day in the trenches.

However, I have reached one paradoxical conclusion that disturbs me. We blame the insurance companies for their bureaucracy and interference in the doctor-patient relationship. We fault government, at all levels, for not prioritizing the fight to establish more humane and cost-effective care, while they almost ignore the very people who deliver it. We chastise big pharma and medical supply companies for their outrageous margins. I get it.

But why *should* they change? Life is good for them. If you are reading this and you work in any of those industries, you would want to keep the status quo. Let us face it: the average person is not so altruistic, especially when money is involved. Hence, the shift will not come from these sectors.

The change must come from us. By "us" I mean ALL clinicians, previously called "providers." I yearn for the day when that term, "provider" is used solely in the insurance industry to refer to the professionals delivering the care to patients. It is fine in that scenario; I just prefer that it not be used by my patients, colleagues, or the public.

The change must also come from those receiving the care -- the patients, which includes all of us. Every healthcare industry professional, whether an insurance exec, big pharma C-suite leader or even a malpractice plaintiff attorney, will consume healthcare at one point. I am certain all of us want it delivered with expertise, efficiency, cost-effectiveness, and compassion. We all deserve the last part. That is what separates our professions from the ones whose primary goal is to earn money, and the reason most doctors participate in a medical mission or at least provide free and indigent care in their community at one time or another. We touched on that only briefly and I could devote a whole book to those experiences with tons of contributors. We must recognize and honor that.

The COVID-19 pandemic has galvanized the medical profession to stand united, demand fair treatment, and regain our proper place in society. We have also seen that the public, the potential pool of patients, has recognized the importance of our role in society. While we are not heroes, the public and even popular media has come to see us through those lenses again.

The question is, how long will this sentiment last? Will it inspire us to seek true healthcare reform? That remains to be answered but long before the pandemic, I was struggling with issues I wanted to bring to light. I wanted to do this in a manner where both groups – the beleaguered clinician and the potential patient – can relate to the issue as brought forth through simple stories. This is my forum and the timing could not be much better.

As I stated unabashedly, I do not have the solution. It will take a combination of bold initiatives to move the needle. This will require not only great ideas but across-the-board collaboration. I believe the genesis will be from the grassroots, from a public who will be roused to demand change. Perhaps this will stem from a 2-nanometer virus but, it is far more likely that recognizing the issues and openly speaking about them will encourage intelligent and motivated entrepreneurs to propose and enact the solutions that are already present. However, we must remove the barriers to adoption. As stated, the current stakeholders have little incentive to change. The public must demand it, debate it on social media, and prioritize it as a goal.

How to achieve that? Education and awareness. The issues my contributors and I have outlined in the preceding chapters will hopefully inspire debate, controversy, and even outrage.

I have read numerous books on our healthcare challenges to gain a bird's eye perspective. To absorb startling facts and figures about the pervasiveness of exorbitant healthcare spending and inefficiencies. I am not an authority, but I do battle the problems every day with my patients. The mere fact that it is difficult to dialogue with some of the trailblazers in healthcare reform is a problem unto itself. I reached out to many of the authors of books, websites, and papers that I read to volunteer as another foot soldier in this struggle. I will say the engagement and response were tepid. It reminded me of similar challenges I have had with my own colleagues in our own microcosm of healthcare in a small city. It is a monumental task and the reason I have become convinced that change will come from the public itself, not our profession, as startling as that may be.

Where Might We Start?

As clinicians, we *must* start collaborating for a change. This means that if there are prudent ideas on how to improve healthcare efficiency and cost-effectiveness, we should embrace them and help each other (imagine that). The current powers controlling healthcare know that we are competitive to a fault, and we need to acquiesce a bit to each other, even when we may not fully agree. I continue to live this at our center in Miami and we would all benefit if we could row the boat together.

We need to understand what the word "value" means. Healthcare bureaucrats frequently throw the catch phrase, Value-based healthcare around without even speaking to the people who could deliver that value. Our OrthoNOW® cofounder, Justin Irizarry loves to quote Warren Buffet when he said, "Price is what you pay. Value is what you get." We are way too focused on arguing about how much care costs, and who is going to pay for it, as opposed to what you get for that unit cost. Hence the ridiculous stories about E.R. care at various prices. Think $500 dollars per stitch for that busted lip.

This brings us directly to the growing concept of price transparency. It nurtures competition and the delivery of value. Yes, many of the players will either adapt or get out of the game. And it should not be a game. An executive order from our nation's President directs all related federal agencies to increase transparency in healthcare pricing. An order is a directive, and not an actual change in the law. Already this order has been challenged by way of lawsuits. Of course. The current stakeholders have a lot to lose but if the public got behind this, we would almost all stand to win. You can already envision that this will go nowhere. But if the public speaks up, and the media cares to let practicing clinicians weigh in, we might see progress. I have commented that the current stewards of our healthcare system are not interested in this dramatic change. This book is one small attempt to force that dialogue.

Transparency will also lay bare the incredible web of intermediaries and obstacles, if you will, within the healthcare delivery process. Revamping the entire notion of authorization will alone dramatically decrease the cost and convoluted nature of providing care. Over decades, I and my orthopedic colleagues have witnessed the presence of numerous, unqualified middlemen within the complex patient journey. Our OrthoNOW® system is just one solution to dramatically change the landscape of initial musculoskeletal care. I have shown how the lack of engagement, whether by insurers, colleagues and even patient groups have not allowed this concept to flourish. Good ideas cannot bring dividends if not adopted, or at least embraced. This is just one example and many more have been brought to light within our OrthoFounders Group. I can only imagine how many like-minded groups within other specialties exist and the similar challenges they must face.

Streamlining care and facilitating that the patient sees the "right clinician at the right time" will significantly diminish costs, not to mention time. We all know time is money. This also assumes that more appropriate care, in the way of tests, diagnostic studies, pharmacotherapy, and even surgical procedures will naturally follow since the suitable physician can deem what is necessary. This assumes ethical practice by those physicians, but with an efficient and transparent process, the unscrupulous can be easily identified. The current system allows them to hide in the weeds and rob our system blind.

Ultimately, we must decide where our priorities lie as a society. We have seen that an immense amount of money is wasted in paying for the cumbersome process of receiving appropriate and timely healthcare. We are willing to pour money into entertainment and consumer goods that suddenly become less relevant when we are sick. When our children or parents get injured, will we evade the opportunists and parasites that siphon off money from the total pool that should go to us, as patients, when the need arises? Will we realize that we need to support and fairly compensate the folks who provide the necessary care, and forego that new plasma TV, aesthetic BOTOX® injection, or meritless lawsuit? The COVID-19 pandemic exposed multiple problems. It remains to be seen if we learn some lessons and begin to shift our priorities and our focus as a people.

It is up to us.

I will present some different perspectives on the concrete changes we can introduce to the healthcare system that might move us in the right direction. As an orthopedist, I identified a problem, namely that patients were not being seen by the right clinician at the right time. Simple concept, right? Well, the execution of a solution, OrthoNOW®, was difficult enough but getting real engagement from the community at multiple levels was the real challenge. Our Co-Founder, Justin Irizarry, will outline the value proposition of our solution that serves a real need.

Before that, I will present recommendations shared by a wide spectrum of healthcare professionals, from therapists to surgeon colleagues to a big hospital executive. They all echo a need for change and present some very compelling ideas that we, the public should consider, discuss in our own circles, and perhaps embrace.

I have had the opportunity to travel to 80 countries, lecture in all seven continents, and humbly observe a grand variety of healthcare systems in action. I do not have one specific recommendation but will tell you that perhaps the single biggest change we can enact in our system is embodied within several countries.

Converting health insurance companies back to non-profit status is perhaps the most impactful change we can make with one fell swoop of legislation.

Let us look at one country which exemplifies this model through the eyes of Mr. T. R. Reid.

The German Healthcare System as a Possible Solution

In his 2010 New York Times bestselling book, *The Healing of America: A Global Quest for Better, Cheaper, and Fairer Healthcare*, author T.R. Reid examines the healthcare systems of industrialized countries around the world. One noteworthy system was founded in Germany by Otto von Bismarck 137 years ago.

Notes Reid, "Always an innovator, Bismarck originated several of the programs that make up the modern welfare state. His Sickness Insurance Law, enacted by the Reichstag in 1883, was the world's first national healthcare system. It was a program of mandatory medical insurance, with premiums paid jointly by employers and workers. For ease of administration, the worker's share was withheld automatically from his pay. To this day, the 1883 structure remains a model for nations around the world. American workers who buy a health insurance plan through their employer,

422 · ALEJANDRO BADIA, M.D., F.A.C.S.

with the premium withheld from their paycheck, are using the Bismarck model of healthcare.

"In its home country today, the Bismarck healthcare system guarantees medical care to just about all 82 million Germans and to millions of 'guest workers,' legal or not, who live in the country. The package of benefits is generous, covering doctors, dentists, chiropractors, physical therapists, psychiatrists, hospitals opticians, all prescriptions, nursing homes, health club memberships, and even vacation trips to a spa (when suggested by a doctor). The quality of care is world-class; Germany stands at or near the top in all comparative healthcare studies. Because the supply of doctors and hospitals is ample, there is no 'queue' for treatment; on measures such as 'waiting time for emergency care' and 'waiting time for elective/non-emergency surgery,' Germans spend less time waiting for care than Americans do. Patients can choose any doctor or hospital, and insurance must pay the bill. And every German has a choice among some two-hundred different private insurance plans, which compete vigorously even though the prices for insurance are fixed.

"It's worth emphasizing that the insurance plans are private entities. The general practitioners who make up the bulk of Germany's medical profession are also private businesspeople, working in private clinics. German hospitals are mainly charity or municipal operations, but there is a growing business in private, for-profit hospital chains. The private insurance plans negotiate prices with the private medical clinics and the hospitals; these are private commercial agreements, with little government input. In many areas of medical practice, there's less government control of medical care in Germany than in the United States."

The serious downside, as the author points out, is that Germany has one of the world's more expensive healthcare systems, consuming nearly 11 percent of the nation's G.D.P. Although higher than other European nations, it is still less than the United States, where we spend 17.7 percent on healthcare for fewer choices and less coverage. To pay for its expensive system, "Germany strictly controls payments to doctors and hospitals, and the system is constantly looking for ways to cut spending. Among other things, German healthcare has far lower administrative costs than the U.S. system. The advent in 2008 of a universal smart card ("the digital health card") has eliminated much paperwork and reduced administrative costs even further.

"As the cost of medicine has risen, the insurance premium has risen as well. Germans pay about 15 percent of their paycheck for health insurance, split between the worker and the employer. That is almost exactly equal to what an American worker and his employer pay in Social Security and Medicare taxes. But the German worker gets a better deal. Most American workers also have to pay a health insurance premium ranging from 2 to 10 percent of pay, in addition to those payroll taxes.

"A private health insurance plan, funded by payroll withholding, that pays hospitals and doctors directly on a fee-for-service basis...sounds very much like American-style employer-based medical insurance. But the German version of Bismarck is different in three fundamental ways:

"1. First and foremost, the sickness funds are nonprofit entities; they exist to pay people's medical bills, not to pay dividends to shareholders. Thus, they don't have the same incentive that the U.S. insurance industry has to limit the people they cover, or to deny claims; in fact, the German insurance plans are required to accept all applicants and to pay any claims submitted by a recognized doctor or hospital. They don't have to pad their premiums to pay for a claims-review bureaucracy or to allow for profit. The result: the sickness funds have about one-third the administrative expenses that are normal in American health insurance. That makes the whole German insurance system much cheaper.

"2. While insurance is purchased and paid for through payroll deduction, Germans don't lose their coverage when they lose their jobs. Government unemployment benefits automatically cover the insurance premium, so the worker has the same insurance coverage while he looks for a new job – no matter how long it takes to find one.

"3. Unlike American workers, who are restricted to the limited selection of insurance plans offered by their employers, Germans can sign up with any sickness fund in the country and can change to a different plan almost anytime they want. To a large extent, the funds all mimic one another. They are all required by law to offer the mandated package of benefits, from cradle to nursing home. Since the premium is a percentage of pay, the premium stays the same, no matter which fund a worker chooses. And yet, there is heated competition among these nonprofit insurance plans. Some compete by promising to pay all clams within five days; some offer benefits beyond the basic package, like exotic Asian therapies or free neonatal nursing care in the home after a baby is born or longer stays in those health spas."

Reid quotes German economist Karl Lauerbach about the German citizen's free choice of any plan and the resulting competition among health insurers: "Americans tend to think the profit motive is the only driver of competition. But our Krankenkassen compete because the executives earn more money, and higher prestige, if they have a larger pool of insured members. So, we have universal coverage, and nobody can be turned down because of a preexisting illness. You have the required package of benefits, so the insurer can't deny a claim for any covered treatment. And then you have this competition to attract more customers."

The Healing of America presented numerous countries' healthcare models through the lens of one journalist who was simply seeking care for an arthritic shoulder. It behooves us to review and analyze these systems with the aim of compiling pros and cons of each to bring real reform to our own American system.

A full review of these is beyond the scope of this book and was amply covered by Mr. Reid. I simply wanted to choose one as a sound example of what the possibilities can be. While I do not fully endorse the German system and have close friendships with many colleagues abroad who express their own reservations about it, it does exemplify one key feature: the pervasive interference, and resultant inefficiencies brought about by for-profit insurance companies exposes a serious conflict of interest. Rather than re-investing cost savings into further care, or even lowering prices, the publicly traded health insurance "businesses" must bring those profits to shareholders and investors. It is anathema to what healthcare should be.

Looking beyond the German model, our contributors bring forth a series of recommendations that we should all consider once we get serious about bringing forth a solution.

PROPOSALS FROM THE TRENCHES

Dr. Scott Sigman - Board-Certified Orthopedic Surgeon
https://scottasigmanmd.com/about-dr-sigman/

"Efficient quality care requires accountability and a collaborative effort. This is where ACO's – Accountable Care Organizations – were born. Essentially, an insurance company will provide the organization a single large sum of money to be used for all medical care and expenses for the population it covers. The entire organization needs to focus on what treatments work and analyze the cost of a certain technique, not just for the episode of care for an individual surgery, but the cost of any long-term lingering effects a treatment may have.

"For example, if the A.C.O. switches to an opioid sparing strategy, the cost of the initial pain management may go from $50 to $400. Yes, there is more cost to the system up front, but by employing an opioid-sparing strategy, you can eliminate all the costs associated with treatment of opioid addiction. The team needs to include doctors, nurses, and hospital and insurance administrators – all working toward a common goal of high-quality, cost-effective medicine.

"Many of these large employer groups are becoming self-insured. While they still use the insurance, it is only at the administrative level. These employer groups seek efficient, high-quality care that allows their employees to return to work and become productive members of society as soon as possible. They want to see the data.

- How much will the entire procedure cost?
- How long will our patients be in the hospital?
- What is the likelihood of a complication or a return to the OR?
- Are you willing to guarantee your work?

"In this effort, they will shop around to make the best possible business decision for their employees' healthcare.

"Transparency is crucial. Depending on what state you live in, or the hospital, one hospital can charge $75,000 for a total knee, while another hospital charges $25,000 for the same operation. So, the question becomes, 'Are you really getting three times more value?' And the answer is, of course not. We can effectively track outcomes. The goal is to provide high quality care that is cost efficient: that is the value equation. It requires teamwork with the approach that people get together, solve problems, create solutions, and eliminate variability.

"You can drive down the cost of these procedures and still get excellent outcomes. But at the same time, technology is expensive. We now use robots in the operating room. I can give you a couple of examples. I use a new patch that we use in the shoulder called the REGENETEN implant. It is made from the Achilles tendon of a cow. The cow DNA is eliminated, and you get a collagen scaffold that we lay over top of the rotator cuff. The implant itself costs $3,000. This seems expensive to the system. However, my patients that undergo surgery two days later are out of a sling, require no opioids and many of them are back to work in less than a week, becoming productive members of society much faster than traditional rotator cuff surgery. Sometimes spending the money up front on improved techniques winds up saving money to the system in its entirety not just the episode of care for the individual patient."

Dr. Sigman presents a utopian concept in healthcare, ACOs, that should work if there is actual innovation in HOW that care is delivered. Much of the focus has been on the profits made by the members which should inspire transformational changes in that care delivery but often suffers from the same challenges that I discussed in collaboration chapter.

I recall the challenges in having them understand, let alone embrace, the value proposition of a specialty center, telling me that a different motivation may be needed. In fact, one of the large ACOs in South Florida was managed by a friend of mine, who sadly passed, and now by a renowned cardiologist and friend, who was also open to discussion, yet nothing transpired. It will take a combination of some visionary physicians, along with good business operators, to bring real change via this platform. Perhaps it will come.

Dr. Sigman also espouses the use of certain technologies and methodologies that indeed can bring major downstream healthcare savings. The challenge is not only colleague adoption, but healthcare systems and certainly the payors, to also recognize this. I have the collagen patch, Regeneten® in my own shoulder, where it was placed weeks ago, and I felt no post-op pain due to the EXPAREL® administration he also discussed. No opiates for me or my patients. However, taking excellent products to the broader marketplace is a bigger task than you would think, due to the obstacles and barriers I discussed throughout this book.

Dr. George Balfour – Hand and Upper Extremity Surgeon
https://www.georgebalfourmd.com/

"Why is healthcare so expensive? We can date the destruction of the American healthcare system to the early 1990s, when all the insurance companies like Blue Cross, Blue Shield and others were converted from not-for-profit mutual companies to for-profit stock companies. At the time, the health insurance CEOs gave themselves a "Happy Day" with billion-dollar bonuses for their conversion. Of the total health care dollar, which is in this country is $3.3 trillion, it is estimated $1.3 trillion is waste and some 10- to- 15 percent goes to profit margins of the insurance industry and the drug industry right off the top. And that works out to be about a half a trillion dollars.

"Another huge cause of waste is the billing and collection system. It takes about eight to 10 percent for my company or any other private physician practice to send out a bill, and another eight to 10 percent for the Blue Cross Blue Shields of this world to deny that bill. I once had a conversation with former presidential candidate Michael Dukakis, who described the experience in Massachusetts, when looking at the billing and collecting system and AIDS. He estimates the waste alone to be on the order of 15 percent – another three-fourths of a trillion dollars.

"E.M.R., which we were all forced to invest in, is a huge contributing factor to skyrocketing healthcare costs. None of these E.M.R. systems talk to each other. It would have been smarter and cheaper for the federal government to buy one system and give it to the entire country. Add the whole country to one system, where we could all read each other.

"It is important for the public to understand that physician fees – which account for no more than 10 percent of the entire healthcare dollar – are not to blame for increased costs. Trying to reduce physician fees is a waste because it is not a high point of the system. If we cut 10 percent of all physicians' fees arbitrarily, we would save one-tenth of one percent. If we cut costs to billing and collections, we would save 15 percent. It is the math that tells us you do not reduce costs in healthcare by looking at physicians or medical care itself. Duplication of studies, for example, while an expense, is not the big issue.

"Therefore, we cure the U.S. healthcare system by focusing on the big problems: excessive profits in the insurance industry. I suggest that we convert them to public utilities, which have controlled profits. We must rein in the excesses, including markedly overpriced medications, which represent a bottom third of the healthcare dollar. To prove it, pick any drug. Look up the cost at the neighborhood pharmacy or pick up a phone and call them to get the price. Then, look it up in Britain or in France and that same drug will cost one-half to one-third of that. One-third of the healthcare dollar in the United States goes to medications. That is $1.3 trillion. Roughly half of that is waste. So, there is another $6 trillion we can save.

"In summary, you do not control healthcare costs by looking at physicians and hospitals, but rather, the profit margins of the big players: health healthcare insurance companies and pharmaceutical companies. They are the heavy hitters. There certainly could be efficiency found in actual medical care; it just will not change the total dollars very much.

There are savings to be made with hospitals. That would add a few percentages. But the biggest dollars can be saved by going after the healthcare insurance companies and the drug companies."

Dr. Balfour echoes what many "providers" feel – that the major cost driver of healthcare is not coming from us in the trenches. He throws some impressive numbers around, but one thing is clear: further cutting reimbursement to the ones who do the work is not only foolish but would not even move the needle in terms of cost savings.

Dr. A.J. DiGiovanni – Retired General and Vascular Surgeon

"At one time, healthcare was an underpaid industry. The hospital returns were poor in terms of what they were able to get from insurance companies in remuneration for patient care. That has improved steadily, and now it is almost inflationary. Some of the inflationary expansion was valid to compensate the underpaid people in medicine, including medical technicians and nurses. Back then, the pay scale was around $270 a month for a nurse, which was about one-half of the going scale for graduate people, whether they were in the industry or otherwise. Today, nurses can make a decent living and they deserve every penny they get.

"The inflation in medicine is partially caused by the fact that there are limited payers now, and a big payer is the government. Once that occurs, inflation just keeps spiraling. I am afraid it is going to spiral even more as it becomes a political football: who is going to give more and more services for less? Well, somebody must pay for that. And it is going to be the subscriber.

"The broader private insurance industry has been narrowed over the years and there are fewer insurance programs that can be purchased outside of Medicare. It's a shame that inflation has spawned like that because it brings other factors into play, like restrictions on the amount of time patients can stay in the hospital and requirements for patients to be admitted to the hospital on the same day of surgery, which in general, is not a good thing.

"It is true that years ago in the 60s and 70s, when hospital stays were relatively inexpensive, there was an overstay commitment. At the time, post-op hernia patients might be in the hospital for five, six, or seven days ...which was really overdone. There was a valid reason to adapt shorter hospital stays to keep the cost of medical care within reasonable limits. But right now, it is too expensive in the hospital. As I mentioned, some of that

expense is necessary to compensate formerly undercompensated personnel. That is an example of a cost increase based on real issues, although
Medicare created inflationary costs. The administrative functions of a hospital expanded, and now there are a billion people working in a hospital
in an administrative capacity.

"When I started at Misericordia Hospital, a 400-bed facility in West
Philadelphia, there was one accountant. One. He had an assistant who
came in after high school. That was the administrative staff at the time.
And things ran smoothly, believe it or not. When the accountant dared to
ask for a raise, they let him go. However, in the years following the passage
of Medicare, twelve types of accountants had to be hired to handle the
complexities that arose in medicine and advanced care.

"Most of the expansion that took place should never have happened.
We have excessive administrative costs that could be curtailed to a great
degree. But when you have single payers like Medicare, there is no way
you can control inflation. Politicians outdo one another in terms of making
promises about what they can do for their constituents to get elected. It
creates even more spiraling inflation.

"I recently came across one of the most ironic headlines I have ever
read in a newspaper: *More Administrators Needed to Keep Costs Down.*
What a ridiculous premise. First, costs are too high because there are too
many of them already. I sometimes quip that if you put a big computer in
central Philadelphia, you could probably manage all Philadelphia hospitals without the administrative expense we have now. That is probably not
true, but on the other hand, expansion of the administrative process has
expanded costs beyond what is necessary. The thing that is irksome is
that it was accepted by Medicare, the governing body, and it all led to
unnecessary personnel at the administrative level.

"We are all paying for these huge salaries. My colleagues and I used
to laugh about seeing retired nurses walking around with clipboards at
meetings. Most of us did not know what the meetings were about, but
they took place all over the hospital. You could look in each of the meeting
rooms and see personnel with clipboards, yet there didn't seem to be a
quantitative relationship about what was going on in the room and what
came out the other end as treatment programs for patients. There was
no correlation.

"I would like to see some of that streamlined and some unnecessary
personnel done away with, so we could at least keep the inflation rate

down. I am sure there is an inborn inflation in everything we do in economics in the United States, but it must be minimized and brought under control in medicine.

"During my first year as an intern, I remember playing Wiffle ball with my colleagues in the intern area because the Catholic hospitals were on strike. They had demanded a modicum of increase from Blue Cross; something like a $31 versus a $28 room rate. Decades later, general inflation has expanded that cost by a factor of 10. The inflation that took place in medicine exceeds inflation in every other industry. The worst part? None of it had to happen. Government involvement created it.

"Readers might ask, "Well, how would you take care of elderly people?" And my answer is that we did take care of elderly patients back then before Medicare. And certainly, I would not be against improving our capability of delivering those services. But I do not think the United States needed this type of government management to dedicate better care to the elder population."

Dr. DiGiovanni takes us back to the golden era of medicine where clinicians were paid fairly, administrators were not adding extreme cost to the system, and the combination of factors allowed doctors to "give back" by simply taking care of the less fortunate or elderly in need. My comments on altruism support that statement and it is the outside interference that paradoxically hinders that action. The focus must return to those doing the work of healing.

Dr. Stefano Lucchina Orthopedic Surgeon, Hand Surgeon, Specialist in Reconstructive Microsurgery, Ticino, Switzerland
www.DrLucchina.com

"Healthcare is expensive because of the excessive requests for diagnostic exams or therapeutic procedures from patients, especially in health systems based on health insurance; the progressive aging of the population; and the excessive number of administrative employees due to the burden of bureaucracy created by politicians and health insurance companies. In the name of false safety, the hospitals conduct too many useless procedures that increase the amount of time and resources required to address easy tasks. Doctors practice defensive medicine and order unnecessary exams. Both in and out of the hospitals, we have too many general practitioners and not enough qualified, specialized doctors to evaluate patients. Pharmaceutical products could be delivered at lower costs, with a shorter number of pills per package.

"To reduce costs in healthcare, we must abolish the system based on private health insurance only. I recommend introducing the entry fee of $30 USD for E.R. cases not belonging to the red code, and an entry fee of $30 USD for every visit or exam, to be paid as "out-of-pocket" at the time of service. We should also reduce the number of "general" doctors in the hospitals and in the cities with the creation of specialized centers that focus on a field of medicine. It is debatable if health insurance or affiliated hospitals should be the filter to forward people to the right centers and people.

"We can also create emergency rooms that focus on different specialties 24 hours a day, or at least from 7 am to 11 pm, and close the emergency rooms from 11 p.m. to 7 a.m. Apart from life-threatening conditions that require an I.C.U., oncology, heart surgery, surgery, etc., the private institutions controlled from an ethical viewpoint by the local medical associations are more efficient and cheaper than public institutions. In many cases they know their patients better and are more patient-focused and friendlier than general practitioners.

"Safety depends on people, not procedures. The real quality and perceived quality of health services are two different things, but the right individual, in the right moment, in the right place – not the institution – is the factor that affects the result. Private health insurance companies are not interested in people's health, only their business."

Dr. Lucchina clearly illustrates that our problems are not solely American. My travels have shown me that most Western, industrialized countries have a growing problem of controlling healthcare costs, although some of this can be attributed to increasing technology and efficacy of treatments – a good thing. The issue, here again, is the burden of bureaucracy and excessive administration. He also argues for increased specialization which seems counterintuitive to some, but I made the case for having the patient see the right clinician at the right time. Hence the specialty emergency rooms that he mentions. The challenge, as usual, is getting those in charge of paying to recognize this. They too will benefit which underscores why this dilemma is fixable.

KRISTIN FORNO, OCCUPATIONAL THERAPIST, NEW MEXICO
www.WildRoseHandTherapy.com

"We need more education and prevention. Our whole culture is conditioned to the quick fix. And we have become a society that is completely dependent on the medical system to fix us. Kids are not taught about healthy food to eat in school. They get the worst – packaged and synthetic foods. The dependency mindset starts from a young age and expands. People resign themselves to a self-determined fate, thinking, 'Oh, my parents had this disease. I'm going to have it, too.' Americans are not empowered when it comes to their health. More prevention would decrease the cost of healthcare, but our healthcare system does not cover it. Insurance does not cover preventative complementary services or treatments like acupuncture, yoga, and meditation, yet all of them contribute to overall wellness.

"I would love to establish a wellness center with several different types of practitioners including acupuncturists, yoga teachers, therapists, Reiki practitioners, and energy healers. That might sound crazy, but all these aspects support our overall mental health. If we had wellness centers that offered these different types of therapies under one roof, it would be so much easier for people to access. Instead of having to go to the physical therapist, to the personal trainer, to the counselor, to the yoga class, etc., everything would all be contained in one wellness center. If we had more of those across the United States, it could possibly start to bring down health care costs. Unfortunately, we seem to be going in the opposite direction, especially with kids, who are much more sedentary these days.

"For example, we must set technology boundaries for ourselves as adults and for kids. Adults have the executive decision-making skills to recognize that we cannot be on social media 100 percent of the time, but kids do not have that executive functioning developed in their brain yet to make that decision. It is easy for parents to be lazy and say, 'Oh, just set them up on the iPad.' But we must be the ones that set those like boundaries for them.

"Many people go to somebody outside of themselves to fix a problem that they could have prevented from happening in the first place by being proactive. Our bodies have an innate capacity for self-healing. In my practice, I see people coming to therapy who could probably be fine on their own. But they almost take advantage of the services provided because they like it so much and they are getting an education. I think there is a craving for it at some level.

"Today, it seems like people are stuck in this cycle of go to the doctor and get the cortisone shot or whatever. It is so temporary. And then they come back after six months to get the cortisone shot again, instead of looking at the root cause of it. On the other hand, it does seem that more and more people are aware of these alternative types of therapies and modalities than they were 20 or 30 years ago. I hope it will cause a shift in terms of insurance coverage because preventing things from happening will help reduce healthcare costs."

Mrs. Forno, an experienced occupational therapist, has the insight to see care from a different lens. She focuses on restoring function, hence realizes that preventive measures are the ideal. Much focus has been on preventive health, and certainly there are some pitfalls that should be recognized. However, the concept of a one-stop shopping wellness center aligns perfectly with the notion that direct access to specialized care can save money on many fronts. The American business community has espoused "corporate wellness" for many years, but much like telemedicine, it was not widely adopted and seemed simply a nice notion. Our "Corporate Well-Being" program through OrthoNOW® similarly interested many in the marketplace, but with few real adopters. This seems to be the experience of many in the industry who seek more adoption so that the resultant benefits may materialize. Again, true engagement and change in behaviors will need to occur before we see major cost savings.

Dr. Laurent Dreyfuss
Emergency Medicine Physician/General Emergency Medicine
Owner/Operator OrthoNOW Biscayne, Miami

"At this point, the biggest problem is that patients are overpaying for their healthcare insurance, as am I. It is almost unaffordable for a family of four when the parents are a teacher and a police officer, for example, if they are lucky to have two good jobs. Patients have every right to obtain decent healthcare whether they pay for it or not...and I am not a socialist by any means. But at the same time, we already have universal healthcare in the United States. Anybody can walk into my emergency room and get care. It does not matter if they have any money in their pocket or not.

"If it is a disaster, for example, you need surgery for appendicitis, you are going to get that surgery. Nobody is going to discharge you. Now, if you have a home and credit cards and you are planning out your future, that $10,000 hospital stay is going to affect you because it is going to take years to pay it off. And you do not want it to impact your credit score. Problem is, I would be willing to bet that most of the people that use our system like a piggy bank do not care about their credit scores or have a mortgage. It does not affect them, so they do not experience a negative outcome from not paying the bill. I am not suggesting we should have stricter outcomes for not contributing, but maybe we should consider some sort of a pool that covers everyone because we are doing it anyway, and it is much more expensive. It is driving up our costs. We already cover people who do not contribute, so we might as well cover them in a more formal way, where everybody has access to health care. Because the problem is that these guys are coming into the hospital because there is no access for them. Where are they going to make appointments for primary care? Where is the money? And then what if you get diagnosed with something; where are you going to go next? Now I need a specialist, I need medication. That is why they end up coming to the hospital. Sometimes the case managers find out that they qualify for Medicare, Medicaid, or some type of assistance. But most of them do not have access. We must find a way to cover them to help contain costs."

Dr. Dreyfuss is truly in the trenches, not only when we consider the sacrifice and selfless risk he and his colleagues faced during the viral pandemic, but on a day-to-day basis. As related during my Bellevue E.R. tales, he confronts the sad spectacle of humanity every day. The classic emergency room frequenter consumes healthcare to rival those in their last few months of life, but on an often-weekly basis. The difference is that most do not contribute to the potty. They expend resources, challenge staff, and often disrupt needed attention to other patients with episodic need. We do not want to confront this problem, yet we all pay for it. It is my answer, when traveling abroad, to the classic charge, "Your American system allows people to go without care and even die in the streets." Yes, our system is not perfect, but it is human – too much so in many cases. Once we contain costs among those who can pay, the savings will allow us to better care for those who use the system in such an abusive and costly manner. Speak to any inner-city physician or E.R. nurse and you will hear the same stories. It is time for us to listen.

John Kastanis, M.B.A., F.A.C.H.E., Hospital Executive

"Commercially insured patients increasingly prefer digital care because of factors related to value, convenience, and customer service. Therefore, healthcare providers who do not have strong primary care presence must find ways to do so or partner with retailers that can fill the gap. For patients with serious illnesses, conditions, or diseases, hospitals should strive to be the destination of choice. Also, with everyone's interest in digital services, hospitals should continue to adopt promising new technologies, especially those focused on population health. These technologies include disease management using predictive analytics and wearables; home-base health care technology and virtual visits with clinicians; supply chain initiatives to improve delivery of pharmaceuticals and medical equipment. All these types of innovations reduce cost in the short and long run, while increasing patient satisfaction and quality of care.

"On the aggregate scale, patients do not understand how a single-payer or Medicare-for-all insurance program will work, nor where the funding will come from. As we have seen national health systems already established in other countries struggling with access, quality, and financial issues, it would be difficult for our nation to try to implement something better.

"Starting with financial challenges, most of us don't realize that each state will have to include more funding for their share of a single payer system, providing care to every resident. In our current payer system, Medicaid services in each state are funded only partially by the Federal government. States with disproportionate numbers of Medicaid beneficiaries already have overburdened expense budgets, particularly the "blue" states that have expanded their Medicaid eligibility requirements, and subsequently have serious budget overruns. With a single-payer system in place, more pressures will develop in providing funding for all state residents. This is the reason so many governors and state legislators have not further pursued this endeavor, as they have in the past. It is not affordable without levying significant new taxes on their constituents.

"As for access and quality of care, most national health systems suffer from lack of capital, resulting in antiquated facilities and no replacement of equipment and technology, while adopting priority waiting lists for patients to get the care they need. In the U.S. we are not accustomed to this type of health care delivery, and we could easily fall behind in quality of care if federal and state funding is curtailed, such as we have seen in Great Britain, Canada, and other rich European countries. Certainly, if a single-payer system is implemented in the U.S., a significant increase in payroll taxes will need to be imposed, and it probably still will not cover the cost of delivering the amount, scope, and quality of care that we are now very used to.

"I think the most important message to the public is that we have an evolving health care system that is less than perfect, but still has many of the best medical centers in the world with many medical advances that are being discovered in record rates. These advances alone will provide different and improved modes of care, prolonging life and improving the quality of the lives we live. We must all be patient and understanding of the fact that our health care delivery system will need to continue its transformation while still grappling with: ongoing financial pressures and the rising costs of care; changing consumer expectations; new disruptive innovators; and empty hospital beds and underused facilities.

"In the meantime, with all the new technologies available to us now and in the future, we must move beyond the current, reactive 'sick care' model to one that is more continuous and preventive. What will get us closer to that more effective model of care includes new technologies, such as: Artificial Intelligence (AI); Wearable devices and quantified health data; Genomic and precision medicine; and Telehealth and virtual care. If hospitals and other healthcare providers prioritize the implementation of these technologies, they have the potential to proactively optimize health and wellness, detect disease at earlier stages and improve the treatment of acute and chronic conditions.

Mr. Kastanis, having run some of the more prestigious hospitals in the American Northeast, makes an excellent point about the American psyche. We will NOT tolerate the waits, inefficiencies and limited technology access that often comes with the classic single payor system. We discussed Canada earlier. Our current inefficiencies are due to the hurdles we have been discussing throughout the book: overblown bureaucracy, hyperregulation and needless complexities such as the cumbersome E.M.R. systems. It is not generally due to deficient funding or lack of political will to serve our needs.

He does address the emerging consumerization of medicine and it will be up to the healthcare systems and clinicians to adopt these effectively. Unbridled competition can bring down costs, but we must unleash the classic American free-market system that Dr. Julio Gonzalez and so many others espouse.

Dr. Mark Rekant – Orthopedic Surgeon
www.Hand2ShoulderCenter.com

"The average person with an Obamacare insurance plan has a $5,000 deductible, which means the first $5,000 of their care is on them anyway. They would be much better off saving that money for themselves. We should mandate health savings accounts through their employers where the employer matches their contribution, instead of the way we do it now.

"Another part of the expense is that healthcare organizations require coverage of every little thing as opposed to the way auto insurance works. If you get a flat tire, your auto insurance does not pay for that. If your windshield shatters and needs to be replaced, your auto insurance does not pay for that. Health insurance should work the same way. For example, if you catch the common cold, the insurance company should not have to have to pay for your visit to the doctor. These changes to health insurance alone would reduce our overall healthcare costs dramatically. If people really understood that health insurance should be reserved for catastrophic problems, like life-saving surgery, a health condition that requires hospitalization, or an emergency room visit for a true emergency, we could reduce costs.

"That would require educating the public that their health insurance plan does not cover the common cold. Or that if you stub your toe, you have got to just deal with it and pay for the doctor visit. When a third-party payer covers mostly every little thing, you do not appreciate the value. But the whole system is messed up because if you do come in with a common cold, the physician who is worried about malpractice must order 18 X-rays. If the patient is also on multiple medications, it becomes even more expensive. It is a cycle that feeds on itself."

Dr. Rekant brings up the integral concept that "free" leads to increased cost and abuse in any system, with healthcare being no exception. You might remember my V.A. E.R. moonlighting experience where vets would come in with a simple chest cold, often at 4 a.m. with no waiting anticipated, simply because it resulted in zero cost to them. Healthcare consumers, i.e. patients, must have some skin in the game and my last physician contributor, Dr. Julio Gonzalez, recently wrote a book, *The Case for Free Market Healthcare* that succinctly argues for just that.

He also points out some glaring inadequacies that are never discussed among the public, yet affect those of us in the trenches, and certainly the patients we serve.

DR. JULIO GONZALEZ – Orthopedic Surgeon
www.OrthoVenice.com

"One important aspect of healthcare that patients are most uninformed and unaware about is the shortage of medicines in the United States. It is overwhelming. There is a shortage of epinephrine, Lidocaine, and Marcaine.™ Some of your essential IV antibiotics are all unavailable from time to time in the United States. Google 'medication shortage list.' There is a pharmaceutical organization that publishes a list and you will find that about 280 are not available in the United States right now. And the most common ones, the most notorious ones are IV medications that have lost their patents, particularly IV oncology drugs.

"The manufacturer will manufacture a medication so long as they get a patent for seven years. They do their R&D which can cost over seven figures. Then they put it out in the market, use it for seven years, and then leave the market because it is not productive for them to continue to supply it. Why? Medicare reimbursement only allows 6 percent profit on any medicine after it comes off the patent list when the patent expires.

"When these guys leave the market, they stop supplying the medicine. At a 6 percent profit margin, no competitor decides to come in, leaving a gap that no one will fill. There is no incentive and an insufficient return on their investment to follow through on a medicine that is no longer patented.

"It is like a third world country. It is shocking. Whenever I give a speech about healthcare and ask the audience if they knew that there was such an intense shortage of medications, not a single person raises their hand. Nobody knows. The only people who do are the doctors and the hospitals. The doctors receive the email through the hospitals informing them that there is a shortage of X, Y, and Z medicines this week in your hospital. And of course, the hospitals must try to procure it. It is a grossly under reported problem for which we must find a solution."

Dr. Gonzalez has perhaps the best birds-eye view of our glaring inefficiencies due to the combined roles that he has served, often concurrently. Besides being a practicing orthopedic surgeon, he is an attorney, a recent Florida state legislator and has served several tours in the military as a flight surgeon. His grasp of public policy, legal challenges and what we face in the trenches of healthcare is nearly unparalleled. He has written 4 books on healthcare and now chooses to focus on a topic barely addressed in this book- the pharmaceutical industry.

Medication spending represents 10 percent of the total US healthcare spend in 2018, a sizeable number considering that huge cost centers, such as hospitals, are 33 percent of the total cost. We have demonstrated the high cost of hospital care but the fact that medication alone is one-third of that indicates this too, is monumental.

Many of my contributors echo the points that have been made throughout the book. There is certainly no one fix solution. It is clear, however, that the true concept of value has been overlooked in the current U.S. healthcare quagmire. We recite the term, "value-based care" without looking beyond this catchphrase and truly defining what that means.

I close this discussion of possible solutions with the astute observations that my OrthoNOW® co-founder, Justin Irizarry, compiled over a decade of struggles to increase adoption of a specialty specific care model that we have proven despite lack of capital and real engagement. He comes from an M&A background on Wall Street, a fresh perspective that was completely devoid of any real healthcare knowledge, let alone experience. I remember thinking, "Perfect." A new, unprejudiced stance is needed to tweak and refine our healthcare system – not completely upend it as some have tried.

We must listen to those in the trenches, while engaging the public at all levels, if we are to preserve and improve the medical care that has been the world's envy for the past century.

Justin Irizarry – Co-Founder of OrthoNOW®, Value-Based Care

"U.S. Healthcare date on spending and patient outcomes is sobering. The United States spends more on healthcare per capita and as a percentage of G.D.P. than its industrialized counterparts. Compared to these same peers, U.S. taxpayers' foot a significantly larger amount of their healthcare bill, and most do not receive subsidized healthcare.

"In the 50-year period from 1960 to 2010, U.S. spending on healthcare increased more than 4.5 times its increase in GDP while spending on healthcare increased a whopping 51 times more than wage increases.

"This must be explained by U.S. patients visiting their doctors more, or staying in the hospital longer when they are admitted, compared to their peers, right? Unfortunately, no. Per capita, the U.S. healthcare patient visits his or her doctor about 4.1 times per year. Compare this to about 13.1 times per year for the Japanese healthcare patient, or 9.7 times per year for the German patient. Likewise, the average length of a hospital stay in the United States is about 30 percent less than that of Germany although the cost of the U.S. hospital stay is 400 percent more than in Germany.

"This would not necessarily be a problem if outcomes in the United States were proportionally better than its peers. But they are not. The rate of a hospital visit for congestive heart failure in the United States is about four times that of Canada and the United Kingdom. The rate of hospital visits for asthma is about 10 times that of the Canada and two times that of the United Kingdom. Similarly, the rate of lower extremity amputations from diabetes per 100,000 population is significantly higher in the United States than any of its developed peers. And overall the life expectancy at birth in the United States is lower than that of Denmark, the United Kingdom, Canada, France, Norway, Switzerland, New Zealand, Korea, and Israel, at the same time that the projected spending per person in U.S. dollars is between 50 percent and 400 percent more than any of the previously mentioned countries

"See the problem? The U.S. healthcare market is spending far too much and receiving far too little. This is not to say that the U.S. healthcare system does not produce excellent outcomes in many areas; in fact, the U.S. healthcare system is still considered the gold standard for certain advanced procedures. But in the arena of basic healthcare, it is failing.

"The U.S. healthcare industry is different than any other industry in the United States specifically because the consumer of the healthcare is different than the party paying for the health care. This leads to what economists call the "principal agent problem": one entity – usually the insurance company – can make decisions and/or take actions on behalf of the patient. Which doctor the patient can see and what procedures the patient can receive, is up to the insurance company. And the clinician treating the patient is often constrained in what he or she would choose to do with the patient. What makes this particularly bad is that the insurance company has a different set of incentives than the patient. The patient cares about the quality of care he or she receives, while the insurance company cares about how much it pays.

"Because of this, we have seen the U.S. healthcare system put a heavy focus on reducing the cost of incidental care by negotiating its contracted rates with clinicians and hospitals. In other words, commercial insurance companies push volume to those organizations with lower and lower prices. But what if that lower-priced care does not solve the patient's issue? What if, instead, it starts the patient down a journey that requires him or her to see multiple doctors, have multiple tests, and delay definitive treatment for months? Isn't the total cost of solving the patients issue what should matter? And considering that, shouldn't the system reward those organizations that deliver the best outcomes at the most competitive total cost of care?

"My point is that price (or cost) does not equal value. And value-based care is what is needed in the U.S. healthcare system. Furthermore, while many people agree that "value" or "value-based care" is needed in the healthcare industry, few people can define value when asked. (In most cases, they just mean "cheap").

"OrthoNOW®'s exclusive focus was on providing value to the patient in the sector of musculoskeletal and orthopedic care. Patients with acute pain, orthopedic or musculoskeletal conditions care about three things: eliminating their pain as fast as possible, treating their underlying condition (so it does not re-occur), and paying a fair price. Therefore, OrthoNOW®'s definition of value was the ratio of [Delivering a convenient and timely treatment that definitively solves the patient's problem, pain, or injury] divided by [the cost of delivering that treatment].

Cost of Delivering that Treatment

"Patients walk in on their terms, receive specialty care, and walk out treated in 70 minutes or less, on average. Its prices are transparent and published on its website. Fair prices are charged – particularly for the quality of care – and are about 1/ 10 that of the emergency rooms. OrthoNOW® democratized access to specialty care, which means it eliminated the need for patients to jump around between doctors, schedule multiple appointments, or pay multiple times. At once, OrthoNOW® turned up the dial on quality of care and turned down the dial on cost. Simultaneously.

"This model is distinctly different than that of a general urgent care center. While general urgent care centers have successfully diverted urgent, but non-emergency cases away from the hospital emergency room, they are ill-equipped to deal with specialty conditions like orthopedics. In general, urgent care centers are good at delivering definitive care to patients with low acuity conditions, such as bronchitis, sore throats, and other infections. But they cannot deliver definitive treatment for high acuity conditions which require specialized clinician training and diagnostic equipment.

"A big reason OrthoNOW® could deliver value is that its entire operation was focused around treating a defined range of conditions. All the clinicians, tools, treatments, business processes, and knowledge needed to treat this range of conditions are co-located in the same center. Furthermore, the OrthoNOW® patient journey begins before the patient is at the center – the company's mobile application allows the patient to auto-matically locate the nearest center, have an Uber pick the patient up and deliver him or her to the center. During the ride, the patient can send check-in information to the front desk, and upload pictures of his or her injury so that the staff is ready to deliver treatment when the patient walks in. This is uncommon elsewhere in the healthcare industry as it is largely organized around specialty. Oftentimes, patients need to see one doctor for an assessment, visit another location for diagnostics testing, return to the first doctor for a summary of the test, and then visit another doctor for treatment."

# # #

The value proposition that Mr. Irizarry describes is straightforward. Whether via an orthopedic care model or any other care delivery standard, the goal is to provide the patient with the care they need, at the time they need it, and minimizing any interference of that process.

Simple as it may seem, further complexities only serve to drive up cost and increase delays. For those of us who serve in the trenches of healthcare, there is little else that matters. Once the public recognizes that, we can roll up our sleeves and provide better care for less cost. Let us get started...

About the Author

Alejandro Badia, M.D., F.A.C.S. has been in the trenches with our broken healthcare system since 1989.

A hand and upper extremity orthopedic surgeon at Badia Hand to Shoulder Center in Miami Florida, Dr. Badia previously served as Chief of Hand Surgery at Baptist Hospital of Miami. He studied physiology at Cornell University and obtained his medical degree at New York University, where he also trained in orthopedics. He runs an active international hand fellowship and previously organized a yearly Miami meeting for surgeons/therapists that was devoted to upper limb arthroscopy and arthroplasty. In 2005, Dr. Badia co-founded the world-renowned Miami Anatomical Research Center (M.A.R.C.), the world's largest surgical cadaveric training lab.

In 2008, he completed the Badia Hand to Shoulder Center, a fully integrated clinical facility for the upper limb also encompassing the Surgery Center at Doral, rehabilitation, and an MRI imaging facility. In 2010, Dr. Badia inaugurated OrthoNOW®, the first walk-in orthopedic care center in South Florida, which later became an officially licensed system. Dr. Badia continues to actively engage healthcare entrepreneurs and surgeons in the United States and abroad, to open immediate orthopedic care facilities.

Contact: alejandro@drbadia.com

References and Resources

Prior Authorization

https://www.ama-assn.org/practice-management/sustainability/why-prior-authorization-was-white-hot-issue-2018

https://www.aafp.org/news/practice-professional-issues/20170609priorauth.html

https://electronichealthreporter.com/prior-authorization-healthcare-primer/

https://getreferralmd.com/2018/04/prior-authorization-problems-healthcare/

https://en.wikipedia.org/wiki/Prior_authorization

https://www.covermymeds.com/main/insights/articles/a-brief-history-of-how-we-got-to-electronic-prior-authorization/

Moral Injury

https://www.statnews.com/2018/07/26/physicians-not-burning-out-they-are-suffering-moral-injury/

https://www.law.upenn.edu/live/files/4602-moralinjuryshayexcerptpdf

Medicare vs. Private Payer Reimbursement

https://healthpayerintelligence.com/news/hospital-payment-disparities-emerge-among-private-payers-medicare

The People's Almanac, David Wallenchinsky and Irving Wallace

https://www.amazon.com/Peoples-Almanac-David-Wallechinsky/dp/0385040601

Stanford Medicine: How an Industry Shifted from Protecting Patients to Seeking Profit

https://stanmed.stanford.edu/2017spring/how-health-insurance-changed-from-protecting-patients-to-seeking-profit.html

Health Maintenance Organization Act of 1973

http://healthoverprofit.org/2017/03/19/for-profit-health-care-used-to-be-illegal/

Escalated Costs of Medication

https://time.com/5564547/drug-prices-medicine/

https://www.theatlantic.com/health/archive/2019/03/drug-prices-high-cost-research-and-development/585253/

E.M.R.

https://www.americanactionforum.org/research/are-electronic-medical-records-worth-the-costs-of-implementation/

https://www.studentdebtrelief.us/news/average-cost-of-medical-school/

https://today.duke.edu/2009/01/sabiston1.html

https://www.amazon.com/Goldfranks-Toxicologic-Emergencies-Robert-Hoffman/dp/0071801847

https://transferwise.com/gb/currency-converter/eur-to-usd-rate?amount=5

https://www.amazon.com/House-God-Samuel-Shem/dp/0425238091

https://www.dailysignal.com/2019/03/11/these-3-doctors-in-congress-diagnose-the-problems-with-medicare-for-all/

https://www.forbes.com/sites/brucejapsen/2019/03/12/two-blue-cross-plans-to-merge-into-national-player/#4a1a09cb236e

https://www.studentdebtrelief.us/news/average-cost-of-medical-school/

https://www.theguardian.com/science/2017/jun/27/profitable-business-scientific-publishing-bad-for-science

If restaurants were run like healthcare.

https://www.youtube.com/watch?v=4M0ooFlJmfk

The Messy Middle: Finding Your Way Through the Hardest and Most Crucial Part of Any Bold Venture - Scott Belsky

https://www.amazon.com/Messy-Middle-Finding-Through-Hardest/dp/0735218072/ref=sr_1_1?ie=UTF8&qid=1547403014&sr=8-1&keywords=the+messy+middle

Current Drug Shortages

https://www.ashp.org/Drug-Shortages/Current-Shortages/Drug-Shortages-List?page=CurrentShortages

https://www.rxlist.com/marcaine-drug.htm

https://www.accessdata.fda.gov/scripts/drugshortages/dsp_ActiveIngredientDetails.cfm?AI=EpiPen%C2%AE+Auto-Injector+and+Epinephrine+Injection%2C+USP+Auto-Injector&st=c&tab=tabs-4&panels=0

https://www.fda.gov/drugs/drug-safety-and-availability/drug-shortages

https://www.fda.gov/drugs/development-approval-process-drugs/frequently-asked-questions-patents-and-exclusivity

https://www.nbcnews.com/health/health-news/u-s-hospitals-fda-grapple-shortages-life-saving-drugs-n1074821

https://infuserveamerica.com/intravenous-antibiotics-old/

https://www.rxlist.com/marcaine-drug.htm

https://www.accessdata.fda.gov/scripts/drugshortages/dsp_ActiveIngredientDetails.cfm?AI=EpiPen%C2%AE+Auto-Injector+and+Epinephrine+Injection%2C+USP+Auto-Injector&st=c&tab=tabs-4&panels=0

https://www.fda.gov/drugs/drug-safety-and-availability/drug-shortages

https://www.fda.gov/drugs/development-approval-process-drugs/frequently-asked-questions-patents-and-exclusivity

https://www.nbcnews.com/health/health-news/u-s-hospitals-fda-grapple-shortages-life-saving-drugs-n1074821

https://infuserveamerica.com/intravenous-antibiotics-old/

https://www.ashp.org/Drug-Shortages/Current-Shortages/Drug-Shortages-List?page=CurrentShortages

https://www.fda.gov/drugs/drug-safety-and-availability/drug-shortages

The Guardian: Is the staggeringly profitable business of scientific publishing bad for science?

https://www.theguardian.com/science/2017/jun/27/profitable-business-scientific-publishing-bad-for-science

Elsevier Fact Sheet

https://libraries.mit.edu/scholarly/publishing/elsevier-fact-sheet/

European University Association

https://eua.eu/component/attachments/attachments.html?task=attachment&id=1691

Journal of Hand Surgery

https://www.jhandsurg.org/

The Wolf of Wall Street

https://www.imdb.com/title/tt0993846/

Volar fixation for dorsally displaced fractures of the distal radius: A preliminary report

https://www.jhandsurg.org/article/S0363-5023(02)27279-2/abstract

AO Foundation

https://www.aofoundation.org/

Seven Summits

https://en.wikipedia.org/wiki/Seven_Summits

BRAVA

https://www.miamibreastcenter.com/brava-breast-enhancement

Med Page Today

https://www.medpagetoday.com/special-reports/exclusives/82743

Hand Re-Attachment Surgery of four Fingers in an elderly man Dr. Alejandro Badia Hand Surgeon

https://www.youtube.com/watch?time_continue=2&v=gw-ykpnUGOQ

Finger Reattachment Surgery Hand & Digits reattachment Operation Dr. Badia Best Hand Surgeon

https://www.youtube.com/watch?v=ZYJ-vb6ZAHA

Duke Today: Legendary Chair Dr. Sabiston Dies

https://today.duke.edu/2009/01/sabiston1.html

Giants in Orthopaedic Surgery: Sterling Bunnell MD

https://www.ncbi.nlm.nih.gov/pmc/articles/PMC3825913/

Healthcare.gov: Affordable Care Act

https://www.healthcare.gov/glossary/affordable-care-act/

Medicare Resources.gov: A Brief History of Medicare

https://www.medicareresources.org/basic-medicare-information/brief-his-tory-of-medicare/

AHA.org: Paul M. Ellwood

https://www.aha.org/oral-history-project/2018-03-29-paul-m-ellwood-jr-md-first-person-oral-history

The Balance.com: Obamacare Pros and Cons

https://www.thebalance.com/obamacare-pros-and-cons-3306059

HCAHP

https://www.hcahpsonline.org/globalassets/hcahps/facts/hcahps_fact_sheet_november_2017.pdf

National Institutes of Health: Moving Beyond Pain as the Fifth Vital Sign

https://www.ncbi.nlm.nih.gov/pmc/articles/PMC5878703/

Joint Commission.org

https://www.jointcommission.org/en/

Centers for Medicare and Medicaid Services

https://www.cms.gov/

CMS Research Statistics

https://www.cms.gov/Research-Statistics-Data-and-Systems/Statistics-Trends-and-Reports/NationalHealthExpendData/NationalHealthAccountsHistorical

Wikipedia: Healthcare in Norway

https://en.wikipedia.org/wiki/Healthcare_in_Norway

American Medical Association: Studies Show Continued Cost Burden to Medical Liability System

https://www.ama-assn.org/press-center/press-releases/ama-studies-show-continued-cost-burden-medical-liability-system

American Museum of Tort Law: Liebeck versus McDonalds

https://www.tortmuseum.org/liebeck-v-mcdonalds/

Forbes.com - Malcolm Gladwell On American Healthcare: An Interview

https://www.forbes.com/sites/robertpearl/2014/03/06/malcolm-gladwell-on-american-health-care-an-interview/#1d4f651578ab

Dr. Kevin, M.D.

https://www.kevinmd.com/blog/2018/08/physicians-dont-just-suffer-burn-out-they-suffer-moral-injuries.html

Dr. Aileen Marie Gonzalez

https://www.aileenmariewellness.com/

Acknowledgments

Dr. Julio Gonzalez
Orthopedic Surgeon, Attorney, Former Flight Surgeon, & Former Florida State Representative, Venice Florida

Dr. Philip Forno
Orthopedic Hand and Upper Limb Surgeon
Santa Fe, New Mexico

Dr. George Balfour
Orthopedic Hand Surgeon
Burbank, California

Dr. Mark Rekant
Orthopedic Hand Surgeon
Philadelphia, Pennsylvania

Dr. A.J. DiGiovanni
Retired General and Vascular Surgeon
Newtown Square, Pennsylvania

Dr. Laurent Dreyfuss
Emergency Room Physician/OrthoNOW® Center Owner
Miami, Florida

Dr. Roger Khouri
Reconstructive Plastic and Hand Surgeon
Coral Gables, Florida

Dr. Jose Lamas
General and Vascular Surgeon
Hialeah, Florida

Dr. Stefano Lucchina
Orthopedic Hand Surgeon
Lucarno, Switzerland

A South Florida Pediatrician
Dr. Juan Manuel Rios-Ruh
Orthopedic Foot and Ankle Surgeon
Madrid, Spain

Dr. Scott Sigman
Orthopedic Sports Medicine Surgeon
Lowell, Massachusetts

Dr. Robert Terrill
Orthopedic Hand and Upper Limb Surgeon
Worcester, Massachusetts

Dr. Gregorio Caban
Podiatric Foot and Ankle Surgeon
Miami, Florida

Dr. Kay Kirkpatrick
Orthopedic Surgeon and Georgia State Senator
Atlanta, Georgia

Dr. Aileen Marie Gonzalez
Registered Pharmacist
Miami, Florida

John Kastanis
Healthcare System Executive/Consultant
New York, New York

Nancy Williams, R.N.
Nurse Case Manager
Miami, Florida

Cindy Papale-Hammontree
Medical Office Manager and Author
Miami, Florida

Uva de Aragon
Author, Retired University Professor, Orthopedic Patient

A Pennsylvania Medical Malpractice Defense Attorney

Kerry Anderson
Restaurant Worker, Orthopedic Patient
Miami-Dade, Florida

Kristin Forno, O.T., C.H.T.
Occupational Hand Therapist
Santa Fe, New Mexico

Lina Peterson, D.P.T
Physical Therapist and Rehab Clinic Manager
West Palm Beach, Florida

Kimberly Light
Regulatory Affairs Executive
BioPro Implants

Tina Rodriguez
Billings and Collections Supervisor
Orthopedic Practice
Doral, Florida

Erica Pacey
Jewelry Designer/Patient

Justin Irizzary
Co-Founder and CFO, OrthoNOW®

CPSIA information can be obtained
at www.ICGtesting.com
Printed in the USA
LVHW041908230223
740255LV00001B/20